EVALUATION
in Occupational Therapy
Obtaining and Interpreting Data

4th Edition

Edited by
Jim Hinojosa, PhD, OT, BCP, FAOTA
Paula Kramer, PhD, OTR, FAOTA

Foreword by
Joan C. Rogers, PhD, OTR/L, FAOTA

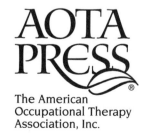

The American
Occupational Therapy
Association, Inc.

AOTA Centennial Vision

We envision that occupational therapy is a powerful, widely recognized, science-driven, and evidence-based profession with a globally connected and diverse workforce meeting society's occupational needs.

Mission Statement

The American Occupational Therapy Association advances the quality, availability, use, and support of occupational therapy through standard-setting, advocacy, education, and research on behalf of its members and the public.

AOTA Staff

Frederick P. Somers, *Executive Director*
Christopher M. Bluhm, *Chief Operating Officer*

Chris Davis, *Director, AOTA Press*
Ashley Hofmann, *Development/Production Editor*

Rebecca Rutberg, *Director, Marketing*
Amanda Goldman, *Marketing Specialist*
Jennifer Folden, *Marketing Specialist*

American Occupational Therapy Association, Inc.
4720 Montgomery Lane
Bethesda, MD 20814
Phone: 301-652-AOTA (2682)
TDD: 800-377-8555
Fax: 301-652-7711
www.aota.org
To order: 1-877-404-AOTA or store.aota.org

Disclaimers

This publication is designed to provide accurate and authoritative information in regard to the subject matter covered. It is sold or distributed with the understanding that the publisher is not engaged in rendering legal, accounting, or other professional service. If legal advice or other expert assistance is required, the services of a competent professional person should be sought.
—*From the Declaration of Principles jointly adopted by the American Bar Association and a Committee of Publishers and Associations*

It is the objective of the American Occupational Therapy Association to be a forum for free expression and interchange of ideas. The opinions expressed by the contributors to this work are their own and not necessarily those of the American Occupational Therapy Association.

ISBN: 978-1-56900-356-5

Library of Congress Control Number: 2014942181

Cover Design by Debra Naylor, Naylor Design, Inc., Washington, DC
Composition by Manila Typesetting Company, Manila, Philippines
Printed by Automated Graphic Systems, Inc., White Plains, MD

Dedication

We dedicate this book to all who are evaluated by occupational therapists and to those who have evaluated us. Evaluation can be daunting, but it promotes learning about the people we serve and about ourselves.

We are very grateful to have the love and support of the following people, who continually help us learn about ourselves:

Steven A. Smith
David L. Hunt
Andrew L. K. Hunt.

—*Jim Hinojosa & Paula Kramer*

Contents

Acknowledgments

We are very proud of the illustrious group of people involved in this project. We extend our heartfelt thanks to all the contributing authors who worked diligently to share their thoughts and ideas in a way that would be useful to students, occupational therapists, and occupational therapy assistants. Also, we offer a special thank you to the spouses, significant others, and families who have supported them during the writing process. We know how grueling it can be!

On every project, there are particular people who stand out for their contributions. On this project, we acknowledge Chris Davis, Director of AOTA Press, and Ashley Hofmann, Development/Production Editor, who guided this project and were supportive throughout. We are always grateful to our colleagues at New York University and the University of the Sciences in Philadelphia, who stimulate our thoughts and help shape our perspective.

Finally, we could not have undertaken this project without the love and caring of our families and significant others. They will always be the center of our lives.

About the Editors

Jim Hinojosa, PhD, OT, BCP, FAOTA, is a professor of occupational therapy in the Department of Occupational Therapy in the Steinhardt School of Culture, Education, and Human Development at New York University in New York. Specializing in pediatrics, he is a strong advocate for family-centered care, believing that everyone benefits when health professionals work closely with families to develop interventions that reflect their needs and values.

Dr. Hinojosa has more than 35 years' experience as an occupational therapist, researcher, and educator. In his role as educator, Dr. Hinojosa has presented and conducted workshops throughout the United States and Canada. He is the coeditor and author of 12 textbooks and has written or published over 200 chapters and articles.

A Fellow of the American Occupational Therapy Association (AOTA), Dr. Hinojosa has served on many of its commissions and boards and was awarded its highest honors, the Award of Merit and the Eleanor Clarke Slagle Lectureship. He also served as director of the American Occupational Therapy Foundation Board and received its Meritorious Service Award.

Paula Kramer, PhD, OTR, FAOTA, is professor and director of the doctoral program in the Department of Occupational Therapy at University of the Sciences in Philadelphia. She has published numerous book chapters and scholarly articles and has coauthored seven textbooks. Dr. Kramer was a former chairperson of the Accreditation Council for Occupational Therapy Education (ACOTE®) and a member of the Board of Directors of the American Occupational Therapy Association (AOTA). She has chaired the Standards Review Committee for ACOTE.®

In recognition of her contributions relating theory to practice, Dr. Kramer was awarded the A. Jean Ayres Award from the American Occupational Therapy Foundation. For contributions to service and education, she was awarded the Award of Merit from AOTA. She is a Fellow of AOTA.

About the Authors

Julie D. Bass, PhD, OTR/L, FAOTA
Professor
Department of Occupational Science and
    Occupational Therapy
Henrietta Schmoll School of Health
St. Catherine University
St. Paul, MN

Helen Bourke-Taylor, PhD, BAppScOT
Senior Lecturer
School of Allied and Public Health
Faculty of Health Sciences
Australian Catholic University
Fitzroy, Victoria
Australia

Ted Brown, PhD, OT(C), OTR
Associate Professor
Department of Occupational Therapy
School of Primary Health Care
Faculty of Medicine, Nursing and Health
    Sciences
Monash University–Peninsula Campus
Frankston, Victoria
Australia

Denise Chisholm, PhD, OTR/L, FAOTA
Associate Professor and Vice Chair
Department of Occupational Therapy
School of Health and Rehabilitation Sciences
University of Pittsburgh
Pittsburgh

Patricia Crist, PhD, OTR, PC, FAOTA
Founding Chairperson and Professor
Department of Occupational Therapy
Northern Arizona University
Phoenix Biomedical Campus
Phoenix

Lenin C. Grajo, EdM, OTR
Assistant Professor
Department of Occupational Science and
    Occupational Therapy
Edward and Margaret Doisy College of Health
    Sciences
Saint Louis University
St. Louis

Lou Ann Griswold, PhD, OTR/L, FAOTA
Associate Professor
Occupational Therapy Department
University of New Hampshire
Durham

Jim Hinojosa, PhD, OT, BCP, FAOTA
Professor
Department of Occupational Therapy
Steinhardt School Culture, Education, and
    Human Development
New York University
New York

Kristie Patten Koenig, PhD, OTR/L, FAOTA
Chairperson and Associate Professor
Department of Occupational Therapy
Steinhardt School of Culture, Education, and
    Human Development
New York University
New York

Paula Kramer, PhD, OTR, FAOTA
Professor and Program Director of the Doctoral
    Program
Department of Occupational Therapy
Samson College of Health Science
University of the Sciences
Philadelphia

Penny Kyler, OT, ScD, FAOTA
Public Health Analyst
U.S. Department of Health and Human Services
Health Resources and Services Administration
Maternal and Child Health Bureau
San Jose, CA

Aimee J. Luebben, EdD, OTR, FAOTA
Professor Emerita
Occupational Therapy Department
University of Southern Indiana
Evansville

Jennifer S. Pitonyak, PhD, OTR/L, SCFES
Vice Chairperson and Assistant Professor
Interim Program Director, Master of
    Occupational Therapy
Department of Occupational Therapy
Samson College of Health Sciences
University of the Sciences
Philadelphia

Charlotte Brasic Royeen, PhD, OTR, FAOTA
Professor
Department of Occupational Science and
    Occupational Therapy
Edward and Margaret Doisy College of Health
    Sciences
Saint Louis University
St. Louis

Fern Silverman, EdD, OTR/L
Program Director and Associate Professor
Occupational Therapy Department
Salus University
Elkins Park, PA

Virginia Stoffel, PhD, OT, BCMH, FAOTA
Associate Professor and Graduate Coordinator
University of Wisconsin–Milwaukee
Milwaukee

Nikhil Tomar, MS
Doctoral Student
Division of Occupational Science and
    Occupational Therapy
University of North Carolina–Chapel Hill
Chapel Hill

Rondalyn V. Whitney, PhD, OTR/L, FAOTA
Assistant Professor
Samson College of Health Science
University of the Sciences
Philadelphia

List of Figures, Tables, Exhibits, Case Examples, and Appendixes

Exhibits

Case Examples

Appendixes

Foreword

Joan C. Rogers, PhD, OTR/L, FAOTA

"Would you tell me, please, which way I ought to go from here?"
"That depends a good deal on where you want to get to," said the Cat.
"I don't much care where—," said Alice.
"Then it doesn't matter which way you go," said the Cat.
"—so long as I get SOMEWHERE," Alice added as an explanation.
"Oh, you're sure to do that," said the Cat, "if you only walk long enough."
—Lewis Carroll, *Alice in Wonderland* (1864/1993, p. 41)

In this conversation, the Cheshire Cat stresses the importance of direction in Alice's journey through Wonderland. Knowing the destination—the goal—is the first step in planning how to get there. In the occupational therapy process—evaluation → intervention → outcome evaluation—the evaluation component provides guidance for where the client "wants to go," the intervention component maps out "how the client will get there," and the outcome evaluation component assesses the extent to which "somewhere" matches the client's destination.

In the American Occupational Therapy Association's (2010) *Standards of Practice for Occupational Therapy, evaluation* is "the process of obtaining and interpreting data necessary for intervention" (p. S107). Regardless of whether evaluation is applied to individuals, groups, or populations, it identifies the problems in occupational status that are to be resolved or ameliorated through occupational therapy interventions, describes the character of those problems, and finally determines (measures) the degree to which the intervention resolved or reduced the problems and achieved the client's goals.

As the starting point of the occupational therapy process, evaluation plays a pivotal role in helping therapists to understand clients, including their goals, priorities, and performance problems. During the evaluation, therapists use interviewing, observation, and testing (standardized and nonstandardized) to compile information about clients' occupational status. In collaboration with clients, therapists then integrate and synthesize this evaluative data into a coherent picture of clients' occupational status, including strengths and weaknesses. Occupation-related problems or potential problems, which become the focus of occupational therapy intervention, are prominent in this picture. Given the complexity of evaluation and its importance in the occupational therapy process, it warrants careful attention and study.

In this age of health care accountability and comparative effectiveness research, evaluation is critical not only for planning interventions and assessing client progress but also, more importantly, for examining the efficacy and efficiency of our interventions. Thus, it is imperative that occupational therapists understand the importance of having psychometrically sound measures and know how to select, administer, and interpret them. A measure that is reliable and valid for use with one clinical population (e.g., arthritis) may not be for another clinical population (e.g., cardiopulmonary disease). A measure that is reliable and valid for characterizing occupational status may not be sufficiently responsive to detect changes in occupational status following occupational therapy interventions and hence would not be a useful outcome measure for the individual client or the aggregate of clients seen in a particular clinical or educational setting.

Therapists need to be able to analyze whether a measure is reliable and valid for use with the clinical populations that are commonly referred to their settings. Importantly, the measure's ability to detect change in occupational status attributable to occupational therapy interventions needs to be determined. If the measure is not responsive to changes in function, then the evaluation data may indicate that the client is not progressing and should be discharged. Thus, there is not only a pragmatic reason to select measures that are psychometrically sound but also an ethical reason—measures that are not reliable, valid, and responsive to changes in occupational status may not provide data that accurately reflect client progress and subsequently lead to denial of services and early discharge.

As more measures used in rehabilitation are based on item response theory, basic familiarity with concepts such as unidimensionality, person–fit analysis, Rasch model, and differential item functioning is needed to support our understanding of tests and measurement. *Evaluation in Occupational Therapy: Obtaining and Interpreting Data, 4th Edition,* is designed to assist therapists to gain facility in measurement concepts and serve as a resource to provide guidance for evaluating where the client "wants to go," to use those data to map out "how the client will get there," and to evaluate occupational therapy outcomes to determine the extent to which "somewhere" matches the client's destination.

References

American Occupational Therapy Association. (2010). Standards of practice for occupational therapy. *American Journal of Occupational Therapy, 64*(Suppl.), S106–S111. http://dx.doi.org/10.5014/ajot.2010.64S106

Carroll, L. (1993). *Alice's adventures in wonderland.* New York: Dover. (Original work published 1864)

Introduction

Jim Hinojosa, PhD, OT, BCP, FAOTA
Paula Kramer, PhD, OTR, FAOTA

More than 20 years ago, American Occupational Therapy Association's (AOTA) Commission on Practice requested the first edition of this book in 1994 to address the importance of the evaluation process in occupational therapy (Hinojosa & Kramer, 1998). Since then, occupational therapists' focus on evaluation has shifted in response to a demand that therapists provide evidence-based interventions, and the second and third editions of this text reflected these changes (Hinojosa, Kramer, & Crist, 2005, 2010). Without valid, reliable, or credible and trustworthy assessments, therapists cannot document outcomes and the efficacy of their interventions.

Changes to the profession, such as progress towards the *Centennial Vision* (AOTA, 2007) and the revision of AOTA's official documents, highlighted the need for this new edition. AOTA recently revised official documents and adopted a revised philosophical base (AOTA, 2012) that emphasizes the importance of occupation and occupational performance. Revised official documents include *Occupational Therapy Practice Framework: Domain and Process* (3rd ed.; *Framework;* AOTA, 2014), *Standards of Practice for Occupational Therapy* (AOTA, 2010b), and the *Occupational Therapy Code of Ethics and Ethics Standards* (AOTA, 2010a).

The Accreditation Council for Occupational Therapy Education (2012) adopted revised standards for an accredited educational program for the occupational therapist for master's degree and doctoral entry-level programs. In the practice settings, there is an increased demand by employers and reimbursers for occupational therapists to have increased competence in selecting, administering, and interpreting assessments. Therapists can no longer do observations, take a few measurements, and call it an evaluation.

Evaluation promotes a greater understanding of the people whom occupational therapy serves. This fourth edition focuses on the occupational therapist as an evaluator and emphasizes evidence-based evaluation as a foundation of occupational therapy best practices. This book presents a comprehensive view of the evaluative process that reflects the needs of professionals as well as the level of content required in postbaccalaureate education. We have included discussions of the various aspects of a comprehensive evaluation, including screening, assessment, reassessment, and reevaluation. Evaluation is presented as part of the total scheme of practice and as a means of supporting the efficacy of interventions.

In this text, authors reaffirm the importance of understanding the person as an occupational being and focus on how the occupational therapist's understanding of human occupation influences evaluation. Authors explore the roles and influences of the examiner on assessment and how he or she affects evaluation and examine the roles of culture and test bias when assessments are not culturally sensitive. Additionally, authors acknowledge the critical importance of understanding the psychometric properties of standardized assessments and the need to interpret assessment data so that it is applicable to practice. The authors also discuss the importance of using nonstandardized assessments to obtain real-life knowledge about the client and his or her participation and engagement in occupations. Finally, the authors explore how an occupational therapist uses evaluation data to determine intervention effectiveness.

This new edition is designed to be compatible with the revised AOTA documents previously mentioned, especially the *Framework* (AOTA, 2014). The text begins with an overview of evaluation and its philosophical and theoretical issues. It next proceeds to discuss critical issues related to practice, such as choosing an assessment, the importance of evaluation in intervention planning, and administration of evaluations. Then types of evaluations are presented, including standardized, nonstandardized, and ipsative evaluations. An overview of psychometrics is presented. Finally, the text addresses some thought-provoking areas, such as the role of ethics in evaluation, the importance of evaluation to evidence-based practice, evaluations of special populations, and others ways that evaluations may be used.

Our intention with this revision is to provide the occupational therapy profession with a much-needed comprehensive book on the occupational therapy evaluation process. The expansion of this text in breadth and depth reflects changes to contemporary evaluation approaches. As therapists, we need to constantly keep best practices in mind and think about not only what the current practice environment wants an evaluation to be but also what we believe a comprehensive evaluation should be.

References

Accreditation Council for Occupational Therapy Education. (2012). 2011 Accreditation Council for Occupational Therapy Education (ACOTE®) standards. *American Journal of Occupational Therapy, 66*(Suppl.), S6–S74. http://dx.doi.org/10.5014/ajot.2012.66S6

American Occupational Therapy Association. (2007). AOTA's *Centennial Vision* and executive summary. *American Journal of Occupational Therapy, 61*(6), 613–614. http://dx.doi.org/10.5014/ajot.61.6.613

American Occupational Therapy Association. (2010a). Occupational therapy code of ethics and ethics standards (2010). *American Journal of Occupational Therapy, 64*(Suppl.), S17–S26. http://dx.doi.org/10.5014/ajot.2010.64S17

American Occupational Therapy Association. (2010b). Standards of practice for occupational therapy. *American Journal of Occupational Therapy, 64*(Suppl.). S106–S111. http://dx.doi.org/10.5014/ajot.2010.64S106

American Occupational Therapy Association. (2012). *Policy manual.* Bethesda, MD: Author.

American Occupational Therapy Association. (2014). Occupational therapy practice framework: Domain and process (3rd ed.). *American Journal of Occupational Therapy, 68*(Suppl. 1), S1–S48. http://dx.doi.org/10.5014/ajot.2014.682006

Hinojosa, J., & Kramer, P. (Eds.). (1998*). Occupational therapy evaluation: Obtaining and interpreting data.* Bethesda, MD: American Occupational Therapy Association.

Hinojosa, J., Kramer, P. & Crist, P. (Eds.). (2005). *Evaluation: Obtaining and interpreting data* (2nd ed.). Bethesda, MD: AOTA Press.

Hinojosa, J., Kramer, P., & Crist, P. (Eds.). (2010). *Evaluation: Obtaining and interpreting data* (3rd ed.). Bethesda, MD: AOTA Press.

CHAPTER 1

Evaluation: Where Do We Begin?

Jim Hinojosa, PhD, OT, BCP, FAOTA
Paula Kramer, PhD, OTR, FAOTA
Patricia Crist, PhD, OTR, PC, FAOTA

Highlights

- Importance of evaluation in occupational therapy
- Definitions of terms used in this book
- Foundational documents for evaluation in occupational therapy
- Evaluation responsibilities of occupational therapists
- Influence of evaluation on intervention planning
- External influences on the evaluation process
- Focus and content of this book.

Key Terms

Accountable evaluation
Assessment
Autonomy and confidentiality
Beneficence
Clinical reasoning
Evaluation
Evaluation report
Evidence-based evaluation
Formative
Health Insurance Portability and Accountability
    Act of 1996
International Classification of Functioning,
    Disability and Health

Nonmaleficence
Occupational performance
Occupational profile
Occupational Therapy Practice Framework:
    Domain and Process
Outcome-focused evaluation
Practice standards
Reassessment
Reevaluation
Scope of practice
Screening
Summative
Team approach

Evaluation is central to the process of occupational therapy intervention, and **clinical reasoning** is central to the process of evaluation. Occupational therapists engage in constant reflection, making choice after choice about which pieces of information are important and which are missing and determining how to obtain the information needed to reach an effective decision. Effective decisions in the evaluation phase lead to a clear intervention plan and, eventually, to improved client outcomes. Aggregating client evaluation information for program evaluation and outcomes studies ultimately leads to effective decisions regarding the overall effectiveness of intervention programs.

After defining the evaluation-related terms used in this book and discussing how evaluation and assessment fit within the context of several important practice-oriented documents, we outline in this chapter the responsibilities of occupational therapists and occupational therapy assistants in the evaluation process. We also discuss the influence of evaluation data on intervention planning and implementation, describe clinical decision making in the evaluation process, and note external influences on the evaluation process. Finally, we provide brief descriptions of some other important concepts in occupational therapy evaluation, including *accountable evaluation*, *evidence-based evaluation*, and *outcome-focused evaluation*.

Specifically, this chapter introduces the foundation and introductory content of the book while the other chapters deepen understanding of the evaluation process. Here, we present an overview of the core professional knowledge and attitudes requisite to being an effective occupational therapy evaluator. This core knowledge prepares one for practice-based evaluation and assessment processes on which any therapist can extend and refine the evaluation process so that it is relevant to specific practice contexts. This text will assist in making informed practice decisions after scanning publications and the literature to uncover resources for context- or condition-specific evaluation processes and valid, reliable assessments.

IMPORTANCE OF EVALUATION IN OCCUPATIONAL THERAPY

Although occupational therapists have always recognized the importance of evaluation, they have used the evaluation process and associated terms inconsistently. In addition, therapists have been guided by the questions,

- What information do I need to gather to determine if there is a need to initiate, continue, or discontinue intervention?
- What are the essential occupational performance and performance components that need evaluation in order to determine meaningful intervention?
- How can I document my accuracy and have confidence in my evaluation outcomes in order to prioritize intervention goals and advocate for my client's engagement in intervention processes?

The answers to each of these questions require therapists to use best practices during evaluation to ensure that they reflect the optimal way of obtaining the necessary information. A lack of attention to gathering the best information possible can lead to an evaluation process that looks *meaningful* (i.e., is valid) but has *low quality* (i.e., has low reliability or defensibility). The emphasis on treatment strategies over evaluation in the occupational therapy literature is reflected in practice. The profession now needs to revisit the concept and practice of occupational therapy evaluation to better determine, describe, and document the client's need for interventions, the results of intervention, and program outcomes.

This process is supported by the recent change in the profession to an evidence-based perspective. Professionals always construct evaluations using processes that reflect their unique professional philosophy and intervention frameworks to arrive at their independent decisions for treatment planning. An essential aspect of evidence-based practice is the valid and reliable evaluation of the client. Additionally, some reimbursement guidelines and legislation require standardized assessments and related data. The occupational therapist must reconcile that although professional association documents emphasize the use of nonstandardized assessments, such as the occupational profile, the requirements of external entities may be different.

The occupational therapist faces a conflict when performing an assessment given the profession's inherent focus on the occupational performance of a client. ***Occupational performance*** is "doing a task related to participation in a major life area" (Forsyth et al., 2014, p. 509). Clearly, occupational performance is difficult to measure, and few standardized assessments are available to measure it. Occupational performance is personal and contextual, and it varies from person to person and setting to setting.

However, many components of occupational therapy practice are measurable and must be measured to demonstrate the need for therapeutic input and the progress and change that are gained through the therapy process. Moreover, in addition to practicing within the guidelines of the profession, occupational therapists also need to practice within legal and reimbursement guidelines. Thus, occupational therapists face a dilemma and a challenge when doing a comprehensive evaluation of a client.

Occupational therapy textbooks that discuss evaluation usually focus on the use of specific assessments, with extensive overviews of proper administration coupled with guidance in interpreting specific findings. These descriptions of the assessments, however, do not address how occupational therapists should use the assessments to obtain a full perspective of the client. This book provides an overview of evaluation as well as a broad and comprehensive exploration of the evaluation process, contributing to the process of clinical reasoning and decision making. It also discusses the professional knowledge and skills underpinning competent decision making in selecting and administering quality evaluation approaches.

DEFINITIONS OF TERMS USED IN THIS BOOK

Screening, evaluation, and *assessment* are terms that have distinct purposes, definitions, and timing. Using these terms interchangeably can cause confusion. In this book, the following definitions are used.

Screening refers to the process of reviewing available data, observing a client, or administering screening instruments to identify a client's (or a population's) potential strengths and limitations and the need for further assessment. Screening results should never be the evaluative basis for

diagnostics, intervention planning, or monitoring. In the American Occupational Therapy Association's (AOTA's; 2010e) *Standards of Practice for Occupational Therapy, screening* is defined as "obtaining and reviewing data relevant to a potential client to determine the need for further evaluation and intervention" (p. S107).

Evaluation refers to the comprehensive process of obtaining and interpreting the data necessary to understand the person, system, or situation. As defined in the AOTA (2010e) *Standards of Practice for Occupational Therapy, evaluation* is "the process of obtaining and interpreting data necessary for intervention. This includes planning for and documenting the evaluation process and results" (p. S107). An occupational therapy evaluation requires synthesis of all data obtained; analytic interpretation of the data; reflective reasoning; and consideration of occupational performance, client factors, performance skills, performance patterns, context and environmental factors, and activity demands (AOTA, 2014).

In the evaluation reports, the therapists document the evaluation process, synthesize all findings, state results, and make recommendations, including the need for intervention. Evaluation reports may also describe potential changes to the intervention plan or summarize the client's performance abilities and limitations at the time of termination from current service.

Reevaluation refers to a formal comprehensive review of a client, system, or situation at some point after the initial evaluation. It may identify any need to modify the intervention plan or change the intervention approaches. According to the *Standards of Practice for Occupational Therapy* (AOTA, 2010e), *reevaluation* is "the process of critical analysis of client response to intervention. This analysis enables the therapist to make necessary changes to the intervention plan" (p. S107). Reevaluation may or may not include the use of assessments or instruments for assessment. When standardized assessments are not used, clinical reasoning and judgment direct intervention decisions that are made as part of the reevaluation process.

Assessment refers to a specific tool, instrument, or systematic interaction (e.g., observation, interview protocol) used as part of an evaluation to understand a client's occupational profile, client factors, performance skills, performance

EXHIBIT 1.1. KEY EVALUATION TERMS

Screening: Reviewing available data, observing a client, or administering screening instruments to identify potential strengths and limitations and the need for formal, targeted assessment.
Evaluation: Interpreting the data to understand the person, system, or situation for intervention planning, intervention progress, or discharge.
Reevaluation: The comprehensive formative review of a client, system, or situation at some point after the initial evaluation.
Assessment: Tool, instrument, or systematic interaction to measure or determine a client's occupational profile, occupational performance, or performance deficits.
Reassessment: Reviewing client performance at any time other than at initial evaluation; it may involve the use of an assessment.

intervention is effective or whether an intervention plan needs to be modified and contributes to reevaluation decision making. Use of the initial assessment during reassessment allows the detection of changes more easily; when using the initial assessment is not appropriate, a therapist may select a new assessment that measures the same construct or performance (Exhibit 1.1).

When one considers the clinical reasoning aspect of the evaluation process, it is helpful to explore some terms from education that can guide one's thinking through the evaluation process. The first term is *formative,* which refers to the process of gathering data so that one can identify what the potential problem areas are with a client. During this process, the therapist forms his or her ideas about what areas need attention and how he or she will begin to approach them. It can also refer to when client data are gathered between the initial data collection and later activities in specific areas to analyze current results and pinpoint observable performance improvement to fine-tune or update the intervention plan.

The second term is *summative,* which refers to the conclusions the therapist draws in the evaluation or the decisions the therapist makes after a course of intervention during the reassessment and reevaluation process. Summative processes also take place during the intervention process to

patterns, and contextual and environmental factors, as well as activity demands that influence occupational performance. Assessments, which vary from basic to complex, are component parts of the evaluation process.

Reassessment refers to the ongoing process of reviewing client performance at any time other than at initial evaluation. It may include the use of standardized or nonstandardized assessments. Reassessment is used to determine whether an

Table 1.1. Distinguishing Between Evaluation and Assessment Processes on the Basis of Use of Evaluation in Education

Initial Assessment	Reassessment	Final Reevaluation or Discharge Summary
Formative: Involves initial data gathering, is ongoing, aims to improve response to intervention	*Summative:* Determine progress and whether goals have been met *Formative:* Determine direction of future intervention; set or modify additional goals	*Summative:* Gauge quality or outcomes of intervention
Process-oriented: Determine how intervention is going or will go forward	*Product-oriented:* Identify what has improved or changed; determine need for more intervention *Process-oriented:* Determine need for and direction of additional intervention	*Product- or outcome-oriented:* Determine what has changed or improved and what requires a change in the intervention
Diagnostic: Identify areas for improvement	*Clinical judgment:* Measure progress, and determine areas for possible future intervention	*Clinical judgment:* Arrive at an overall measure of final condition's performance or function

determine the need to change or modify the approach being taken. Summative processes also occur at the end of an intervention to judge the outcomes or results of services. A summative evaluation is usually a global analysis of all assessment results—initial, formative, or final—using clinical reasoning and decision making to synthesize findings. Based on the use of formative and summative evaluation in education, Table 1.1 provides the foundation for distinguishing between these evaluation and assessment processes. The evaluation sequence is illustrated in a different manner in Figure 1.1.

The consistent use of terms can help the occupational therapy profession to communicate internally with greater efficacy. In turn, this practice will increase occupational therapists' and occupational therapy assistants' understanding of the evaluation and assessment processes and broaden the body of knowledge in this area. Note that some professions continue to use these terms interchangeably and that some define *evaluation* and *assessment* differently than we have defined them here.

Data Gathering (Formative)

Initial Evaluation With Initial Assessments (Summative)

Establish baseline function; diagnose or plan intervention

Reevaluation With Reassessments (Formative)

Determine response to change and need for changes in intervention goals

Reevaluation or Discharge Summary With Summative Assessments

Document the outcomes or results from intervention that is being discontinued

---

Figure 1.1. Evaluation sequence.
Source. J. Hinojosa. Used with permission.

FOUNDATIONAL DOCUMENTS FOR EVALUATION IN OCCUPATIONAL THERAPY

Occupational therapy evaluation has changed over the years, and the profession currently embraces several core constructs. The importance of occupation as a component of health and performance is a key concept to address in a comprehensive evaluation. Meaningful, successful occupations are grounded in a person's ability to function. The focus of a comprehensive evaluation is identifying the client's strengths, skills, weaknesses, and limitations. Because evaluation is directed toward deciding what the occupational therapist will do with the client, the client must be embraced as an essential part of the evaluation process. These core constructs are at the heart of several key documents that have important implications for occupational therapy evaluation.

Occupational Therapy Practice Framework: Domain and Process

The *Occupational Therapy Practice Framework: Domain and Process* (3rd ed.; AOTA, 2014; *Framework*) describes the occupational therapy process as having three steps: (1) evaluation, (2) intervention, and (3) outcomes. The discussion of the evaluation process in the *Framework* includes the occupational profile and an analysis of occupational performance, two important components of an occupational therapy evaluation. Within the analysis of occupational performance, the therapist may use both standardized and nonstandardized assessments.

The *Framework* does not identify screening as a step in the evaluation process, but it does take place in standard practice and, in our view, is one key element of the evaluation process. The result of a screening provides "trigger points of concern" to the therapist, suggesting the direction and need for more comprehensive and formal evaluation areas. Moreover, screening data provide direction for the selection of a theory-based guide for choosing assessments.

The **occupational profile** presented in the *Framework* is based on the fundamental philosophical belief in the importance of human occupation and client-centered care. This summary of occupational history, patterns of daily living, interests, values, and needs (AOTA, 2014) provides a perspective that should always be part of the occupational therapy evaluation and intervention. Additionally, an important point recognized in the *Framework* is that the occupational therapist's knowledge and skills and available evidence guide his or her clinical reasoning for the selection and application of various theories and frames of reference throughout the evaluation process (AOTA, 2014). However, missing from the *Framework's* discussion of evaluation is a consideration of real-world practicality. In some settings, there may not be enough time to compile a thorough occupational profile as the *Framework* describes it. In this book, we propose that the occupational profile is a legitimate occupational therapy assessment but is also a process and that it may be used over time, throughout both the evaluation and treatment phases of client-centered intervention, rather than purely as an assessment.

In the *Framework,* the analysis of occupational performance is a step in the evaluation process during which the therapist identifies the client's needs, problems, and concerns. Occupational performance is analyzed through collecting and interpreting information through assessment methods and measures that observe, discover, and quantify factors that support or hinder occupational performance (AOTA, 2014).

In a comprehensive evaluation, an occupational therapist must use multiple assessments, including standardized and nonstandardized, to have sufficient data to plan intervention. The ideas in this book are built on the principle that, in best practice, the therapist uses multiple assessments when evaluating a client, always considering the client's occupational history and goals.

Scope of Practice Documents

Professional associations, legislative acts, and common practice generally define the **scope of practice**. The purpose of a scope of practice document is to define both the parameters of a profession and what practitioners do on a day-to-day basis. Moreover, the scope of practice document defines the parameters for decision making, thereby setting limits on practice. Thus, these documents influence accepted evaluation and intervention processes for the profession (AOTA, 2004, 2010c; Clark, Polichino, & Jackson, 2004; Moyers & Dale, 2007).

Common practice also serves to determine the scope of practice of a profession. Regardless of the external influences, demands, or standards, the professional never abdicates the ethical responsibility for delivering quality intervention reflecting findings from evaluation processes as the basis for clinical reasoning.

AOTA's (2010c) official scope of practice document specifies what an occupational therapist should evaluate (Exhibit 1.2) but does not discuss the process of evaluation or the specific assessments occupational therapists might select. It is written to be consistent with the second edition of the *Framework* (AOTA, 2008). According to the scope of practice document, an occupational therapist evaluates the following four factors that affect activities of daily living, instrumental activities of daily living, education, work, play, leisure, and social participation:

1. Client factors, including body functions (e.g., neuromuscular, sensory, visual, perceptual, cognitive) and body structures (e.g., cardiovascular, digestive, integumentary, genitourinary systems);
2. Habits, routines, roles, and behavior patterns;
3. Cultural, physical, environmental, social, and spiritual contexts and activity demands that affect performance; and
4. Performance skills, including motor, process, and communication/interaction skills (AOTA, 2010c, p. S71).

EXHIBIT 1.2. AREAS EVALUATED ACROSS THE LIFESPAN IN OCCUPATIONAL THERAPY

- Activities of daily living
- Instrumental activities of daily living
- Occupations, including education, work, play, leisure, and social participation
- Client factors and body functions
- Habits, routines, roles, and behavior patterns
- Cultural, physical, environmental, social, and spiritual contexts
- Performance skills. (AOTA, 2010c, p. S71)

Emerging areas include diversity (individual and context), rest, and sleep.

The document also discusses the importance of the occupational therapy evaluation being client-centered. The scope of practice position paper identifies that the occupational therapist develops an occupational profile and analyzes the client's ability to participate and complete everyday life activities to determine the need for and priorities of intervention (AOTA, 2010c).

The Guide to Occupational Therapy Practice (Moyers & Dale, 2007) describes the occupational therapy evaluation process and is consistent with the second edition of the *Framework* (AOTA, 2008). Moyers and Dale defined *evaluation* as developing an occupational profile and analyzing occupational performance. The occupational profile is to occupational therapy what the medical history is to medicine and the social history is to social work. For the profile, the occupational therapist explores the client's past with a specific focus on that client's meaningful occupations throughout his or her life and especially in the recent past. From an occupational therapy perspective, understanding a client and the direction for intervention is dependent on what occupations are meaningful to him or her and what occupations are critical to his or her health and well-being for the future.

The therapist analyzes occupational performance to gain an understanding of the client's ability to complete ADLs, IADLs, education, work, play, leisure, and social participation. The analysis requires an examination "among performance skills and patterns, contexts and environment, general activity demands, and client factors" (Moyers & Dale, 2007, p. 23).

When the evaluation is complete, the occupational therapist develops an occupational performance statement based on all the collected data. This statement influences evaluation processes in the following ways:

- Prioritizing areas of occupational performance needs and activities
- Measuring occupational performance skills (motor, cognitive, communication, and interaction) and occupational performance patterns (roles, habits, rituals, and routines) related to prioritized activities
- Gauging the impact of person factors (body structure and function, spirituality, beliefs, and values)

- Appraising the influence of contextual and environmental supports and barriers (culture, physical, social, personal, temporal, or virtual). (Moyers & Dale, 2007, p. 30)

Although *The Guide to Occupational Therapy Practice* (Moyers & Dale, 2007) describes the important aspects of an occupational therapy evaluation, how theoretical perspectives may influence evaluation or intervention is not addressed. To be effective, assessments should be selected that reflect the specific theoretical model or frame of reference that is chosen to guide the evaluation process, intervention planning, and implementation.

Standards of Practice for Occupational Therapy

One of AOTA's most important responsibilities to society and to the profession is to establish **practice standards** (Exhibit 1.3). Practice standards define the minimum requirements for performance and quality of care by occupational therapists and occupational therapy assistants delivering daily practice across all settings. Employers, clients, peers, and the general public use these standards to assess the appropriateness and quality of services received. Any performance or quality of care below these standards is incompetent practice.

According to AOTA's (2010e) *Standard of Practice for Occupational Therapy*, the occupational therapy assistant participates in the evaluation process under the direction of the occupational therapist. Furthermore, "An occupational therapy assistant contributes to the screening, evaluation, and re-evaluation process by implementing delegated assessments and by providing verbal and written reports of observations and client capacities to the occupational therapist in accordance with federal and state laws, other regulatory and payer requirements, and AOTA documents" (AOTA, 2010e, p. S107). Thus, an occupational therapist may delegate aspects of specific assessments to be administered by the occupational therapy assistant.

Both the therapist and the assistant share the responsibility to ensure that the assistant is competent enough to administer the specific assessment assigned. However, although the process may be collaborative, the supervising therapist is

---

EXHIBIT 1.3. EVALUATION PRACTICE STANDARDS FOR THE OCCUPATIONAL THERAPIST AND THE OCCUPATIONAL THERAPY ASSISTANT

Occupational therapy assistant:
- Participates in the evaluation process under the direction of the occupational therapist.
- Contributes to the screening, evaluation, and reevaluation process by implementing delegated assessments.
- Provides verbal and written reports of observations and client capacities to the occupational therapist in accordance with federal and state laws, other regulatory and payer requirements, and AOTA documents.

Occupational therapist:
- Supervises and may delegate aspects of specific assessments to be administered by the occupational therapy assistant.
- Is responsible for:
  - Selecting specific assessments;
  - Initiating and completing the evaluation;
  - Interpreting the data; and
  - Developing the intervention plan.

Occupational therapist and occupational therapy assistant:
- Work collaboratively during evaluation.
- Share the responsibility to ensure that the occupational therapy assistant is competent to administer the specific assessment assigned.
- Show compliance with practice and competency standards.

Note. From AOTA (2010d, 2010e).

---

ultimately responsible for selecting specific assessments, initiating and completing the evaluation, interpreting the data, and developing the intervention plan (AOTA, 2010e). Both the therapist and the assistant have professional responsibility to show and maintain compliance with the *Standards of Practice for Occupational Therapy* (AOTA, 2010e) and *Standards for Continuing Competence* (AOTA, 2010d).

The current AOTA (2010e) *Standards of Practice for Occupational Therapy* have one standard related to screening, evaluation, and reevaluation (Exhibit 1.4), whereas the 2011 Accreditation Council for Occupational Therapy Education (ACOTE®) *Standards for an Accredited Educational Program for the Occupational Therapist and Occupational*

Therapy Assistants (ACOTE, 2012) further divided evaluation into separate standards for screening and evaluation. In Exhibit 1.5, we propose additional standards to ensure competent performance of assessment and evaluation, using ideas from the American Psychological Association (2010), the American Counseling Association (2005), and the Council for Exceptional Children (2004).

Accredited Educational Programs for the Occupational Therapist

Occupational therapy education prepares occupational therapists and occupational therapy assistants for their therapeutic responsibilities. According to the 2011 ACOTE Standards (ACOTE, 2012), occupational therapy doctoral and master's students are required to learn to select, administer, and interpret standardized and nonstandardized tests and assessments. These assessments must be culturally relevant and have a theoretical base. Additionally, the process should be based on individual needs as well as those of populations.

As mentioned earlier, occupational therapy assistants need to be able to collect assessment data under the supervision of and collaboration with the occupational therapist. They may use a variety of standardized and nonstandardized assessments under these guidelines (ACOTE, 2012).

According to the 2011 ACOTE Standards (ACOTE, 2012), the entry-level occupational therapist, both at the doctoral and master's level, is to be able to select appropriate assessments for screening and evaluation using standardized formats for the administration and interpretation of the evaluation data. Potential bias interpreting standardized assessments is to be eliminated and, if not, reported regarding potential influence on results. Additionally, the occupational therapist should consider evidence-based practice in the use of assessments and prepare documentation that meets local, state, and federal guidelines for accountability and reimbursement when documenting need for services (ACOTE, 2012). Both the occupational therapist and the occupational therapy assistant should understand and act on expected evaluation roles, responsibilities, and parameters for each other.

When multiple professional guidelines coexist, inconsistences might be found. To guide

---

EXHIBIT 1.4. AOTA STANDARDS OF PRACTICE FOR OCCUPATIONAL THERAPY: STANDARD II: SCREENING, EVALUATION, AND REEVALUATION

1. An occupational therapist is responsible for all aspects of the screening, evaluation, and re-evaluation process.
2. An occupational therapist accepts and responds to referrals in compliance with state or federal laws, other regulatory and payer requirements, and AOTA documents.
3. An occupational therapist, in collaboration with the client, evaluates the client's ability to participate in daily life by considering the client's history, goals, capacities, and needs; the activities and occupations the client wants and needs to perform; and the environments and context in which these activities and occupations occur.
4. An occupational therapist initiates and directs the screening, evaluation, and re-evaluation process and analyzes and interprets the data in accordance with federal and state law, other regulatory and payer requirements, and AOTA documents.
5. An occupational therapy assistant contributes to the screening, evaluation, and re-evaluation process by implementing delegated assessments and by providing verbal and written reports of observations and client capacities to the occupational therapist in accordance with federal and state laws, other regulatory and payer requirements, and AOTA documents.
6. An occupational therapy practitioner uses current assessments and assessment procedures and follows defined protocols of standardized assessments during the screening, evaluation, and re-evaluation process.
7. An occupational therapist completes and documents occupational therapy evaluation results. An occupational therapy assistant contributes to the documentation of evaluation results. An occupational therapy practitioner abides by the time frames, formats, and standards established by practice settings, federal and state law, other regulatory and payer requirements, external accreditation programs, and AOTA documents.
8. An occupational therapy practitioner communicates screening, evaluation, and re-evaluation results within the boundaries of client confidentiality and privacy regulations to the appropriate person, group, organization, or population.
9. An occupational therapist recommends additional consultations or refers clients to appropriate resources when the needs of the client can best be served by the expertise of other professionals or services.
10. An occupational therapy practitioner educates current and potential referral sources about the scope of occupational therapy services and the process of initiating occupational therapy services.

Source. From AOTA (2010e). Standards of practice for occupational therapy. *American Journal of Occupational Therapy, 64*(Suppl.), S107–S108. http://dx.doi.org/10.5014/ajot.2010.64S106. Copyright © 2010 by the American Occupational Therapy Association. Reprinted with permission.

---

professional behavior, the therapist is responsible to attend to all guidelines in combination and to keep up with changes in or additions to expectations. Minor differences or omissions can currently be found in professional behavior expectations related to screening, occupational profiles, and occupational therapist supervision of an occupational therapy assistant delivering assessment parts or input in intervention planning parts of assessment.

Occupational Therapy Code of Ethics and Ethics Standards

Occupational therapists and occupational therapy assistants must abide by the *Occupational Therapy Code of Ethics and Ethics Standards* (AOTA, 2010b), which are "an aspirational document to guide occupational therapists, occupational therapy assistants, and occupational therapy students toward appropriate professional conduct in all aspects of their diverse roles" (AOTA, 2010a). The *Code of Ethics* contains three key ethical principles related to evaluation and assessment: (1) beneficence, (2) autonomy and confidentiality, and (3) nonmaleficence (AOTA, 2010b; Table 1.2).

Beneficence

Beneficence is the ethical principle that a professional shall demonstrate concern for the well-being and safety of clients and should not put them at risk or harm. All tests have biases because of gender, educational level, socioeconomic background, ethnic background, cultural background, geographic environment, or medical status that must be acknowledged. Selection of the least biased assessment appropriate for a particular person is required.

For example, if an occupational therapist receives a referral to evaluate a person with right

EXHIBIT 1.5. PROPOSED STANDARDS TO ENSURE COMPETENT PERFORMANCE OF ASSESSMENT AND EVALUATION

Screening

1. An occupational therapist observes a potential client, reviews available records, or administers screening instruments to identify a client's or population's potential strengths and limitations and the need for an evaluation.

Evaluation

1. An occupational therapist is responsible for choosing appropriate assessments for the evaluation of the client. Therapists select assessments that do not discriminate against people because of race, color, creed, culture, gender, language preference, religion, national origin, age, political practices, family or social background, sexual orientation, or disability status.
2. An occupational therapist uses assessments whose reliability and validity have been established with the population being tested. The therapist should explicitly state the strengths and limitations of the results and interpretation when validity and reliability have not been established for a population being tested. An occupational therapist uses only the assessments for which he or she has appropriate knowledge, expertise, and skills and is competent in administering. An occupational therapist never allows unqualified people under his or her supervision to administer tests for which they do not have appropriate training and experience.
3. An occupational therapist explains, before administering any assessment, the purpose of the evaluation. Furthermore, the therapist outlines the purpose of each assessment and explicitly states how the results will be used.
4. An occupational therapist administers and adapts or uses assessments that are appropriate and consistent with the research and scores and interprets assessment results in the manner intended by the developer or publisher of each assessment.
5. An occupational therapist is responsible for the appropriate scoring, interpretation, and use of assessment. An occupational therapist ensures the accuracy and appropriateness of the evaluation summary. The therapist completes evaluation summaries within the time frames, formats, and standards established by the professional practice settings, government agencies, external accreditation programs, and third-party payers. Evaluation summaries reflect the guidelines for assessment interpretation provided by the developers or publishers of the assessments used.
6. An occupational therapist writes an evaluation report that explicitly reflects a synthesis of all data obtained, analytic interpretation of the data, reflective clinical reasoning, and consideration of contextual factors. Evaluation reports document the evaluation process, synthesize all findings, and state results and recommendations, including the need for initiation of or changes in intervention.
7. An occupational therapist and an occupational therapy assistant respect the boundaries of client confidentiality. They maintain the confidentiality of information, except when information is released with specific written consent and within statutory confidentiality requirements.

Note. Drawn from using ideas from the American Psychological Association (2010), the American Counseling Association (2005), and the Council for Exceptional Children (2004).

hemiplegia, the therapist first needs to find out about the person's age, gender, culture, and other relevant factors in order to choose an appropriate assessment that will accurately reflect the person's performance. Using multiple assessments to obtain a more accurate picture of performance variations may reduce test bias. Therapists frequently find that a combination of standardized and nonstandardized instruments, together with observations and clinical judgment, provides a reasonably accurate overall portrait of a client's strengths and limitations.

The evaluation report should present a balanced perspective of the client's occupational performance, identifying his or her strengths and areas of concern. Conclusions made by the therapist in the report should be directed toward helping the client rather than labeling the client in a way that might be harmful.

Autonomy and confidentiality

The principle of **autonomy and confidentiality** addresses clients' rights and the occupational therapists' and occupational therapy assistants'

Table 1.2. Ethical Principles Related to Occupational Therapy Evaluation

Ethical Principle	Code of Behavior	Relevance to Occupational Therapy Evaluation
Beneficence	Concern for the well-being and safety of clients to avoid potential risk or harm	• Prevent bias in testing • Use whatever tests are needed to obtain an accurate picture of client performance and function
Autonomy and confidentiality	Being respectful of the client's independence and protecting the right of privacy	• Secure clients' information to ensure privacy • Uphold HIPAA protections • Accurate, comprehensive evaluation reporting
Nonmaleficence	Not doing harm to the client at any time during evaluation and intervention	• Evidence-based, reflective selection of assessments • Comparison of test results with valid norms • Documenting deviations from standardized test procedures and impact on results • Being competent in all procedures required by the assessment

Note. HIPAA = Health Insurance Portability and Accountability Act of 1996.

responsibility to respect clients and keep clients' information private. Therapists must protect the confidential nature of all information obtained from a client during the screening and evaluation process. The **Health Insurance Portability and Accountability Act of 1996 (HIPAA)** further reinforced confidentiality protections.

In most cases, the evaluation process is not complete until the findings have been written up in an evaluation report or evaluation summary. These reports should be concise yet comprehensive and should include only honest and accurate information. Evaluation data should be interpreted using a theoretical framework and the therapist's knowledge and expertise in working with the population.

Nonmaleficence

The ethical principle of *nonmaleficence* refers to the importance of not doing harm to the client at any time during evaluation and intervention through careful selection of assessments. When occupational therapists use standardized and nonstandardized assessment with clients whose characteristics differ from those of the intended testing population, the results may not be comparable or even valid, and areas identified as deficits may not actually be deficits.

Occupational therapists are expected to be competent in the administration and interpretation of an assessment before using it with a client. To achieve such competency, therapists need to study and practice assessments, including adhering to the manualized administration procedures, ensuring the psychometric properties are upheld, and following expected interpretation guidelines for reporting results. Some assessments require certification, postprofessional continuing education, or even an additional academic degree. Examples of advanced-level assessments include the Sensory Integration and Praxis Tests (Ayres, 1989) and the Assessment of Motor and Process Skills (Fisher & Jones, 2012).

International Classification of Functioning, Disability and Health

The World Health Organization (WHO) has worked diligently to facilitate the use of universal language regarding disability across countries and cultures. The most current revision to the *International Classification of Functioning, Disability and Health (ICF;* WHO, 2001) uses a disability model and readily understood labels that go beyond the traditional medical model by focusing on a social model of health and participation (Hinojosa, Kramer, Royeen, & Luebben, 2003). The *ICF* provides parameters for gaining a comprehensive understanding of the person in two areas—functioning and disability—and introduces the concept of *participation,* which is increasingly discussed in our profession as an important practice consideration to address the whole client (WHO, 2001).

One of the intended applications of the *ICF* is "as a clinical tool—in needs assessment, matching treatments with specific conditions, vocational assessment, rehabilitation and outcome evaluation" (WHO, 2001, p. 5). Evaluation consistent with *ICF* principles has a broad perspective, including an exploration of the interaction between the person and the context. Additionally, the *ICF* proposes that a comprehensive evaluation of a person may be needed for his or her needs and abilities to be understood (WHO, 2001).

EVALUATION RESPONSIBILITIES OF OCCUPATIONAL THERAPISTS

Effective evaluators have a comprehensive knowledge of the domain of concern of the profession, human development and individual variation, statistics, tests and measurements, and the concepts of *activities* and *occupation*. Additionally, occupational therapists have to be skilled in interacting with clients to elicit information and judge their performance and the quality of their response. Therapists need to be competent in administering a broad repertoire of assessments. When using a specific assessment, therapists should know its strengths and limitations, psychometric properties, and applicability to specific situations.

Another important influence on the type and focus of evaluation is the client. It is incumbent upon occupational therapists to listen to the client and respond appropriately. The client may have specific concerns or expectations; for example, a client may want to be independent in bathing and toileting but is content to receive help with dressing. In this case, therapists have two options: (1) to evaluate and address only the performance areas of concern to the client or (2) to educate the client about how identified areas might be improved or enhanced through therapy. Clients always have the right to accept or refuse evaluation or intervention. They also have the right to know the outcomes of

> Effective evaluators know the domain of concern of the profession, human development and individual variation, statistics, tests and measurements, skilled interaction, and the concepts of *activities* and *occupation*.

specific assessments, so therapists should review the results with clients and answer any questions they may have. Finally, when interpreting the results of the evaluation, therapists need to put the data within the context of the client's personal view of his or her life, interests, environment, and chosen occupations.

Each of the chapters that follow is written to deepen readers' knowledge regarding these major essential topics to fully engage the evaluator's roles and functions in occupational therapy practice. The following is an overview of the essential considerations in being an evaluator.

> Another important influence on the type and focus of evaluation is the client. It is incumbent upon therapists to listen to the client and respond appropriately.

Occupational therapists need to understand the circumstances of the evaluation and how they influence the selection of assessment. These circumstances include the time and space available for testing, the service delivery model, the purpose of the evaluation, and other evaluations being administered to the client. Therapists also need to have the expertise and skills to administer the chosen assessments and, once the assessments have been administered, to interpret the data.

Data interpretation involves combining data from various sources and determining which data are important and how the data fit, both with the domain of concern of occupational therapy and with the role of occupational therapy within the setting. Therapists must then document their findings in a format that is appropriate to the setting and that highlights points clearly and concisely so all persons involved can understand the issues.

In addition to documenting the evaluation, therapists often need to convey the findings to the client, his or her family or caregivers, and other professionals. This communication should be clear and accurate, appropriate to the audience, and conducive to providing the best services for the person within and between provider groups and agencies.

INFLUENCE OF EVALUATION ON INTERVENTION PLANNING

Once occupational therapists have completed a screening or a thorough review of the client's educational or health records, they decide how to proceed with the evaluation. The assessments used in the evaluation process will affect the intervention process and approach. Sometimes, therapists know what theory or frame of reference would be appropriate for a client just by reading a chart or interviewing the client. Other times, there is limited information available to help determine which theoretical approach would be the best to follow.

During the process of evaluation, occupational therapists continually review the assessment data and make decisions and judgments based on the information. The process is intensive and dynamic, requiring reflective practice, constant thinking and decision making as the client completes each assessment. As the therapist reviews the data from each assessment, he or she decides how to proceed, and each decision leads to another set of choices regarding the next steps. The experienced therapist's clinical decisions flow smoothly and indubitably.

> The assessments used in the evaluation process will affect the intervention process and approach. The process is intensive and dynamic, requiring reflective practice, constant thinking, and decision making as the client completes each assessment.

The entry-level therapist needs to become familiar with a wide variety of assessments, including the development of skills in using these assessments, to become a competent evaluator. Both experienced and entry-level therapists use reflective practice approaches to learn through critically analyzing responses to their interventions to continually deepen and improve their assessment skills.

Other clinical constraints influence clinical decision making during evaluation. Practice settings typically allow little time for evaluation and, at times, third-party payers or certain settings such as schools prescribe the assessments to be used. In addition, an institution may have a set protocol for evaluation that is required for every client, regardless of his or her individual needs. In such situations, the therapist's evaluation decisions are greatly influenced by outside factors. It is imperative that therapists develop their skills and competence so that they can adequately justify their actions and decisions in evaluations.

Evaluation Report

Because the purpose of the **evaluation report** is to communicate information to others, occupational therapists need to know the target audience when constructing the report. The client may need a report that is written with an educational focus, a physician may need medical data presented in a succinct manner, and a third-party payer may require documentation to show that the situation meets the criteria for reimbursement. Thus, more than one summary may need to be written for the same client. Reports should be proofread carefully to ensure that they are clearly written for the intended audience and errorless, using a professional style; the report is often the first impression therapists make and therefore warrants skillful execution. Likewise, therapists must ensure that documentation is accurate, legally defensible, unalterable by others, and secure.

Evaluation reports should indicate that assessments used are standardized for the individual client or population and are reliable and valid. Moreover, if the test is used for a different population or age group, the rationale for usage should be clearly explained along with the strength and limitations of the assessment for this population.

> Evaluation reports, like all professional documentation, should be proofread carefully to ensure that they are clearly written for the intended audience and errorless, using a professional style; the report is often the first impression therapists make and therefore warrants skillful execution.

Accountable Evaluation

Accountable evaluation starts with an evaluation process based on an occupational profile followed by the choice of specific assessments that are standardized; reliable; valid; suitable for the specific client or client group; and acceptable to other professionals, consumers, and third-party payers. Accountability concerns are reflected through the form and content of the evaluation report and the degree to which the report is evidence based or outcome focused.

> Accountable evaluation starts with an evaluation process based on an occupational profile and the choice of specific assessments that are standardized; reliable; valid; suitable for the specific client or client group; and acceptable to other professionals, consumers, and third-party payers.

These assessments or processes are defensible in terms of professional standards and best practice, and they reflect the domain of concern of the profession. Because of the nature of occupational therapy, all evaluations should include an occupational profile that describes a client's occupations, contextual information, and client-centered priorities. When a client is unable to express his or her ideas, the occupational profile may be generated with information from care providers, significant others, and other professionals. Full accountability requires that an evaluation provide an accurate assessment of the client's performance, skills, and deficits, combined with his or her personal needs and goals, in a manner that is generally acceptable in the context of that client's life.

Evidence-Based Evaluation

Evidence-based evaluation requires sufficient facts about the client, the assessments, and the evaluation process to support appropriate decision making. Using a reflective process, occupational therapists consider what the particular client needs and explore the literature for guidance about best practice. The literature can help therapists identify the assessments most often used in the relevant type of situation, as well as the value and rigor of those assessments (intended purposes, reliability, and validity).

As part of this process, therapists are required to scrutinize their own clinical experiences and integrate them with information gleaned from the literature regarding the assessments, client characteristics, and the context of the evaluation. During this reflective process, the therapist considers those assessments in which he or she is competent and that meet the age and suspected strengths and deficits of the client. This reflective process should result in a well-thought-out plan for evaluation.

> The literature can help therapists identify the assessments most often used in the relevant type of situation, as well as the value and rigor of those assessments (intended purposes, reliability, and validity). These should be the assessments of choice rather than the assessments with which the therapist is most comfortable.

Outcome-Focused Evaluation

Outcome-focused evaluation is the process of evaluating a client on the basis of his or her desired outcomes. This process requires occupational therapists to use reverse thinking and to begin with the client's identified needs, desires, and limitations. Once clients have identified their preferred outcome of treatment (through an interview or an occupational profile), therapists need to determine what type of evaluation will measure the achievement of those desired outcomes. Clients' desired outcomes guide therapists' judgment during evaluation and throughout treatment.

Another type of outcome-focused evaluation can take place before discharge from occupational therapy services. The discharge evaluation data are compared with initial evaluation results to describe the client's level of performance improvements or change relative to the stated expectations at the beginning of intervention. Not only must therapists consider whether or not the desired outcome was reached, but they must also carefully reflect on whether the initial goals were realistic and whether the process used was effective enough to achieve the desired results. At the end of this process, therapists may determine that different assessments should be used either for initial evaluation in the future or for determining outcome performance.

Team Approach

Occupational therapy practitioners commonly use a **team approach** to plan and implement interventions. Often, occupational therapy evaluation reports are part of a larger comprehensive team evaluation. Sharing hypotheses with the team may provide an enhanced view of the client. Individual members of the team contribute a different perspective on the client as a result of their own evaluation process, and information gained from the collaborative process can provide a more complete picture of the client's abilities and disabilities. The team will discuss which assessments each member will use and the purpose of each to ensure that unnecessary duplication is avoided and that assessments provide complementary data regarding the client's abilities and disabilities.

> Each member of the team contributes a different perspective on the client as a result of his or her own evaluation process, and information gained from the collaborative process can provide a more complete picture of the client's abilities and disabilities. The sum is greater than each part individually.

In addition, it is helpful for team members to keep their findings and interpretations confidential until all members have completed their evaluations; when multiple professionals evaluate the client, it can be helpful for each to come to his or her own conclusions individually before the team meets collectively. This strategy can prevent one member from being swayed by the hypotheses of another, thus helping the team avoid an inaccurate conclusion. This strategy can also help the team identify variations in the client's performance from one evaluation session to another.

EXTERNAL INFLUENCES ON THE EVALUATION PROCESS

At times, the type or focus of the evaluation is determined externally. The institution may require that an evaluation include one or more specific assessments; for example, a hospital may require that all clients on their inpatient unit be evaluated using Functional Independence Measure (FIM™; Granger, Hamilton, & Sherwin, 1986) and the Bay Area Functional Performance Evaluation (Williams & Bloomer, 1987). Alternatively, a service delivery model may require that the evaluation have a specific focus; for example, a school system typically requires an evaluation with a focus on educational relevancy or a screening to provide early identification of students with potential learning difficulties.

In other circumstances, a referral may suggest or require a specific type of evaluation, such as a referral for occupational therapy following joint replacement surgery. Regardless of whether occupational therapists have a choice in the evaluation process or the assessments used, they have a professional responsibility to make sure that the overall evaluation meets the needs of the client, reflects the domain of concern of occupational therapy, and is relevant to the programming and intervention services that will be offered.

> Regardless of whether occupational therapists have a choice in the evaluation process or the assessments used, they have a professional responsibility to make sure that the overall evaluation meets the needs of the client, reflects the domain of concern of occupational therapy, and is relevant to the programming and intervention services that will be offered.

When completing an occupational profile, an informed client often brings his or her own concerns, ideas, and expectations about what the evaluation process will include and what outcomes he or she expects. Occupational

therapists may agree with the client's perspective or may have differing views about what the evaluation should entail. It is critical that therapists involve the client and consider his or her point of view. Open discussion about the evaluation process, the use of the results, and the concerns of both parties can be a large step forward in developing a rapport that will serve as the basis for a positive therapeutic relationship.

Therapists can inform clients that therapists likely cannot interpret the specific results from an assessment session immediately because they need time to consider the meaning of overall assessment results first. Through a collaborative process, therapists and clients work toward reaching a consensus on the evaluation, its focus, and what it will include. Forthright discussion and willingness to consider each other's perspectives enable mutual trust to develop, and a trusting relationship is the foundation for future intervention.

FOCUS AND CONTENT OF THIS BOOK

The focus of this book is the evaluation and assessment of people seeking occupational therapy services. Although the authors mention specific assessments and processes in some chapters to illustrate their points, no chapter presents or reviews the use of specific assessments or evaluations with specific populations. Occupational therapists are responsible for choosing the appropriate assessments from all those available to provide the data they need to make sound clinical judgments. One goal of this book is to explore evaluation as a vehicle for determining the need for intervention and for developing or changing intervention plans. This book will not deal with the complex topic of non-client-related evaluations that occupational therapists engage in, such as systems facilities, or programmatic evaluations. However, systematic and well-planned evaluation that is congruent with the goals of each occupational therapy program provides valuable data for these other very important types of evaluation as well.

A critical element of this book is its emphasis on the process of evaluation rather than on the assessments for evaluation. An understanding of the entire evaluation process will help occupational therapists better determine the need for intervention, establish an appropriate treatment plan, and determine the results of intervention.

Moreover, the ongoing process provides therapists with an understanding of when and how to modify the intervention plan on the basis of ongoing clinical reasoning and monitoring of intervention effectiveness. Collaboration with the client is essential to ensure that the intervention has the desired effect of enabling him or her to engage in meaningful occupation. Once they thoroughly understand the various concepts foundational to evaluation, therapists are in a better position to choose the most appropriate assessments for the situation at hand.

Chapter 2, "Philosophical and Theoretical Influences on Evaluation," continues the discussion of the general theoretical issues in evaluation begun in this chapter. It describes the philosophical basis of evaluation and its relationship to occupational therapy theory and, in particular, to frames of reference. It also provides an overview of the evaluation process. Chapters 3 through 6 center on the use of assessments throughout the evaluation process: Chapter 3, "Assessment Identification and Selection," provides a process for identifying and selecting assessments to use in practice; Chapter 4, "Practical Aspects of the Evaluation Process," discusses evaluation issues in today's complex practice environment; and Chapter 5, "Evaluation in the Intervention Planning Process," discusses the use of evaluation in the intervention planning process. Chapter 6, "Administration of Evaluation and Assessment," discusses the administration of evaluation and assessment, and Chapter 7, "Contextual Evaluation to Support Participation," explores the influence of context on the client and the evaluation process. Subsequent chapters discuss the use of nonstandardized assessments (Chapter 8, "Nonstandardized Testing"); the psychometrics of standardized assessments, including reliability and validity (Chapter 9, "Standardized Testing: Psychometrics"); and the scoring and interpretation of assessment results (Chapter 10, "Standardized Testing: Scoring and Interpretation of Results").

Chapter 11, "Interpretation and Documentation," presents discussions of the critical areas of data interpretation and documentation of evaluation results. Chapter 12, "Reassessment and Reevaluation," investigates reassessment and reevaluation in depth. Evaluation issues with special populations are addressed in Chapter 13, "Evaluating Special Populations," and the ethical implications of evaluation are outlined in Chapter 14, "Ethical Implications in Evaluation." Chapter 15, "Use of Evaluation Data to Support Evidence-Based Practice," discusses the use of evaluation data to support evidence-based practice, and Chapter 16, "Additional Uses of Evaluation Data," describes other uses of evaluation data, including outcomes measurement, research, and program development.

SUMMARY

Evaluation is a primary aspect of the occupational therapy process. Although many ways of conceptualizing practice exist, occupational therapists generally approach the evaluation of clients by starting with an assessment of an aspect of the profession's domain of concern. Comprehensive evaluation requires that occupational therapists assess all aspects of the domain of concern as they relate to the individual client. In the occupational therapist's role as an evaluator, he or she must comply with AOTA's current standards of practice, the *Occupational Therapy Code of Ethics and Ethics Standards*, and sound professional judgment. The occupational therapy assistant participates in the evaluation process under the direction of the occupational therapist.

The process of evaluation is complex and challenging. Both knowledge and skill on the part of the therapist are required. Entry-level academic education provides a core understanding of evaluation in general; however, this education is just the beginning. To gain proficiency in evaluation, occupational therapists must continually learn new assessments, develop mastery of a variety of assessments, reflect on the relevancy of generally used assessments, understand the various roles that the client plays in the evaluation process, and examine the literature regarding all aspects of evaluation. This text provides the foundational knowledge on evaluation to competently engage in test and measurement processes as an occupational therapist.

QUESTIONS

1. Explain why an occupational therapist should not develop an intervention plan based on screening data alone.
2. What is the difference between *reassessment* and *reevaluation*? Why is it important to differentiate between these two concepts?
3. The authors state that a supervising therapist may delegate specific assessments to be administered by an occupational therapy assistant. How would a therapist justify the delegation of this responsibility?
4. How would the current AOTA standards of practice influence your conceptualization and administration of an evaluation?
5. Identify the consistencies and inconsistencies in the various documents regarding the role and activities associated with occupational therapy evaluation discussed in this chapter.
6. Examine the occupational profile and analysis of occupational performance. Describe how you would use these elements as part of an evaluation. What critical elements would you add to make it a comprehensive evaluation?
7. Identify the basic characteristics and benefits of a good evaluation program.
8. What are the potential problems or challenges that arise when a therapist does not implement evaluation for individuals, the system, or setting?

References

Accreditation Council for Occupational Therapy Education. (2012). 2011 Accreditation Council for Occupational Therapy Education (ACOTE®) standards. *American Journal of Occupational Therapy, 66*(Suppl.), S6–S74. http://dx.doi.org/10.5014/ajot.2012.66S6

American Counseling Association. (2005). *ACA code of ethics.* Retrieved from http://www.counseling.org/Resources/aca-code-of-ethics.pdf

American Occupational Therapy Association. (2004). Assistive technology within occupational therapy practice. *American Journal of Occupational Therapy, 58,* 678–680. http://dx.doi.org/10.5014/ajot.58.6.678

American Occupational Therapy Association. (2008). Occupational therapy practice framework: Domain and process (2nd ed.). *American Journal of Occupational Therapy, 62,* 625–683. http://dx.doi.org/10.5014/ajot.62.6.625

American Occupational Therapy Association. (2010a). Enforcement procedures for the occupational therapy code of ethics and ethics standards. *American Journal of Occupational Therapy, 64*(Suppl.), S4–S16. http://dx.doi.org/10.5014/ajot.2010.64S4

American Occupational Therapy Association. (2010b). Occupational therapy code of ethics and ethics standards (2010). *American Journal of Occupational Therapy, 64*(Suppl.), S17–S26. http://dx.doi.org/10.5014/ajot.2010.64S17

American Occupational Therapy Association. (2010c). Scope of practice. *American Journal of Occupational Therapy, 64*(Suppl.), S70–S77. http://dx.doi.org/10.5014/ajot.2010.64S70

American Occupational Therapy Association. (2010d). Standards for continuing competence. *American Journal of Occupational Therapy, 64*(Suppl.), S103–S105. http://dx.doi.org/10.5014/ajot.2010.64S103

American Occupational Therapy Association. (2010e). Standards of practice for occupational therapy. *American Journal of Occupational Therapy, 64*(Suppl.), S106–S111. http://dx.doi.org/10.5014/ajot.2010.64S106

American Occupational Therapy Association. (2014). Occupational therapy practice framework: Domain and process (3rd ed.). *American Journal of Occupational Therapy, 68*(Suppl. 1), S1–S48. http://dx.doi.org/10.5014/ajot.2014.682006

American Psychological Association. (2010). *Ethical principles of psychologists and code of conduct with the 2010 amendments.* Retrieved from http://www.apa.org/ethics/code/index.aspx

Ayres, A. J. (1989). *Sensory integration and praxis tests.* Los Angeles: Western Psychological Services.

Clark, G. F., Polichino, J., & Jackson, L. (2004). Occupational therapy services in early intervention and school-based programs. *American Journal of Occupational Therapy, 58,* 681–685. http://dx.doi.org/10.5014/ajot.58.6.681

Council for Exceptional Children. (2004). *Professional standards.* Retrieved from http://www.cec.sped.org/Standards/Ethical-Principles-and-Practice-Standards

Fisher, A. G. & Jones, K. B. (2012). *Assessment of Motor and Process Skills* (7th ed., rev.). Fort Collins, CO: Three Star Press.

Forsyth, K., Taylor, R. R., Kramer, J. M., Prior, S., Richie, L., Whitehead, J., . . . Melton, J. (2014). The Model of Human Occupation. In B. A. B. Schell, G. Gillen, & M. E. Scaffa (Eds.), *Willard and Spackman's occupational therapy* (12th ed., p. 505–526). Baltimore: Lippincott Williams & Wilkins.

Granger, C. V., Hamilton, B. B., & Sherwin, F. S. (1986). *Guide for use of the uniform data set for medical rehabilitation.* Buffalo, NY: Buffalo General Hospital, Department of Rehabilitation Medicine.

Health Insurance Portability and Accountability Act of 1996, Pub. L. 104–191, 45 C.F.R. § 160, 164.

Hinojosa, J., Kramer, P., Royeen, C. B., & Luebben, A. (2003). The core concept of occupation. In P. Kramer, J. Hinojosa, & C. B. Royeen (Eds.), *Perspectives in human occupation: Participation in life* (pp. 1–17). Philadelphia: Lippincott Williams & Wilkins.

Moyers, P., & Dale, L. (Eds.). (2007). *The guide to occupational therapy practice* (2nd ed.). Bethesda, MD: AOTA Press.

Williams, S. L., & Bloomer, J. (1987). *Bay Area Functional Performance Evaluation administration and scoring manual* (2nd ed.). Palo Alto, CA: Consulting Psychologists Press.

World Health Organization. (2001). *International classification of functioning, disability and health.* Geneva: Author.

CHAPTER 2

Philosophical and Theoretical Influences on Evaluation

Paula Kramer, PhD, OTR, FAOTA
Jim Hinojosa, PhD, OT, BCP, FAOTA

Highlights

- Philosophical influences on evaluation
- Beginning the evaluation process
- Choosing the frame of reference
- Therapist perspectives, theory, and practice.

Key Terms

Biases
Bottom-up approach
Clear choice
Client
Concepts
Contextual approach
Contextual factors
Evaluation process
Evaluation summary
Exploratory approach

Frame of reference
Idiosyncratic approach
Perspective
Philosophical beliefs
Population
Postulates
Reassessment
Screening
Theories
Top-down approach

Each occupational therapist has a set of philosophical assumptions and beliefs based in part on those of the profession, acquired through education, and in part on personal experiences, especially those gained in his or her professional career. These assumptions and beliefs influence the way a therapist does evaluation, the assessments he or she chooses, the theories he or she uses, and the approaches he or she applies to intervention. Some therapists follow particular models, others use distinct paradigms, and still others use specific frames of reference. In all of these perspectives, evaluation is an essential part of practice. This chapter focuses on the links among philosophy, theory, and practice as they influence evaluation and provides an overview of the evaluation process.

PHILOSOPHICAL INFLUENCES ON EVALUATION

The fundamental **philosophical beliefs** influence what occupational therapists and occupational therapy assistants consider important and guide their actions. These philosophical beliefs collectively form the unique philosophical foundations of the profession. Therefore, occupational therapy's philosophical beliefs have a strong influence on therapists' actions, including how they perform evaluation and provide intervention. The following foundational beliefs for occupational therapy were first attributed to William Rush Dunton Jr. in a retrospective article (American Occupational Therapy Association [AOTA], 1967):

- Occupation is as necessary to life as food and drink.
- Every human being should have both physical and mental occupation.
- All should have occupations that they enjoy or hobbies—at least two, one outdoor and one indoor.
- Sick minds, sick bodies, and sick souls may be healed through occupation.

Although various authors have updated these basic beliefs (e.g., Kielhofner, 2009; Mosey, 1996), the core is still the same: Occupation is necessary to a healthy, meaningful life (AOTA, 2012; Baum & Christiansen, 2005; Kielhofner 2009).

One conceptualization of the profession's philosophy (Mosey, 1996) reflects this in terms of its view of the person and his or her rights. Occupational therapists and occupational therapy assistants believe that a person

- Has the right to a meaningful existence;
- Is influenced by the biological and social nature of the human species;
- Can be understood only within the context of family, friends, community, and cultural group membership;
- Has the need to participate in a variety of social roles and to have periodic relief from participation;
- Has the right to seek his or her potential through personal choice within the context of accepted social constraints; and
- Is able to reach his or her potential through purposeful interaction with the human and nonhuman environments.

Occupational therapists thus believe that clients have the right to make choices and to be active participants in the therapeutic process. The importance of the client's collaboration in the evaluation process is discussed throughout this book. Evaluation begins with the client and considers his or her life experiences, life roles, interests and occupations, age, cultural background, and context. The client's own view of what is important and his or her own perceived strengths and limitations are essential to the evaluation process in occupational therapy.

Additionally, occupational therapists have strong beliefs about the importance of occupations and activities, including that people are naturally active beings (i.e., have an occupational nature) and that occupation is necessary to society and culture. Kielhofner (2009) proposed that occupation is a basic need for people, a source of meaning in their lives, and a domain of human behavior. These constructs influence the way occupational therapists look at people, the ways they evaluate clients, and the areas in which they intervene. Thus, an occupational therapy evaluation always considers the person's

> Throughout evaluation, a therapist must take into consideration the multiple factors that influence intervention outcomes for an individual client. The first, and most important, factor is the needs of the particular client and the desired outcomes of that person and his or her family (Law, 1998).

- Biological and individual development,
- Cultural and social context,
- Relationship with family and significant others,
- Engagement in meaningful occupations,
- Quality of occupational performance, and
- Unique occupations in relationship to their physical and psychological development.

A fundamental belief of the profession is the importance of occupation and occupational performance. Fisher (2013), in refining her Occupational Therapy Intervention Process Model, discussed the importance of evaluation focusing on occupation. She made a clear distinction among the following terms: *occupation-centered*, *occupation-based*, and *occupation-focused*. Exhibit 2.1 includes her definitions of each term. Fisher maintained that although the initial assessment may not be occupation focused, it is occupation based. During the interview, the therapist focuses on the person's occupations and how they are realized in his or her life. According to Fisher, the performance analyses component

---

EXHIBIT 2.1. SUMMARY OF THE DEFINITIONS OF THE TERMS
OCCUPATION CENTERED, OCCUPATION BASED,* AND *OCCUPATION FOCUSED

How we guide our reasoning and our subsequent actions

Occupation-centered	To adopt a profession-specific perspective—a world view of occupation and what it means to be an occupational being—where occupation is placed in the center and ensures that what we do is linked to the core paradigm of occupational therapy

What we do and how we do it in research, education, and practice

Occupation-based	To use occupation as the foundation—to engage a person in occupation (i.e., the performance of chosen daily life tasks that offer desirable levels of pleasure, productivity, and restoration and unfold as they ordinarily do in the person's life) as the method used for evaluation and/or intervention
Occupation-focused	To focus one's attention on occupation—to have occupation as the proximal (i.e., immediate) focus of the evaluation or the proximal intent of the intervention

Source. From "Occupation-Centered, Occupation-Based, Occupation-Focused: Same, Same or Different?" by A. G. Fisher, 2013, *Scandinavian Journal of Occupational Therapy, 20,* p. 167. Copyright © 2013 by Taylor & Francis. Used with permission.

---

of the evaluation, which may use standardized assessments, should be both occupation based and occupation focused (see Exhibit 2.1).

Basic philosophical beliefs influence the way an occupational therapist conducts an evaluation. A therapist operationalizes his or her beliefs, values, and biases when evaluating clients. However, a therapist should consider best practice and keep personal values and biases in check to perform an effective client-centered evaluation. Personal beliefs, values, and biases, which influence an individual therapist, are separate from the beliefs and values of the profession. A therapist should develop an awareness of his or her beliefs, values, and biases so that they do not interfere with his or her choice of assessments and interpretation of the results.

We propose the following six principles as best reflecting the philosophy of the occupational therapy profession regarding evaluation and as being fundamental to an effective evaluation process:

1. Evaluation, in the form of screening, starts when the occupational therapist first receives information about the client or population and continues until the client is discharged from therapy.

2. Evaluation of a client always considers his or her perspective as well as those of the family, significant others, and caregivers with the client's permission.

3. Specific meaningful information about the client or population is best acquired through interviews, assessments, and observation of occupational performance.

4. Therapists need to be aware that assessments have potential biases that may influence their usefulness and appropriateness with clients, groups of people, or populations and how these biases may affect assessment results.

5. Contextual factors may influence a client's performance on assessments.

6. Evaluation is an ongoing process in which the therapist is continually gathering information about the client.

BEGINNING THE EVALUATION PROCESS

When the occupational therapist first makes contact with a potential client, the **evaluation process** has begun. The first step of the evaluation process is to screen the client using data collected from referral information, recorded observations, and knowledge of the possible sequelae of the client's diagnosis. If the occupational therapist determines that occupational therapy services may be needed, the process continues with a thorough review of available data.

The therapist begins this dynamic interactive process with the client through an interview with the client to gain foundational information about the occupational focus of the client. This interview will also determine the most appropriate assessments for use in that particular situation. The administration of assessments and the data collected continue to be part of the process between the therapist and the client. Both parties shape the evaluation through their input, interaction, and responses to each other and to the assessments or activities. Although the therapist may start with a formalized assessment, the process is fluid and may take many different directions.

A therapist spends much effort evaluating his or her clients, striving to do so effectively and efficiently to obtain all the information necessary with optimal reliability and validity. The formal evaluation provides a baseline measurement of the client's performance. Using this baseline, with ongoing reassessment, the therapist determines the client's specific needs for intervention and continually observes whether the client is making progress and whether a change in programming is needed. Thus, once an initial evaluation is done, **reassessment** takes place throughout the intervention. At regular intervals, a therapist conducts reevaluations to ensure that the intervention plan is meeting the identified goals.

This overview of evaluation emphasizes that evaluation begins with the first contact with the client and continues until he or she is discharged from therapy. The **evaluation summary** should include a comprehensive description of the client's occupational roles, client factors, performance skills, performance patterns, context and environment, and activity demands that influence his or her occupational performance.

The occupational therapy philosophy provides a continual underpinning for practice, making the profession's contribution to society unique. This philosophy defines who the occupational therapist is and what is his or her focus. The profession's philosophical belief in the importance of occupation-based, client-centered care should guide a therapist's practice, determining what the therapist will assess and how he or she will intervene.

Perspective of the Client, Family, Significant Others, and Caregivers

An essential element of the evaluation is to address the client's **perspective** and his or her desired outcomes for intervention. A client cannot be evaluated in isolation, however, and it is important in a client-centered approach to consider the client's wishes regarding the involvement of family members, significant others, and caregivers. These individuals are additional sources of data who may give the therapist another perspective on the client and his or her ability to engage in meaningful activities, as long as the therapist has the permission of the client. The therapist interprets information from these sources using clinical reasoning and judgment to gain a total picture of the client.

Written evaluations need to be complete enough to provide others with all important information about the total person, his or her lifestyle, and the occupations and activities that are important to him or her. Evaluation summaries should not discuss just one client factor, performance skill, performance pattern, or contextual factor that influences a person's occupational performance and should reflect the client's strengths as well as any limitations. Occupational therapy evaluation narratives should reflect the values of the profession in providing an integrated snapshot of the client's life.

Reassessments throughout the intervention process should capture the focus of intervention and the functional changes that occur as the intervention progresses. Reassessment data may be gathered routinely through various sources, including family members, significant others, and other professionals who interact with the client. The goal of intervention—progress toward meaningful, relevant goals—will be reflected in the data about the client's daily life activities.

Client or Population Assessment

The data collected from assessments are specific to the **client** or **population.** Client data offer insight into who he or she is, what occupations are important to him or her, and what the client's performance skills are. Data collected from client assessments are personalized, reflecting the fact that no two people have the same strengths, needs, or expected outcomes from intervention.

For a population, assessments offer a greater understanding of a group as comprised of members, its unique characteristics that identify it as a population, the health needs and life patterns of the group, and the specific activities in which members engage. Assessments and the interpretation of the population data should also provide some insight into the activity needs of the population and the supports needed to participate in society. Some characteristics may be common across groups, but the data also will reflect the unique identity of each group, including differing values, strengths, limitations, and performance goals.

The data that an occupational therapist collects should be within the occupational therapy scope of practice and should shed light on how to facilitate engagement in personally meaningful activities and occupations that will fulfill life roles. Once a therapist interprets the data, the therapist may find that he or she needs more information from additional assessments or from other professionals and team members.

Assessment Biases

Assessments have potential **biases** that may influence their applicability, usefulness, and appropriateness with selected groups of people. All assessments have some degree of bias. The most obvious biases are based on culture, gender, age, lifestyle, health status, geographic area, and socioeconomic status. With standardized assessments, the bias may result from the use of a homogeneous population when standardizing the assessment. It also may come from certain items that are specific to one cultural group or gender or to a particular region of the country.

Another type of bias is personal or examiner bias, resulting from personal beliefs or feelings of the evaluator that are conscious or unconscious (Goldyne, 2007; King-Thomas, 1987). One type of examiner bias is based on expectations. If the client is wearing soiled clothes, for example, the examiner may expect that the client will not do well on the evaluation, and his or her unconscious actions or attitudes may influence the results. Everyone has some prejudices but may not be aware of them and how they affect the way they view others. Although it is difficult to acknowledge and explore one's own prejudices, it is important to do so to prevent these prejudices from interfering with one's professional judgment (Campinha-Bacote, 2003; Jeffreys, 2006).

Additionally, an occupational therapist may have preconceived notions about client characteristics based on his or her professional background and experiences. When a therapist reads a diagnosis in a chart, for example, he or she may expect to see certain characteristics that may or may not be present. A therapist needs to be aware of what he or she is actually observing to guard against being deceived by expectations. Although reading a chart and becoming familiar with the client's history are part of good practice, a therapist needs to avoid letting that information influence his or her own data gathering and conclusions.

Influence of Contextual Factors on Assessment Performance

Occupational therapy is concerned with the functional performance of the client in his or her daily life, including not only what the client can or cannot do but also how he or she functions within the context of his or her environment. When using assessments, a therapist must think about the **contextual factors**—the physical, social, cultural, and temporal influences of the context on the client's performance. A therapist must also examine potential contextual supports for and barriers to the client's performance (Dunn, Brown, & Youngstrom, 2003). As Dunn and her colleagues noted, a person reacts to contextual variables in unique ways. For one person, background music might be distracting, whereas for another, it might be relaxing. A group setting might be stimulating for one young adult but might be contributing to social anxiety for another. When interpreting data from assessments, the therapist must consider whether contextual factors affected the client's performance.

Ongoing Data Gathering Through Reassessment

The occupational therapist or occupational therapy assistant continually monitors the client's responses to intervention and gathers data about any changes in behaviors or performance. The ongoing reassessment that continues throughout intervention is more informal than the initial evaluation, adjusting to the needs and demands of the intervention process. Data from various sources are used to ascertain whether the intervention is working toward achieving the established short-term goals. Progress is identified by comparing the baseline evaluation data against any ongoing reassessment data obtained. Family, significant others, and additional professionals may provide valuable reassessment data.

The principle of reassessment requires that the occupational therapist and the occupational therapy assistant continually reflect on what happens during the intervention and identify changes in the client's behaviors or performance skills. When a therapist and assistant determine that reassessment data indicate that the intervention program needs to be changed or modified, they should engage in a collaborative discussion to modify the plan.

Theory's Role in Evaluation

In addition to an understanding of the influence of philosophical beliefs on the evaluation process, it is critical to explore the effect of theory on this process. Philosophical beliefs guide, to some extent, those theories that are applicable to or appropriate for the profession to use. The theories that an occupational therapist chooses to guide practice must be congruent with the philosophical perspective of the profession.

Theories are a collection of concepts, definitions, and postulates that help professionals make predictions about relationships between events. *Concepts* are labels describing phenomena that have been observed; the meanings of concepts are their definitions. The stated relationships between two or more concepts are *postulates* (Kramer & Hinojosa, 2010). The person or people who develop a theory identify and define the concepts and state the postulates, thus determining the scope and parameters of the theory. A theory organizes information and explains the relationships between ideas and observed events in a logical, understandable manner. A theory links the various concepts, definitions, and principles in a coherent way around a central theme or organizing principle. Theories are critical to the foundation of any type of intervention and therefore are basic to evaluation.

Occupation therapists treat deficits in occupational performance. Theories guide intervention, and when occupational therapists choose assessments, they are guided by theory. Some examples of the use of theory in intervention are obvious. For example, during the screening process of observing a child, the therapist might see behaviors indicative of a sensory processing problem. This observation would lead the therapist to consider the possibility of using a sensory processing theory and then choose assessments related to a sensory dysfunction, such as the Sensory Profile (Dunn, 1999), the Sensory Integration and Praxis Tests–Revised (Ayres, 2003), or the Bruininks–Oseretsky Test of Motor Proficiency (Bruininks & Bruininks, 2005). On the basis of the screening findings, the therapist would then decide exactly which theory he or she would use to develop an appropriate intervention for the child.

In another example, when the therapist is observing a male adult with tremors, the therapist might have a more general idea of which theory to use. The clinical reasoning process might be that tremors are usually neurological and therefore may not be remediated in treatment, so the theory used for intervention would be compensatory rather than remedial. The assessments chosen would be related to determining the client's specific occupational performance deficits and his desires for improved functioning. There are various assessments that the therapist might use.

Regardless of what theories will be used in intervention, the therapist needs to select assessments that measure some aspects of occupational performance. An occupational therapist could choose assessments that are applicable to the client and would fit the client's contextual factors that influence his or her occupational performance. In reality, some assessments focus on specific areas that fit neatly with the theories and philosophical beliefs important to occupational therapy, whereas many others relate to the profession's concerns but were developed using other theoretical orientations.

Although theory is important in the choice of assessments, other factors also influence which assessments are used. Some assessments are used because they are popular. Others assessments are used because other professions value them. Some are used because they are standardized, and standardized data are required by certain settings. Some are used because an institution, regulations, or particular service delivery models require that they be used. Under these circumstances, the occupational therapist has the additional responsibility to translate the assessment results into the domain of concern of the profession.

The application of theory to practice is a complex process. The therapist is obliged to take ideas that are abstract and apply them at a level at which they can be used functionally. There are several acceptable ways of conceptualizing occupational therapy practice. In each, evaluation is an important component and serves as the basis for intervention. Some of the more common conceptualizations are frames of reference (Kramer & Hinojosa, 2010; Mosey, 1970, 1996), conceptual models of practice (Dunn, 2011; Ikiugu, 2007; Kielhofner, 2008), and occupation-based frameworks for practice (Baum & Christiansen, 2005; Brown, Stoffel, & Munoz, 2011). All of these vehicles allow a therapist to use theory as the basis for his or her evaluations and interventions. In this book, we use frames of reference as the way of conceptualizing practice to illustrate the evaluative process.

A **frame of reference** is an acceptable vehicle for organizing theoretical material in occupational therapy and translating it into practice through a functional perspective. A frame of reference provides a linking structure between theory and practice (Dunn, 2011; Kramer & Hinojosa, 2010; Mosey, 1996) and draws from one or more theories to provide a basis for what will occur throughout the intervention process. Based on the theoretical information, a frame of reference addresses specific behaviors or physical signs that are considered functional and specific behaviors or physical signs that are considered dysfunctional (Mosey, 1992, 1996). A therapist often uses more than one frame of reference to address a client's distinctive therapeutic needs.

Inherent within a theoretical perspective or frame of reference may be a ***top-down approach,*** which looks at the person's occupations first; a ***bottom-up approach,*** which looks at the components of tasks that are interfering with performance first; or a ***contextual approach,*** which looks at the contextual effects on performance. The theory and the available assessments that are consistent with the theory then help to define the evaluation process. The therapist's personal predilections should not guide the choice of assessments. Many more assessments are component-driven than driven by occupations or contextual issues.

Regardless of whether the therapist selects a top-down, bottom-up, or contextual approach, it is incumbent on him or her to explore all of these areas to gain a comprehensive view of the client. One perspective is generally primary during the intervention process, but effective intervention usually combines all three approaches.

CHOOSING THE FRAME OF REFERENCE

Theory and practice need to be continually linked and related to the client. Screening provides the first opportunity to decide which theory or theories will guide practice with a particular person. If the screening provides enough information to decide on a theoretical approach, then the therapist has a theoretical direction for evaluation and intervention. However, if the screening does not yield sufficient information to choose a theoretical approach, then the therapist may need to use additional assessments to gain more information about the client and determine an appropriate approach. Whenever a therapist develops an intervention plan, it must be based on sound evidence and guided by theory. The theory selected predicts the consequences of intervention.

Screening Stage

Screening plays a critical role in the choices that a therapist makes in evaluating the client. Data from the screening process have an ongoing effect on the evaluation and intervention process. Sometimes, just by reading a chart or interviewing a client, a therapist knows what theory or frame of reference would be appropriate for the client. When a therapist determines during a screening that a specific frame of reference is appropriate, he or she proceeds to administer assessments that are consistent with that frame of reference.

For example, if a therapist screens a file of a young man with a hand fracture of his nondominant hand caused by a fall from his bicycle, the therapist may decide to use a biomechanical frame of reference. Based on this decision, the therapist proceeds to administer assessments consistent with this approach (e.g., range of motion, manual muscle testing).

When a frame of reference is not immediately apparent, a therapist can use specific screening assessments or data collection strategies to gather more information about the client and his or her occupational performance needs. The purpose of screening is to obtain an overview of the person's needs, strengths, limitations, and environment; it is not meant to be a comprehensive evaluation. Screening may involve an observation of the client, a chart review, medical and developmental history, information gained from the parents or care providers, or data gathered by other professionals involved with the client. The following are examples of standardized and nonstandardized screening assessments that can help the therapist identify an appropriate frame of reference:

- Screening Test for Evaluating Preschoolers (FirstSTEp™; Miller, 1993b)
- Denver II Developmental Screening Test (Frankenburg et al., 1991)
- Ayres Clinical Observations of Neuromuscular Integration (Ayres, 1976)
- Family Observation Guide (Hinojosa & Kramer, 2008)
- Activity Configuration (Mosey, 1986)
- Model of Human Occupation Screening Tool (Parkinson, Forsyth, & Kielhofner, 2006)
- Occupational Performance History Interview Version 2.1 (Kielhofner, 2004).

A screening is usually complete when the therapist has enough information to recommend whether the client needs to receive occupational therapy services and to determine an appropriate frame of reference or intervention approach if services are required.

The screening data provide the therapist with a preliminary picture of the client and a potential view of what occupational therapy might offer. While reflecting on the screening data, the therapist decides whether the needs of the client relate to the domain of concern of occupational therapy and, if so, how to proceed with the evaluation using the assessments that will be most appropriate for the setting and to obtain the data needed. If the therapist decides that occupational therapy is not necessary, the client is discharged from occupational therapy and, if indicated, the therapist refers the client to another service.

Assessment Stage

When selecting the assessments to use in the comprehensive evaluation, there are three possibilities (Figure 2.1): (1) The therapist has enough information from the screening to choose a frame of reference to guide evaluation and intervention; (2) the therapist needs to use an exploratory approach to determine which way to proceed in evaluating the client; or (3) the therapist with expertise decides, given the client's specific problems, that he or she must use an idiosyncratic approach to evaluation.

The therapist chooses assessments that will identify the presence of functional and dysfunctional behaviors and physical signs as described by the selected frame of reference. Some frames of reference are associated with specific assessments; with others, it is up to the therapist to determine which assessment will best be able to identify the presence of the behaviors or physical signs. The same theories should underlie both the assessments and the treatment approach to ensure that they are congruent.

Clear choice of a frame of reference

When a clear theoretical approach is evident from the screening data, the occupational therapist has a **clear choice** of a frame of reference and chooses an assessment based on that approach (Figure 2.2). Many frames of reference or theoretical approaches are associated with one or more assessments that are consistent with that theoretical perspective (see Case Example 2.1).

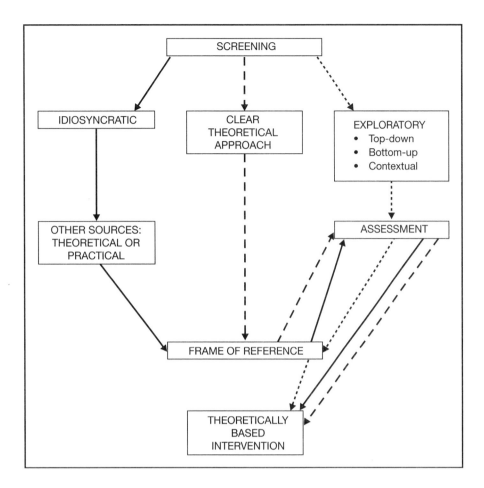

Figure 2.1. Diagram of three approaches to evaluation that lead to theoretically based intervention.
Note. Individual approaches are presented in Figure 2.2, which shows a clear choice of a frame of reference (the long dotted line in this figure), and Figure 2.3, which shows the exploratory approach (the small dotted line in this figure).
Source. J. Hinojosa. Used with permission.

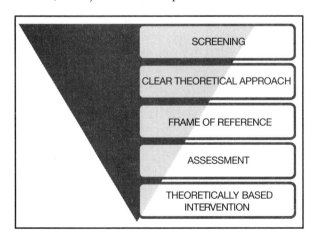

Figure 2.2. Occupational therapy process when presented with a clear choice of a frame of reference.
Source. J. Hinojosa. Used with permission.

CASE EXAMPLE 2.1. CLEAR CHOICE OF A FRAME OF REFERENCE

Sharon was a 16-month-old with high distal tone in both upper extremities and severely delayed developmental milestones. Her diagnosis was cerebral palsy with spasticity. A review of Sharon's medical chart provided the therapist with extensive information. The therapist also observed Sharon for a period of time and then held her, finding low proximal tone and high distal tone. After this screening, the therapist selected a postural control approach with handling and decided to use the neurodevelopmental frame of reference (Barthel, 2010). During the assessment, along with a more extended observation of Sharon's ability to interact with toys and other aspects of her environment, the therapist used the Alberta Infant Motor Scale (Piper & Darrah, 1994) to assess Sharon's gross motor abilities. Once the therapist determined the specific delays, she could proceed to develop a plan for intervention.

Exploratory approach to evaluation

After the screening, if the therapist does not have a clear theoretical direction for how to proceed in the evaluation process, he or she might consider taking an **exploratory approach.** This broad approach to evaluation includes, if possible, a more in-depth interview with the client to determine specific personal goals and to explore physical, psychosocial, and environmental issues (and their component parts) that may prevent those goals from being met. It is essential to understand the client's perspective on why these goals cannot be met at this time.

Within the exploratory approach, the therapist may start in many places: from the top down, by exploring the client's meaningful occupations (see Case Example 2.2); from the bottom up, by exploring the underlying components of meaningful tasks (see Case Example 2.3); or from a contextual perspective, by exploring environmental issues (see Case Example 2.4; Hinojosa & Kramer, 1998; Ideishi, 2003; Weinstock-Zlotnick & Hinojosa, 2004). The therapist's intent is to understand the client and the identified problems and to determine a theoretical approach or frame of reference for intervention (Figure 2.3).

Although a therapist might begin an evaluation with one approach, a comprehensive evaluation

---

CASE EXAMPLE 2.2. TOP-DOWN APPROACH

Joe, age 48 years, was 1-week postcerebrovascular accident and was medically stable. He was referred to occupational therapy for a complete evaluation and potential intervention. The therapist read the medical documentation as part of the screening process and met with Joe. Joe's concerns and the data the therapist collected from the screening directed her to focus on activities of daily living (ADLs). The evaluation explored Joe's ability to feed, bathe, toilet, and dress himself. Through functional activities and specific assessments, including the Canadian Occupational Performance Measure (Law et al., 1998) and the Performance Assessment of Self-Care Skills–Revised (Rogers & Holm, 1994), the therapist determined that Joe had a problem with the performance area of ADLs. She evaluated specific components of his performance (i.e., bottom-up approach), such as manual muscle testing and range of motion, to gain more information about how a body structure deficit might be affecting this area of occupation. Then, with consideration to the context, the therapist was able to develop a plan for intervention.

CASE EXAMPLE 2.3. BOTTOM-UP APPROACH

Mariko, age 4 years, was referred to occupational therapy because of suspected developmental delay. After reading the referral documentation and getting an overview of the child as a person through a discussion with her care providers, the occupational therapist decided to assess Mariko's gross and fine motor skills, muscle tone, movement patterns, and manipulation skills using a standardized assessment, the Miller Assessment for Preschoolers (MAP; Miller, 1993a). Once the therapist identified those components of performance that were interfering with Mariko's functional abilities through clinical observation and the data obtained from the MAP, the therapist ascertained which areas of occupation were affected. Following this step, and considering the context, the therapist was able to develop a plan for intervention.

CASE EXAMPLE 2.4. CONTEXTUAL APPROACH

Muhammad, age 72 years, was recovering from an aneurysm that had resulted in mild motor deficits. He was referred to occupational therapy for an ADL evaluation before being admitted to a skilled nursing facility (SNF). After reading the referral documentation, the occupational therapist decided to assess Muhammad's performance of ADLs, considering in the process both his wants and what he would need to do in the SNF. The therapist interviewed Muhammad and observed the SNF. It was found that before his hospitalization, Muhammad lived alone and he now was fearful of returning to his apartment.

Given his age and lifestyle, along with his newly acquired disability, he felt that he would be more comfortable in the SNF, which had an assisted-living residence to which he could move if his condition improved. He chose this particular setting because he believed that it was respectful of his cultural background and he would feel comfortable with the people there. The therapist used the data from the assessment of the context as the background for the assessment of the areas of occupation and the components of performance. Using all the data, the therapist was able to develop an intervention plan for Muhammad that focused on developing his ability to function within the SNF with the potential of an eventual move to a less restrictive environment.

---

requires the therapist to continually analyze the data and to consider all approaches—top-down, bottom-up, and contextual—before a comprehensive evaluation is complete. The therapist's clinical reasoning skills may indicate that a change in focus is warranted to address the issues that arise from the individual client. Using the data he or she has

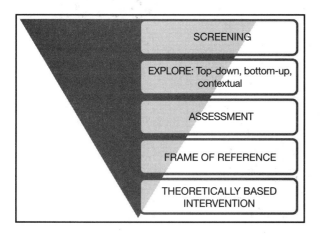

Figure 2.3. Exploratory approach to evaluation.
Source. J. Hinojosa. Used with permission.

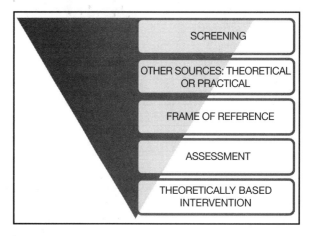

Figure 2.4. Idiosyncratic approach to evaluation.
Source. J. Hinojosa. Used with permission.

collected, the therapist selects an appropriate theoretical perspective to guide intervention.

Idiosyncratic approach

An occupational therapist with advanced knowledge and expertise sometimes screens a client whose data are unique. The presenting picture of such clients is not consistent with known frames of reference or traditional problems seen in occupational therapy. When a therapist moves into nontraditional or emerging areas of practice, develops a new program area, or begins work with a new population not generally seen in occupational therapy, he or she may encounter such clients. This situation also may occur when new phenomena are seen in a clinical environment, such as postpolio syndrome or the aging process in extended life. The type of evaluation approach needed for such clients is an **idiosyncratic approach.** Rather than starting with traditional assessments, the therapist may need to look to other sources and professions for theoretical perspectives to use as a basis for developing an appropriate theoretical base to guide intervention. Once the theoretical base is articulated, it provides the foundation for selecting appropriate assessments for the evaluation of these clients.

In some cases, other professions and disciplines have already dealt with this problem or have theories that relate to this problem that allow the occupational therapist to combine that knowledge with the unique view of occupational therapy (Figure 2.4). This type of evaluation is complex and should not be the role or responsibility of the novice therapist (see Case Example 2.5).

CASE EXAMPLE 2.5.
IDIOSYNCRATIC APPROACH

Jane, age 16 years and obese, was having difficulty relating to her peer group, resulting in depression, social isolation, and acting-out behaviors. She had been receiving ongoing psychological help for 3 years and had been involved in an occupational therapy group, but she showed little response and stopped receiving treatment. Jane was referred again to occupational therapy to try a different approach involving exploration of her self-image and obesity to promote more appropriate social behaviors.

Because there is no articulated frame of reference identified with working with adolescent obesity, the therapist needed to search for theoretical information outside of occupational therapy. The therapist explored literature on lifestyle reengineering, cognitive–behavioral therapy, and theories related to locus of control. Once the therapist identified particular constructs that might relate to Jane, she proceeded to identify assessments that would provide information to develop a plan for intervention. Although the therapist was not using occupational therapy literature or assessments, she was able to develop an idiosyncratic approach to providing occupational therapy evaluation of this client. Once the therapist chose a frame of reference, she explored the evaluation data to determine appropriate goals for Jane. These goals were the foundation of the intervention plan.

Although the idiosyncratic approach sounds different and complex, occupational therapists have addressed unique client issues in this way for years. When occupational therapists first started working with clients with HIV/AIDS, postpolio syndrome, and autistic spectrum disorders, they used an idiosyncratic approach to evaluation.

Theory in Intervention Planning and Implementation

Throughout the course of evaluation, an occupational therapist interprets data and draws conclusions. This reasoning process is ongoing throughout the evaluation process. Once the evaluation is complete, the therapist has a wealth of information to use in developing an intervention plan. If he or she has not already chosen a particular frame of reference, at this time the therapist must choose a theoretical approach to lay the foundation for the development of goals and creation of a comprehensive intervention plan for the client.

When planning the intervention, the therapist is generally heavily influenced by the context of care and payers for services. However, the therapist must ensure that the evaluation completed is consistent with the frame of reference he or she has chosen. The therapist must develop goals and interventions based only on the data he or she has gathered. Additionally, the therapist has to ensure that the needs of the client, the therapist's professional responsibilities, and the ethics of his or her actions are consistent with the requirements of the setting and the availability of payment.

An enormous amount of information is collected during the evaluation of a client, and its scope and complexity can be overwhelming. The therapist's goal is to synthesize the data and interpret them to develop appropriate goals consistent with the frames of reference. A therapist often uses more than one frame of reference to address a client's distinctive therapeutic needs to enhance occupational performance.

Interpretation of evaluation data requires that a therapist bring all the findings together to create a profile of the client as an occupational being in his or her life context. With this visualization of the client, the therapist conscientiously selects key long- and short-term goals that reflect an integration and synthesis of all the evaluation data and, when possible, the needs and aspirations of the client. The goals should be realistic, functional, and achievable, based on clear baseline data. Finally, the number of goals should be limited to major goals that are

reasonable given the intervention approach and the frequency of sessions. We recommend that a therapist develop no more than six long-term goals. When using more than one frame of reference, each frame of reference should have at least one long-term goal.

The initial evaluation is complete when the therapist writes the evaluation summary. An evaluation summary is important to both the client and the third-party payer. Reports should be a documentation of findings and not a lecture on the selected frame of reference. Evaluation reports should be concise and provide a sound argument for occupational therapy services based on the synthesis of the evaluation data. Test scores should be provided to support the therapist's interpretations.

Therapists should be careful not to overinterpret data and should check all scores for accuracy. Reports should include clear descriptions of baseline data that describe a client's behaviors and performance deficits. Hinojosa and Foto (2004) described the importance of evaluation summaries for communicating information in a succinct and effective manner. They suggested that all evaluation summaries avoid jargon and be proofread for misspellings, grammatical errors, and awkward sentences. They described a comprehensive evaluation summary as one that

- Identifies key information considered when preparing the report, including age, diagnosis, and referral information;
- Lists all tests administered and reports how they were administered;
- Identifies factors influencing the client's performance;
- Records actual test scores and interpretation of the data, disclosing any concerns about cultural issues or test bias;
- Presents a clear description of the client's performance and behaviors;
- Reports findings that provide an objective baseline of the client's performance deficits and abilities; and
- Documents baseline data that provide a clear picture of the client's overall functional level and that can be used to assess the efficacy of the intervention plan.

THERAPIST PERSPECTIVES, THEORY, AND PRACTICE

Other factors important throughout the evaluation process are the occupational therapist's skills and his or her perspective. Each person acquires a different set of skills based on what he or she has been formally and informally taught, what he or she has learned, what his or her experiences have been, and who he or she is. Although most occupational therapists have been taught a consistent body of knowledge, it may have been presented from different orientations and organized in different manners. For example, all professional educational programs base their content on the *2011 Accreditation Council for Occupational Therapy Education (ACOTE®) Standards* however, this content may be taught using different orientations (ACOTE, 2012); and emphasizing different areas. Some programs may focus on specific treatment techniques, whereas others may accent the clinical reasoning process. In addition, although occupational therapists may be taught the same content, individual differences mean that therapists learn and interpret material differently. Based on individual experiences and training, a therapist may identify a favorite frame of reference that he or she prefers to use more frequently.

Finally, the therapist's practice setting also influences the choice of frame of reference. For example, some frames of reference may be impossible to implement within a home-based, school-based, or community setting or hospital. Although all the factors mentioned may influence the choice of a frame of reference, the client's needs should be given primary consideration.

SUMMARY

Occupational therapy is based in philosophy; therefore, the process of evaluation has a strong philosophical basis, and each assessment combines a philosophical basis with a theoretical orientation. The assessments used must be consistent with the occupational needs of the client. The evaluation process is complex and requires clinical reasoning so the therapist can adequately identify the needs and concerns of the client and the areas that require

intervention. Frames of reference provide a vehicle for theory-directed interventions.

QUESTIONS

1. Identify 3 personal philosophical beliefs about human development and performance. Are they consistent with those found in this chapter? In what ways are they similar or different?
2. When would it be most appropriate to include a significant other in the evaluation process? What factors might preclude involving the significant other in this process?
3. Reflect on an experience in which you were evaluated. Can you identify any biases (positive or negative) that you experienced or sensed during the evaluation that might have affected the outcome? Do you think that you have any biases that might affect your ability to evaluate another person?
4. The authors purport that theory should influence the choice of an assessment. Identify 2 assessments, and then identify the theories, frames of reference, or models of practice that provide the foundation for these assessments.
5. Explain the difference between a top-down approach and a bottom-up approach to evaluation. In what ways are they similar and in what ways are they different?

References

Accreditation Council for Occupational Therapy Education. (2012). 2011 Accreditation Council for Occupational Therapy Education (ACOTE®) standards. *American Journal of Occupational Therapy, 66*(Suppl.), S6–S74. http://dx.doi.org/10.5014/ajot.2012.66S6

American Occupational Therapy Association. (1967). Presidents of the American Occupational Therapy Association (1917–1967). *American Journal of Occupational Therapy, 21,* 290–298.

American Occupational Therapy Association. (2012). *Policy manual.* Bethesda, MD: Author.

Ayres, A. J. (1976, March). *Clinical observations of neuromuscular integration: Administration of the Southern California Sensory Integration Tests* [certification course]. Conference sponsored by the Center for the Study of Sensory Integrative Dysfunction, Valhalla, NY.

Ayres, A. J. (2003). *Sensory integration and Praxis Test manual*. Los Angeles: Western Psychological Services.

Barthel, K. A. (2010). A frame of reference for neuro-developmental treatment. In P. Kramer & J. Hinojosa (Eds.), *Frames of reference for pediatric occupational therapy* (3rd ed., pp. 187–233). Baltimore: Lippincott Williams & Wilkins.

Baum, C. M., & Christiansen, C. (2005). Person–environment–occupation–performance: An occupation-based framework for practice. In C. Christiansen, C. M. Baum, & J. Bass-Haugen (Eds.), *Occupational therapy: Performance, participation, and well-being* (3rd ed., pp. 243–266). Thorofare, NJ: Slack.

Brown, C., Stoffel, V., & Munoz, J. P. (2011). *Occupational therapy in mental health: A vision for participation*. Philadelphia: F. A. Davis.

Bruininks, R., & Bruininks, B. (2005). *Bruininks–Oseretsky Test of Motor Proficiency* (2nd ed.). Minneapolis: NCS Pearson.

Campinha-Bacote, J. (2003). *The process of cultural competence in the delivery of healthcare services: A culturally competent model of care*. Cincinnati: Transcultural C.A.R.E. Associates.

Dunn, W. (1999). *Sensory Profile: User's manual*. San Antonio: Psychological Corporation.

Dunn, W. (2011). Using frames of reference and practice models to guide practice. In W. Dunn (Ed.), *Best practice occupational therapy for children and families in community settings* (2nd ed., pp. 39–72). Thorofare, NJ: Slack.

Dunn, W., Brown, C., & Youngstrom, M. J. (2003). Ecological model of occupation. In P. Kramer, J. Hinojosa, & C. B. Royeen (Eds.), *Perspectives in human occupation: Participation in life* (pp. 222–263). Philadelphia: Lippincott Williams & Wilkins.

Fisher, A. G. (2013). Occupation-centered, occupation-based, occupation-focused: Same, same or different? *Scandinavian Journal of Occupational Therapy, 20*, 162–173. http://dx.doi.org/10.3109/11038128.2012.754492

Frankenburg, W. K., Dodds, J., Archer, P., Bresnick, B., Maschka, P., Edelman, N., & Shapiro, H. (1991). *The Denver II Developmental Screening Test*. Denver: Denver Developmental Materials.

Goldyne, A. J. (2007). Minimizing the influence of unconscious bias in evaluations: A practical guide. *Journal of the American Academy of Psychiatry and the Law, 35*, 60–66.

Hinojosa, J., & Foto, M. (2004). Occupational therapy documentation for reimbursement. *Sensory Integration Special Interest Section Quarterly, 27*, 1–3.

Hinojosa, J., & Kramer, P. (1998). Evaluation: Where do we begin? In J. Hinojosa & P. Kramer (Eds.), *Occupational therapy evaluation: Obtaining and interpreting data* (pp. 1–15). Bethesda, MD: American Occupational Therapy Association.

Hinojosa, J., & Kramer, P. (2008). Integrating children with disabilities into family play. In D. L. Parham & L. S. Fazio (Eds.), *Play in occupational therapy for children* (2nd ed., pp. 321–334). St. Louis: Mosby/Year Book.

Ideishi, R. I. (2003). The influence of occupation on assessment and treatment. In P. Kramer, J. Hinojosa, & C. B. Royeen (Eds.), *Perspectives in human occupation: Participation in life* (pp. 278–296). Baltimore: Lippincott Williams & Wilkins.

Ikiugu, M. N. (2007). *Psychosocial conceptual practice models in occupational therapy: Building adaptive capacity*. St. Louis: Mosby/Elsevier.

Jeffreys, M. R. (2006). *Teaching cultural competence in nursing and health care: Inquiry, action and innovation*. New York: Springer.

Kielhofner, G. (2004). *A user's manual for the Occupational Performance History Interview (Version 2.1) OPHI–II: Model of Human Occupation Clearinghouse*. Chicago: University of Illinois, Department of Occupational Therapy.

Kielhofner, G. (2008). *Model of Human Occupation: Theory and application*. Baltimore: Lippincott Williams & Wilkins.

Kielhofner, G. (2009). *Conceptual foundations of occupational therapy practice* (4th ed.). Philadelphia: F. A. Davis.

King-Thomas, L. J. (1987). Responsibilities of the examiner. In L. J. King-Thomas & B. J. Hacker (Eds.), *The therapist's guide to pediatric assessment* (pp. 11–18). Boston: Brown.

Kramer, P., & Hinojosa, J. (2010). *Frames of reference for pediatric occupational therapy* (3rd ed.). Baltimore: Lippincott Williams & Wilkins.

Law, M. (1998). Client-centered occupational therapy. In M. Law (Ed.), *Client-centered occupational therapy* (pp. 1–18). Thorofare, NJ: Slack.

Law, M., Baptiste, S., Carswell, A., McColl, M. A., Polatajko, H., & Pollock, N. (1998). *Canadian Occupational Performance Measure* (3rd ed.). Ottawa: CAOT Publications ACE.

Miller, L. J. (1993a). *Miller Assessment for Preschoolers*. San Antonio: Psychological Corporation.

Miller, L. J. (1993b). *Screening Test for Evaluating Preschoolers (FirstSTEP™)*. San Antonio: Psychological Corporation.

Mosey, A. C. (1970). *Three frames of reference for mental health*. Thorofare, NJ: Slack.

Mosey, A. C. (1986). *Psychosocial components of occupational therapy*. New York: Raven Press.

Mosey, A. C. (1992). *Applied scientific inquiry in the health professions: An epistemological orientation.* Rockville, MD: American Occupational Therapy Association.

Mosey, A. C. (1996). *Applied scientific inquiry in the health professions: An epistemological orientation* (2nd ed.). Bethesda, MD: American Occupational Therapy Association.

Parkinson, S., Forsyth, K., & Kielhofner, G. (2006). *User's manual for the Model of Human Occupation Screening Tool (MOHOST) (Version 2.0).* Chicago: University of Illinois, Department of Occupational Therapy.

Piper, M. C., & Darrah, J. (1994). Alberta Infant Motor Scale: Construction of a motor assessment tool for the developing infant. In M. C. Piper & J. Darrah (Eds.), *Motor assessment of the developing infant* (pp. 25–35). Philadelphia: W. B. Saunders.

Rogers, J. C., & Holm, M. B. (1994). *Performance Assessment of Self-Care Skills–Revised (PASS) (Version 3.1)* [Unpublished functional performance test]. Pittsburgh: University of Pittsburgh.

Weinstock-Zlotnick, G., & Hinojosa, J. (2004). Bottom-up or top-down evaluation: Is one better than the other. *American Journal of Occupational Therapy, 58,* 594–599. http://dx.doi.org/10.5014/ajot.58.5.594

CHAPTER 3

Assessment Identification and Selection

Julie D. Bass, PhD, OTR/L, FAOTA

Highlights

- Identifying assessments
- Describing the need for an assessment
- Locating existing assessments that meet current needs
- Analyzing the quality of an assessment: Formal method assessment
- Ethical issues related to selection and use of assessments.

Key Terms

Characteristics of interest
Databases
Documentation
Ethical issues
Expert critiques
Intended purposes
Locating existing assessments

Methodical approach
Population of clients
Practical needs
Qualifications
Resources
Standards for Educational and Psychological Testing

This chapter introduces a process for identifying and selecting assessments for use in occupational therapy practice. Major sources of information on assessments in occupational therapy and other disciplines are identified. This chapter also includes a summary of assessment criteria and a discussion of various practical and ethical issues related to the use of assessments.

Identifying and selecting the best assessments for evaluation are important steps in the occupational therapy process. Using a formal process to choose assessments is one of the best mechanisms for ensuring that the outcome of an evaluation and intervention is efficient and effective and that the use of an assessment is fair (American Psychological Association [APA], Joint Committee on Testing Practices, 2004).

Identifying assessments that meet the purpose of the evaluation process requires a **methodical approach** that includes knowing what you are looking for, where to look, and how to look. Many strategies can help in this process, and selecting a specific assessment requires a careful examination of existing tools and instruments. This examination includes determining the strengths and weaknesses of the assessment in terms of specific criteria and finding a recommendation about how the assessment should be used in a particular setting.

Occupational therapists need to be cautious and rigorous when selecting assessments for a client. Therapists should not simply use what is currently available in the setting. They must be confident that the specific assessment is appropriate for assessing the client. When therapists decide that they need to adapt an existing assessment or develop an instrument, they need to follow sound test construction design to ensure the credibility of the instrument. If these guidelines are not followed and the instrument is adapted or modified, therapists are not providing best practice in occupational therapy. In addition, it may jeopardize the professional standing of occupational therapy where it is used.

IDENTIFYING ASSESSMENTS

Identifying assessments that meet the needs of an evaluation involves

> To identify and select an assessment for evaluation, describe your needs, find existing assessments that meet the needs, and analyze the quality of the available assessments.

- Determining the need for a specific assessment in the evaluation process;
- Locating and examining information about existing assessments that describes their intended purpose, characteristics, quality, and use in evaluation; and
- Identifying a few assessments that seem to match the practice need and drawing up a plan to analyze and compare them in a more deliberate manner. This last step results in the selection of a specific assessment for the evaluation process.

DESCRIBING THE NEED FOR AN ASSESSMENT

In almost every practice setting, there comes a time when a therapist needs to select an assessment as part of an evaluation process. Before reviewing available assessments, the therapist must begin with some reflection on the overall need for an assessment in a particular situation.

Therapists should consider several broad areas of needs, such as

> To identify your need for an assessment, consider person–environment–occupation characteristics to be measured, intended uses or purposes, population of clients, qualifications of the users, and practical factors.

- Description of the overall need for an assessment and the characteristics of interest and importance,
- Intended uses for the assessment,
- Population of clients to be evaluated using this assessment,
- Qualifications or characteristics of the user of the assessment, and
- Other practical considerations.

Characteristics of Interest and Importance

There are several approaches to describing the **characteristics of interest** and importance in an assessment. Several chapters in this text and others have introduced ideas to help occupational therapists reflect on the characteristics and purposes of evaluation. The Person–Environment–Occupation (PEO) and other occupational therapy practice models have received increasing attention in the literature as organizing frameworks for evaluation.

Conceptual, practice, and health models provide alternative approaches to identifying the focus of occupational therapy evaluation. Finally, classification systems such as the *International Classification of Functioning, Disability and Health* (*ICF*; World Health Organization [WHO], 2001) aim to propose an international language that is helpful in describing individual status.

Models that address person, environment, and occupation as essential constructs (Baum & Christiansen, 2005; Dunn, Brown, & Youngstrom, 2003; Kielhofner, 2007; Law et al., 1996; Mathiowetz & Bass-Haugen, 1994; Trombly, 1995) and other occupational therapy practice models provide an important foundation for identifying different factors that a therapist must consider when selecting an assessment. The characteristics of interest and importance in an assessment generally include a description of the person's characteristics, the contextual and environment characteristics, and the person's occupations or occupational performance.

PEO and other occupational therapy practice models also provide the necessary terminology for accessing the literature and may suggest related terms or key words found in other sources. For example, a therapist might be interested in measuring performance in activities of daily living (ADLs) for a given client in a given situation. The PEO model might include the concept of *ADLs* in its description. Other conceptual models might use different terms while still emphasizing the importance of this occupation. They might use terms such as *self-care, daily living skills, self-maintenance,* and *functional performance* to describe basic components of everyday life.

Conceptual and practice perspectives also provide guidelines for evaluation. Occupational therapy uses concepts, models, theories, and frames of reference to describe ideas that influence the conceptual and practice foundations of the profession. Individual therapists, and most practice settings, adopt beliefs or perspectives that guide clinical reasoning and the occupational therapy process. Regardless of the perspective adopted, therapists must always remember that the unique contribution of occupational therapy is occupational performance (Baum & Law, 1997).

Conceptual and practice perspectives may originate either outside occupational therapy or within the domain of occupational therapy. Reed and Sanderson (1999) described 10 models of health commonly used in occupational therapy practice: biomedical, biopsychosocial, chronicity, holistic, milieu, health education and prevention, health development, wellness, normality, and rehabilitation. Numerous models of occupational therapy also have been described and may be organized by domains of concern (Reed & Sanderson, 1999) that include adaptation, context or ecology, occupation or activity, occupational performance and competence, developmental, prevention, productivity, play and leisure, sensorimotor, cognitive, psychosocial, and professional development.

For example, a therapist may be interested in evaluating the biomechanical characteristics (a sensorimotor domain of concern) that support or limit a person's occupational performance after a hand injury. An examination of this perspective on performance may lead to assessments related to joint range of motion and physical endurance.

Classification systems provide another option for describing the characteristics measured by an assessment. The *ICF* (WHO, 2001) has become an important tool for characterizing people and the environments in which they live. The primary classification areas of the *ICF* are body structure, body function, activity, participation, and contextual factors of the person and environment.

For example, an occupational therapist who needs to assess support systems for occupational performance might find it helpful to look at the subcategories under "Support and Relationships" in the *ICF*. Other systems used by occupational therapists include the *Occupational Therapy Practice Framework: Domain and Process* (3rd ed.; American Occupational Therapy Association [AOTA], 2014). The National Center for Medical Rehabilitation Research (1993, 2006) and the Institute of Medicine (1997) have introduced alternative classifications and models to characterize the complex characteristics of the person–environment–occupation relationship. Enacting any one of these systems in practice guides the therapist's assessment, focusing the identification and selection process.

Intended Purposes or Uses

After identifying the characteristics of interest and importance, the next step in describing the need for an assessment is determining the assessment's **intended purposes** or uses. Initially, it may help to think about the purposes or uses in words that depict a specific situation. For example, one therapist might need an assessment of functional and community mobility for the purpose of discharge planning with a client. In another scenario, an occupational therapy researcher might need an assessment of executive cognitive function to support theory development in Alzheimer's disease research.

A broad summary of the intended purposes or uses of an assessment will help identify the need in a given situation (Dunn, 2005). Three purposes of assessments are often described in the literature: (1) description, (2) decision making, and (3) theory building. Assessments used for description clarify and define a person's current needs or performance abilities. If an assessment is needed for decision making, the purpose may be to select interventions, predict future performance, or demonstrate outcomes of services, along with an array of other decisions based on assessment and evaluation results. Theory-building assessments may be part of larger research agendas that support development of the occupational therapy and occupational science knowledge base.

When the intended purpose or use of an assessment involves decision making, the therapist should consider the nature of the decisions that will be made using the assessment (Law, King, & Russell, 2005). In some situations, the results of assessment may be part of decisions that greatly affect people's lives. In occupational therapy, the outcomes of evaluation may contribute to decisions about where a person should live, the driving status of an older person, classroom placement for a child, qualification for specific services, the ability to return to work after an injury, or a person's need for guardianship. In such cases, it is critical to uphold high standards for selecting assessments (Plake, 2002).

Description of Populations and Clients

Along with identifying the personal characteristics of interest in the evaluation process, it is also important to describe the general **population of clients** who will be evaluated. The population may be described in terms of age, certain demographic characteristics, clinical conditions, or special needs. This step in defining the needs for a practice setting is necessary because most assessments have been developed for specific populations. When trying to locate assessments, information on the characteristics of the population or functional performance to be evaluated will help identify more targeted assessments.

User Qualifications

When examining the need for an assessment in a specific setting, it is important to consider the **qualifications** of the therapists who will be using the assessment. Users of occupational therapy evaluations have four primary responsibilities: (1) administration, (2) scoring, (3) interpretation, and (4) reporting. These responsibilities may be carried out by one person or by different people who contribute to the evaluation process. Several questions can be asked to clarify the qualifications of the users:

- What is the training and educational background of the therapists with respect to the assessments?
- What is the experience of the therapists in the specific evaluation area?
- What level of expertise do the therapists have in administration, scoring, and interpretation in general, as well as specific to the selected assessment?
- What professional standards have been established for evaluation in this area?
- What resources are available to obtain additional training in these assessments, if needed?

Some professional associations and test publishers have specific standards related to user qualifications for assessments (College of Occupational Therapists of Ontario, 2007; Turner, DeMers, Fox, & Reed, 2001). These standards should be referred to when describing the qualifications of therapists in a specific setting. In addition, some tests such as the Sensory Integration and Praxis Tests (Ayres, 1989) and the Assessment of Motor and Process Skills (Fisher & Jones, 2012) require special certifications to perform them accurately. A therapist will not be using best practice if he or she is using such tests without certification.

Practical Considerations

When selecting an assessment, the therapist must consider all the **practical needs** of the setting in which the assessment will be administered, including the format, cost, and time available for an assessment. The available options for the format of an assessment may include observation or performance-based tests, self-reporting, and written or verbal questionnaires. Some assessments may not cost anything, requiring only the permission of the author. Other assessments may require the purchase of the test itself and an ongoing budget for the training of test users or the acquisition of test booklets, assessment kits, and software.

The time required for the overall evaluation process also must be considered. Some assessments can be completed in a single session, whereas other assessments include an extensive battery of subtests to obtain a complete picture of a person's performance and therefore take a more extended period of time. Also, some assessments might need to be completed over several sessions to get the most accurate picture of the client.

LOCATING EXISTING ASSESSMENTS THAT MEET CURRENT NEEDS

The description of the need for an assessment, as discussed earlier, should be documented and should guide the strategies used for the next step, **locating existing assessments** that meet this need. Several strategies are available for locating information on assessments relevant to occupational therapy.

Investigate Occupational Therapy and Occupational Science

One strategy is to consider disciplines or professions that may have an interest in measuring the identified characteristics. Naturally, occupational therapy and occupational science are the first areas to investigate. *OTSearch* (a database available through the American Occupational Therapy Foundation), *OTseeker* (an Internet site and database that focuses on evidence-based practice in occupational therapy), occupational therapy sourcebooks (e.g., Asher, 2014; Hemphill-Pearson, 2008; Law, Baum, & Dunn, 2005; Mulligan, 2003; Paul & Orchanian, 2003), and textbooks in occupational therapy are important tools for finding occupational therapy assessments. Psychology, education, and medicine are secondary areas that may have assessments relevant to occupational therapy.

Use References

A second strategy is to consider the sources of information on assessments themselves. Libraries have reference books (e.g., *Mental Measurement Yearbook* [Geisinger, Spies, Carlson, & Plake, 2007]), databases (e.g., Health and Psychosocial Instruments from Behavioral Management Database Services), journals, textbooks, and other materials that can help locate and critique assessments. The Internet has a wide array of sites that provide information on assessments (APA, 2009). There are also publishers that specialize in tests and assessments and have developed reputations for marketing measurements with a certain focus, such as Western Psychology Services (Torrance, CA) and Pearson Education (Upper Saddle River, NJ).

Explore Professional Associations and Netwroks

A third strategy is to use professional connections and networks to keep abreast of changes in assessment and evaluation; these resources may include professional associations, governmental agencies, professional colleagues, and experts in the field. A good identification strategy includes using more than one resource to compare independent reviews.

Reed and Sanderson (1999) reported that occupational therapists use more than 300 assessments in occupational therapy practice. Despite this large number, it is critical that occupational therapists explore sources outside of occupational therapy and occupational science.

> Therapists should always consider instruments within their own profession first and then expand to exploring assessments from related professions that have interest in the area.

Additionally, Reed and Sanderson (1999) described knowledge resources for occupational therapy as including biological sciences, social sciences, humanities and the arts, applied sciences (medicine, nursing, physical therapy, social work, and speech pathology), engineering and technology, orthotics and prosthetics, business and management, government, and vocational rehabilitation. The *Blueprint for Entry-Level Education* (AOTA, 2010a) and the *Occupational Competence Model* (Polatajko, 1992) also suggested searching within disciplines relevant to

- The person (e.g., psychology, biology, kinesiology/human movement, philosophy, neuroscience, human ethnology),
- The environment (e.g., architecture, forestry, ecology, geography, sociology, political science, economics, social policy), and
- An occupation's interaction with the person, the environment, or both (e.g., career development, leisure studies, psychology of play, sports psychology, anthropology, archeology, human geography, human ecology, sociology).

Identify Major Databases or Resources

Numerous **databases** or **resources** may be helpful in locating assessments. Exhibit 3.1 provides a summary of the most common resources in occupational therapy, psychology, education, and medicine. In most disciplines, reference books or databases contain lists and brief descriptions of tests and assessments for relevant domains. These reference books and databases are important tools for obtaining both general and specific information on existing assessments. The

---

EXHIBIT 3.1. SOURCES OF INFORMATION FOR ASSESSMENTS

Occupational Therapy

- *Assessments in occupational therapy mental health: An integrative approach* (2nd ed.; Hemphill-Pearson, 2008)
- CanChild Centre for Childhood Disability Research (http://www.canchild.ca/en/)
- *Measuring occupational performance: Supporting best practice in occupational therapy* (2nd ed.; Law, Baum, & Dunn, 2005)
- *Occupational therapy assessment tools: An annotated index* (4th ed.; Asher, 2014)
- *Occupational therapy evaluation for children: A pocket guide* (Mulligan, 2003)
- OTSearch (American Occupational Therapy Foundation; http://www.aotf.org/resourceswlwlibrary/otsearch.aspx)
- OTseeker (http://www.otseeker.com/)
- *Pocket guide to assessment in occupational therapy* (Paul & Orchanian, 2003)

Psychology

- APA Science Directorate (http://www.apa.org/science/programs/testing/find-tests.aspx)
- *Measures for psychological assessment: A guide to 3,000 original sources and their applications* (Chun, Cobb, & French, 1975)
- Mental Measurements Yearbook (http://buros.unl.edu/buros/jsp/search.jsp)
- *Psychware sourcebook* (Krug, 1987)
- PsycINFO (http://www.apa.org/pubs/databases/psycinfo/index.aspx)
- PsycTests (http://www.apa.org/pubs/databases/psyctests/)
- *Tests: A comprehensive reference for assessments in psychology, education, and business* (8th ed.; Maddox, 2008)

Education

- ERIC/AE Digest (www.ericdigests.org/1996-1/test.htm)
- Test collection (Educational Testing Service, http://www.ets.org/test_link/about)

Medicine/Rehabilitation

- CINAHL (http://www.ebscohost.com/academic/cinahl-plus-with-full-text)
- Cochrane Library (www.cochrane.org/)
- Health and Psychosocial Instruments (HAPI; www.ovid.com/site/catalog/DataBase/866.jsp)
- InCam Outcomes Database (http://www.outcomesdatabase.org/)
- National Quality Forum (http://www.qualityforum.org/Home.aspx)
- NIH Toolbox (http://www.nihtoolbox.org/Pages/default.aspx)
- Patient Reported Outcomes Measurement Group (http://phi.uhce.ox.ac.uk/home.php)
- PubMed (http://www.ncbi.nlm.nih.gov/pubmed)
- Rehabilitation Measures Database (http://www.rehabmeasures.org/default.aspx)

information provided often includes a description of the assessment, the publisher, supporting research studies, measurement characteristics, and critiques by experts in the field. These resources are helpful for both novice and experienced therapists who want an efficient and effective way of obtaining key information on assessments.

Therapists unfamiliar with these sources of information should initially consult a reference librarian to access these sources and identify other strategies for finding assessments. Some institutions have medical libraries with reference librarians to assist with information location and access. Most academic libraries provide instructions, guides, and website addresses that are helpful for a new user of these sources.

The ability to access information will change rapidly in the future with general access through library databases and search engines such as Google Scholar. Some library databases have specific limiters that may be selected when conducting a search. For example, PsycINFO (TM: Tests and Measures) and ERIC (Tests/Questionnaires) limiters restrict the results of the search to include publications on specific measures used in studies. When using databases that do not have these limiters, consider including a string of assessment keywords (e.g., assessment OR measur* OR test OR outcome) along with the topic keywords when conducting a search. Some libraries and databases provide tutorials that can help therapists develop advanced skills in searching for assessments in peer-reviewed publications.

ANALYZING THE QUALITY OF AN ASSESSMENT: FORMAL METHOD ASSESSMENT

A search for existing assessments may often lead to several matches that meet the needs of a specific situation. The next stage in the selection process is to analyze the overall quality of each assessment using standards and criteria associated with good measurement tools. The **Standards for Educational and Psychological Testing** (American Educational Research Association [AERA], APA, & National Council on Measurement in Education [NCME], 1999) provide guidelines for evaluating the quality of tests and testing practices. Although it may be difficult for occupational therapists to meet all of these guidelines, they present a model toward which the profession should strive. Most assessment ratings, or critique forms and guidelines, are similar to or based on these standards (Bass-Haugen, 1989; Law, 2008; Reed & Sanderson, 1999; Tickle-Degnen, 2008). The standards include four parts:

> To critique an assessment, consider test construction and evaluation, test use, particular applications, and administrative procedures.

1. Technical standards for test construction and evaluation,
2. Professional standards for test use,
3. Standards for particular applications (including a section on testing people with handicapping conditions), and
4. Standards for administrative procedures (including scoring and interpretation).

Assessment analysis begins with the acquisition of available **documentation** on the assessment. Several resources should be obtained before beginning a critique of an assessment: the technical manual (if available), published summaries and critiques of the assessment, and published research on the assessment. Documentation of the resources used to analyze the quality of an assessment is important because the quality and utility of an assessment may change over time as it is developed further. A therapist may not select an assessment at one point in time because of its overall quality; however, if it evolves into an assessment that meets specific needs of the evaluation, the therapist may decide to use it.

A formal method of analysis involves two primary steps: (1) a description of the assessment as it relates to practice needs and (2) the evaluation of the overall quality of the assessment (Exhibit 3.2). The description of the assessment includes the characteristics of interest and importance, the purpose, the population or clients, user qualifications, and practical considerations. The evaluation of the overall quality of the assessment requires the examination of

- The technical manual,
- The method of assessment development and administration,
- Scoring and scales and norms used for interpretation,

EXHIBIT 3.2. FORMAL METHOD FOR ANALYZING AN ASSESSMENT

	Sources of Information	Characteristics and Summary	Critique	Recommendations and Comments
Name and publication information				
Characteristic				
Purpose				
Population or clients				
User qualifications Practical considerations				
Technical manual Development and administration				
Scores, scales, and norms				
Reliability				
Validity				
Overall				

- Reliability evidence, and
- Validity evidence.

The *Standards for Educational and Psychological Testing* (AERA, APA, & NCME, 1999) and other guidelines provide specific criteria for each of these analysis areas. For example, the National Center for Education Statistics (2002) states that the development of an assessment must abide by an explicit set of specifications. These specifications must be clearly documented so that the development of the assessment can be replicated. Examples of specifications include the purpose of the assessment, the domain or constructs, the outline for the format, the number of items, time requirements, the context, participant characteristics, psychometric properties, the administration, scoring procedures, and the reporting of results.

Testing standards are especially important when high-stakes decisions are made on the basis of the assessment. For such uses, especially in educational settings, it is critical that the assessment be evaluated in terms of the alignment to test specifications, the opportunity to learn, freedom from bias and sensitive

situations, developmental appropriateness, score consistency and reliability, and appropriateness of mastery-level cut points (Plake, 2002).

Therapists should make good use of **expert critiques** to complete an analysis of an assessment, evaluate technical standards, and determine proper and improper use. Sourcebooks and critical reviews in the literature provide expert critiques of commonly used assessments. These critiques summarize the quality of an assessment in key areas and provide recommendations on how the therapist should use the assessment in practice. Tracking the dates of recently published critiques and studies can give the therapist an indication of an assessment's stage of development and how the assessment has been used in practice, theory development, and outcomes research.

Completion of formal analyses of several assessments can help the therapist identify the best assessment for a given situation or setting. It also makes the therapist aware of the appropriate uses for an assessment and the cautions that he or she must take, given its limitations. These types of summary statements and recommendations about an assessment should be incorporated into the information given during the evaluation process and shared in appropriate ways with both the health care team and the client.

ETHICAL ISSUES RELATED TO SELECTION AND USE OF ASSESSMENTS

Ethical dilemmas occur at every stage of the evaluation process, which is why professional associations adopt and enforce codes of ethics and standards of practice that guide evaluation and practice (AOTA, 2010b, 2010c). Three **ethical issues** will be noted here as they relate to the selection and use of assessments. Other responsibilities and values related to ethics and best practice in evaluation are described in other chapters of this text.

Unauthorized Use

One pertinent ethical issue relates to the unauthorized use of published and copyrighted assessments. In the past, it was common practice in many health care and education settings to simply copy test manuals and test scoring forms from original publications. It is the responsibility of the assessment user to purchase published assessments directly from the publisher. If an assessment is copyrighted but is not available through a publisher, the user must contact the author and obtain permission in writing to use the assessment (APA, 2009).

Qualifications of Assessment Users

A second ethical issue relates to the selection of assessments that may not be a good match with the qualifications of the assessment users. Some organizations (American Counseling Association, 2003) provide specific criteria on the qualifications of test users, including knowledge and skills in the following areas:

- Professional practice and relevant theory supporting an assessment
- Testing theory
- Measurement concepts and statistics
- Ability to review, select, and administer appropriate assessments

- Administration and scoring in relation to a specific assessment's purposes
- Impact of diversity on accuracy
- Responsible use of assessments and evaluation in diagnosing, predicting future ends, and planning intervention.

If the therapist's current qualifications are not adequate for a given assessment, several options may be considered. Therapists may obtain and maintain the additional knowledge and skills required to use the assessment. Sometimes qualifications include earned academic degrees, professional credentials, or certification to administer a specific assessment. Alternatively, another assessment with similar characteristics and fewer user restrictions may be chosen, or the assessment may be used for only limited purposes (e.g., screening) with clearly identified cautions against misuse and as part of a larger evaluation process.

Adapting Assessments to Fit Needs

A third ethical dilemma arises when the therapist cannot find any existing assessments in the literature for the needs in a specific practice setting. Unfortunately, a common practice is to "do your own thing" and create or adapt an assessment that seems to fit the situation. Routinely adopting this approach can set in motion dangerous practices for administering, scoring, and interpreting assessments.

Adapting a standardized assessment will not yield a standard score and may not give the user appropriate information. Keep in mind that assessment and evaluation are powerful tools that either support or refute occupational therapy outcomes; occupational therapy recommendations to clients and other professionals; and the credibility of occupational therapy practice in the larger health care, social services, and educational systems in which therapists work. The creation or use of "home-grown" assessments, or the adaptation of existing assessments, should be rare in occupational therapy practice and should be accompanied by disclaimers that warn others against inappropriate application and caution interpretation of the results. It is important that major decisions and recommendations regarding clients are never based on these types of assessments alone.

SUMMARY

Assessment identification and selection is an important component of the evaluation process. It is a critical step in the effort to ensure that the results of evaluation are accurate and that the outcomes of interventions are effective and efficient. This chapter introduced a three-stage process for selecting assessments, including reflection on the needs in practice, identification of existing assessments that meet those needs, and critical analysis to evaluate the strengths and limitations of assessments and to determine the best assessment for a given situation. Using a formal method to identify and select assessments is one of the best ways to develop confidence in the assessments chosen for evaluation and to gain a professional reputation for excellence in evaluation.

QUESTIONS

1. When planning an assessment for a particular client with a stroke, what parameters would you use to choose an assessment? What parameters would be different if the client were a 3-year-old child with Down syndrome?

2. How does setting or context influence assessment selection?

3. Three purposes of assessment are description, decision making, and theory building. Explain each of these and how they relate to occupational therapy.

4. Go to an online assessment database, select a performance area, and find 3 appropriate assessments for use with an adolescent client.

5. What are the ethical issues related to creating your own assessment method to meet a particular situation? How could you avoid this ethical dilemma?

6. A therapist has suggested that you use a particular assessment for an evaluation. How would you analyze the quality of this assessment? How would you handle the situation if you determined that it was not a quality assessment?

References

American Counseling Association. (2003). *Standards for qualifications of test users.* Alexandria, VA: Author.

American Educational Research Association, American Psychological Association, & National Council on Measurement in Education. (1999). *Standards for educational and psychological testing.* Washington, DC: Author.

American Occupational Therapy Association (2010a). Blueprint for entry-level education. *American Journal of Occupational Therapy, 64,* 186–194. http://dx.dio.org/10.5014/ajot.64.1.186

American Occupational Therapy Association. (2010b). Occupational therapy code of ethics and ethics standards (2010). *American Journal of Occupational Therapy, 64*(Suppl.), S17–S26. http://dx.doi.org/10.5014/ajot.2010.64S17

American Occupational Therapy Association. (2010c). Standards of practice for occupational therapy. *American Journal of Occupational Therapy, 64*(Suppl.), S106–S111. http://dx.doi.org/10.5014/ajot.2010.64S106

American Occupational Therapy Association. (2014). Occupational therapy practice framework: Domain and process (3rd ed.). *American Journal of Occupational Therapy, 68*(Suppl. 1), S1–S48. http://dx.doi.org/10.5014/ajot.2014.682006

American Psychological Association, Joint Committee on Testing Practices. (2004). *Code of fair testing practices in education.* Washington, DC: Author. Retrieved from http://www.apa.org/science/fairtestcode.html

American Psychological Association. (2009). *FAQ/Finding information about psychological tests.* Retrieved from http://www.apa.org/science/faq-findtests.html

Asher, I. E. (Ed.). (2014). *Asher's occupational therapy assessment tools: An annotated index* (4th ed.). Bethesda, MD: AOTA Press.

Ayres, A. J. (1989). *Sensory integration and praxis tests.* Torrance, CA: Western Psychological Services.

Bass-Haugen, J. (1989, October). *Identifying and critiquing measurement tools in clinical practice.* Preconference Institute at the Annual Meeting of the Minnesota Occupational Therapy Association, Minneapolis.

Baum, C. M., & Christiansen, C. H. (2005). Person–Environment–Occupation–Performance: An occupation-based framework for practice. In C. H. Christiansen, C. M. Baum, & J. Bass-Haugen (Eds.), *Occupational therapy: Performance, participation and well-being* (3rd ed., pp. 242–266). Thorofare, NJ: Slack.

Baum, C. M., & Law, M. (1997). Occupational therapy practice: Focusing on occupational performance. *American Journal of Occupational Therapy, 51,* 277–288. http://dx.doi.org/10.5014/ajot.51.4.277

Chun, K.-T., Cobb, S., & French, J. R. P. (1975). *Measures for psychological assessment: A guide to 3,000 original sources and their applications.* Ann Arbor, MI: Survey Research Center, Institute for Social Research.

College of Occupational Therapists of Ontario. (2007). *Standards for occupational therapy assessments.*

Retrieved from http://www.coto.org/pdf/Standards_for_Occupational_Therapy_Assessments.pdf

Dunn, W. (2005). Measurement issues and practices. In M. Law, C. Baum, & W. Dunn (Eds.), *Measuring occupational performance: Supporting best practice in occupational therapy* (2nd ed., pp. 21–32). Thorofare, NJ: Slack.

Dunn, W., Brown, C., & Youngstrom, M. J. (2003). The Ecology of Human Performance: A framework for considering the effect of context. In P. Kramer, J. Hinojosa, & C. Brasic Royeen (Eds.), *Perspectives in human occupation: Participation in life* (pp. 222–263). Baltimore: Lippincott Williams & Wilkins.

Fisher, A. G., & Jones, K. B. (2012). *Assessment of motor and process skills* (7th ed.). Fort Collins, CO: Three Star Press.

Geisinger, K. F., Spies, R. A., Carlson, J. F., & Plake, B. S. (2007). *Mental measurements yearbook* (17th ed.). Lincoln, NE: Buros Institute of Mental Measurements.

Hemphill-Pearson, B. (2008). *Assessments in occupational therapy mental health: An integrative approach* (2nd ed.). Thorofare, NJ: Slack.

Institute of Medicine, Committee on Assessing Rehabilitation Science and Engineering, Division of Health Sciences Policy. (1997). *Enabling America: Assessing the role of rehabilitation science and engineering.* Washington, DC: National Academy Press.

Kielhofner, G. (2007). *Model of Human Occupation: Theory and application* (4th ed.). Baltimore: Lippincott Williams & Wilkins.

Krug, S. E. (1987). *Psychware sourcebook.* Kansas City, MO: Test Corporation of America.

Law, M. (2008). Appendix F: Outcome Measures Rating Form guidelines. In M. Law & J. MacDermid (Eds.), *Evidence-based rehabilitation: A guide to practice* (2nd ed., pp. 381–386). Thorofare, NJ: Slack.

Law, M., Baum, C., & Dunn, W. (Eds.). (2005). *Measuring Occupational Performance: Supporting best practice in occupational therapy* (2nd ed.). Thorofare, NJ: Slack.

Law, M., Cooper, B. A., Strong, S., Stewart, D., Rigby, P., & Letts, L. (1996). The Person–Environment–Occupation model: A transactive approach to occupational performance. *Canadian Journal of Occupational Therapy, 63,* 9–22. http://dx.doi.org/10.1177/000841749606300103

Law, M., King, G., & Russell, D. (2005). Guiding therapist decisions about measuring outcomes in occupational therapy. In M. Law, C. Baum, & W. Dunn (Eds.), *Measuring occupational performance: Supporting best practice in occupational therapy* (2nd ed., pp. 33–44). Thorofare, NJ: Slack.

Maddox, T. (2008). *Tests: A comprehensive reference for assessments in psychology, education, and business* (8th ed.). Austin, TX: Pro-Ed.

Mathiowetz, V., & Bass-Haugen, J. B. (1994). Motor behavior research: Implications for therapeutic approaches to central nervous system dysfunction. *American Journal of Occupational Therapy, 48,* 733–745. http://dx.doi.org/10.5014/ajot.48.8.733

Mulligan, S. (2003). *Occupational therapy evaluation for children: A pocket guide.* Baltimore: Lippincott Williams & Wilkins.

National Center for Education Statistics. (2002). *NCES statistical standards.* Retrieved from http://nces.ed.gov/statprog/2002/stdtoc.asp

National Center for Medical Rehabilitation Research. (1993). *Research plan for the National Center for Rehabilitation Research* (NIH Publication No. 93-3509). Washington, DC: U.S. Government Printing Office.

National Center for Medical Rehabilitation Research. (2006). *National Center for Medical Rehabilitation Research NICHD: Report to the NACHHD Council January 2006.* Washington, DC: U.S. Government Printing Office. Retrieved from http://www.nichd.nih.gov/publications/pubs_details.cfm?from=&pubs_id=5049

Paul, S., & Orchanian, D. (2003). *Pocket guide to assessment in occupational therapy.* Clifton Park, NY: Delmar.

Plake, B. (2002). Evaluating the technical quality of educational tests used for high-stake decisions. *Measurement and Evaluation in Counseling and Development, 35,* 144–152.

Polatajko, H. J. (1992). Naming and framing occupational therapy: A lecture dedicated to the life of Nancy B. *Canadian Journal of Occupational Therapy, 59,* 189–200. http://dx.doi.org/10.1177/000841749205900403

Reed, K. L., & Sanderson, S. N. (Eds.). (1999). *Concepts of occupational therapy* (4th ed.). Baltimore: Lippincott Williams & Wilkins.

Tickle-Degnen, L. (2008). Communicating evidence to clients, managers, and funders. In M. Law (Ed.), *Evidence-based rehabilitation: A guide to practice* (2nd ed., pp. 263–295). Thorofare, NJ: Slack.

Trombly, C. A. (1995). Occupation: Purposefulness and meaningfulness as therapeutic mechanisms (1995 Eleanor Clarke Slagle Lecture). *American Journal of Occupational Therapy, 49,* 960–972. http://dx.doi.org/10.5014/ajot.49.10.960

Turner, S. M., DeMers, S. T., Fox, H. R., & Reed, G. M. (2001). APA's guidelines for test user qualifications: An executive summary. *American Psychologist, 56,* 1099–1113. http://dx.doi.org/10.1037/0003-066X.56.12.1099

World Health Organization. (2001). *International classification of functioning, disability and health.* Geneva: Author.

CHAPTER 4

Practical Aspects of the Evaluation Process

Denise Chisholm, PhD, OTR/L, FAOTA

Highlights

- Screening
- Referral
- Assessments
- Environment
- Time
- Teamwork
- Materials
- Documentation
- Accountability
- Occupational therapy assistants
- Professional development.

Key Terms

Accountability	Mood
Assessments	Occupational therapy assistants
Confidentiality	Physical factors
Documentation	Preparing clients
Effective communication	Professional development
Emotional factors	Referral
Employees	Reimbursement models
Environment	Right to privacy
Fair treatment	Screening
Independent contractors	State laws
Journal club	Team
Materials	Time-related factors
Mentor	

The increased demands of today's practice environments require that an occupational therapist perform evaluations more effectively and efficiently. Evaluation is a complex process that guides occupational therapy intervention and, as such, is an essential component in the provision of high-quality services. Many practical issues related to performing an occupational therapy evaluation can either facilitate or challenge the efficacy and efficiency of the process.

This chapter outlines practical information for the occupational therapist to use to evaluate clients that comprehensively focuses on the priority issues using quality assessments in the shortest amount of time. Unfortunately, there is no magic recipe; however, an occupational therapist with a working knowledge of the evaluation process can use strategies that maximize efficacy and efficiency.

This chapter addresses "real-world" practical aspects that affect the evaluation process, including screening, referral, assessments, environment, time, teamwork, materials, documentation, accountability, participation of occupational therapy assistants, and professional development. Most of these issues are applicable across practice environments. However, when appropriate, specific information related to the unique aspects of specific occupational therapy practice settings is provided.

SCREENING

Many practice settings (e.g., acute care, skilled nursing, long-term-care facilities, schools) include **screening** before or as a component of the evaluation process. Screening determines the need for further evaluation. Although the screening of a potential client is typically not a reimbursable service, it can be highly valuable in determining the need for referrals for clients requiring occupational therapy evaluation and intervention, which are reimbursable services. For these reasons, a therapist must carefully consider the amount of time and effort dedicated to screening, with the goal of performing screening as efficiently as possible.

The first step is to determine the reasonable or approved time frame for the completion of the screening of a potential client for the specific practice setting or facility. Many facilities have a guideline of one unit of service (15 minutes).

The next step is to review available data and interview, observe, or administer a screening instrument to the potential client to determine the need for an occupational therapy evaluation. If obtaining and reviewing data take longer than 15 minutes, the client almost certainly needs a comprehensive evaluation for occupational therapy services (Exhibit 4.1). A general rule is if the therapist cannot unequivocally determine the client could not benefit from occupational therapy services through the screening, then the therapist should initiate completing a comprehensive evaluation.

State laws and regulatory codes may address screening, so it is essential that occupational therapists know the rules and regulations in their state. Therapists should have a copy of or quick access to the state laws and regulatory requirements applicable to their facility and practice setting.

REFERRAL

The implementation of occupational therapy services for most practice settings is based on receipt of a referral. A *referral* is a written order for a specific service. Referral procedures vary on the basis of state laws and the regulatory requirements of the facility or practice setting. Occupational therapists must accept and respond to referrals in compliance with state laws and regulatory codes. Therefore, therapists must be familiar with and have a working knowledge of the laws and regulatory codes that affect practice and understand the interpretation of the rules. Often, the definitions and rules are different for direct services versus indirect services, consultation, and screening. For example, in Pennsylvania, a referral is not required for an evaluation:

EXHIBIT 4.1. HELPFUL HINTS FOR SCREENING

- Screening determines the need for evaluation.
- Screening is typically not a reimbursable service.
- Screening can be highly valuable in generating referrals for reimbursable services.
- The time frame for screening is usually no more than 1 unit of service (15 minutes) or a reasonably short time.

An occupational therapist may enter a case for the purposes of providing indirect services, consultation, evaluating an individual as to the need for services. . . . Implementation of direct occupational therapy to an individual for a specific medical condition shall be based on a referral from a licensed physician, licensed optometrist, licensed podiatrist, licensed certified registered nurse practitioner or licensed physician assistant. (Commonwealth of Pennsylvania, 2012, Section 14, Practice and Referral, p. 10)

Occupational therapists must be familiar with the current laws and regulations of the state where they practice, because these may change or be revised, and changes in other laws affect current laws. For example, when the Occupational Therapy Practice Act (Commonwealth of Pennsylvania, 2012) in Pennsylvania was written originally in 1982, occupational therapists were able to accept referrals from only licensed physicians and podiatrists. However, over the years, the law was amended to include licensed optometrists, and, most recently, in 2012, licensed nurse practitioners and physician assistants were added to the list of professionals who may refer patients for occupational therapy services in Pennsylvania. Similar licensure changes have occurred in other states.

When examining the laws, rules, and regulations, a therapist should identify those sections related to the evaluation process (i.e., referral, evaluation, screening, occupational therapy assistants, supervision). Often, because of the complexity of the language, it is helpful to discuss these documents with colleagues, including those within the facility and those in the same or similar practice settings.

The goal is to have a working knowledge of the documents that govern occupational therapy practice. To do so, therapists must establish a system for obtaining updates and revisions. When a therapist is unsure about the meaning or interpretation of the content, he or she should address questions to the boards or agencies overseeing the laws and regulations.

A licensed physician usually writes referrals for occupational therapy services. State laws may also address oral orders (i.e., if and when a referral in the form of an oral order can be accepted)

and identify other professionals from whom an occupational therapist can accept a referral (e.g., licensed optometrist, licensed podiatrist, certified registered nurse, physician assistant). Therapists should read each referral form carefully and ensure they address all pertinent areas in the evaluation process and associated documentation.

Therapists also must ensure the professionals ordering services understand the unique focus of occupational therapy. It is the responsibility of each therapist to ensure that referral sources understand that the focus of occupational therapy services is on *occupations,* that is, the "activities that people engage in throughout their daily lives to fulfill their time and give life meaning" (American Occupational Therapy Association [AOTA], 1997, p. 865). Referrals must accurately reflect the services being ordered. When they do not, the therapist needs to identify education opportunities and implement strategies to facilitate the ordering of appropriate services (Exhibit 4.2).

The following is specific information related to the initiation of services in pediatric practice settings:

- A child's parents or guardians must give permission for an occupational therapy evaluation.
- In the educational setting, a referral usually addresses education issues. The therapist has to be in compliance with the federal law, and the state rules and regulations may differentiate between the need for services to address an educational issue versus a medical need, and may not require a referral to address problems related to educational issues.

EXHIBIT 4.2. HELPFUL HINTS FOR REFERRAL

- Procedures vary on the basis of state laws and facility regulatory requirements.
- An order for occupational therapy services is usually written but may be oral if permitted by laws and regulations.
- Referrals are typically written by a physician; however, they may be written by other professionals as identified by laws and regulations.
- Referrals should accurately reflect the occupational therapy services of the specific practice setting.

ASSESSMENTS

There are many **assessments** occupational therapists can use in the evaluation process. The difficulty is finding the best ones to address the needs of the client and practice setting. The specific assessments—the tools, instruments, or systematic interactions (e.g., observation, interview protocol) used in the evaluation process—should address occupational therapy's unique focus on occupational performance and factors that support occupational performance. Therapists select assessments based on the demographic (e.g., diagnoses, ages, discharge destinations) and occupational performance needs of the client population by considering and prioritizing the relevant occupations, client factors (e.g., body functions, body structures), performance skills and patterns, and environmental factors.

Additionally, therapists consider the influence of factors related to the practice setting, including reimbursement sources. From this combined information, therapists identify a list or inventory of potential assessments that measure the occupational performance needs of the typical client. From the multitude of possible assessments, therapists determine the best assessment or assessments to use with a specific client (Exhibit 4.3).

EXHIBIT 4.3. DETERMINING THE BEST ASSESSMENTS FOR YOUR CLIENT POPULATIONS AND SETTINGS

- Identify demographic and clinical characteristics (occupational performance problems and strengths) of client population and factors related to the practice setting.
- Analyze assessments that may meet the needs of the client population and practice setting (create a "long list" of assessments).
- Identify the best assessments that meet the needs of the client population and suit the practice setting (create a "short list" of assessments).
- Obtain the most current edition of the manual and materials for the assessments on the short list.
- Choose the assessments from the short list that best meet the individual client's needs.
- Review and revise the short list of best assessments on an annual basis and obtain new assessments or new editions of assessments as needed.

Therapists need to examine a range of factors when determining the best assessments to use during the evaluation process with the clients in their practice setting. The most effective assessment selection method is for two or more therapists to reach agreement through analyzing, discussing, and carefully considering the following information for each assessment:

- Purpose (what the assessment is intended to measure)
- Theoretical basis
- Psychometric integrity (test–retest and interrater reliability and internal consistency; face, criterion-related, construct, and content validity)
- Population (age, diagnosis, abilities, limitations)
- Setting (environmental requirements for use and maintenance)
- Degree of measurable objective data obtained
- Costs (purchase, training, use, maintenance)
- Time issues (training and administration; setup and cleanup; documentation of results)
- Client perception of assessment
- Utility (in conjunction with assessments used by other disciplines on the team).

The process for selecting the most appropriate assessment for a particular client becomes more intuitive and proficient with increased clinical experience. However, both novice and expert therapists can benefit from using assessment resources. The fourth edition of *Asher's Occupational Therapy Assessment Tools: An Annotated Index* (Asher, 2014), which contains profiles of nearly 600 instruments, is useful to therapists choosing appropriate assessments for clinical practice or research purposes. A few other resources are *Occupational Therapy Evaluation for Children: A Pocket Guide* (Mulligan, 2013), *Occupational Therapy Evaluation for Adults: A Pocket Guide* (Vroman & Stewart, 2013), *Measuring Occupational Performance: Supporting Best Practice in Occupational Therapy* (Law, Baum, & Dunn, 2005), and *Willard and Spackman's Occupational Therapy* (Schell, Gillen, & Scaffa, 2014).

Another valuable resource that connects therapists to other therapists in their practice areas is AOTA's Special Interest Sections (SISs). The SIS *Quarterly* newsletters and discussion forums are resources for identifying assessments in specific practice areas (i.e., developmental disabilities, early intervention and school, gerontology, home and community health, mental health, physical disabilities, sensory integration, technology, work and industry). AOTA also offers publications (e.g., *American Journal of Occupational Therapy*, *OT Practice*) and an extensive collection of products (e.g., assessments, books, CDs, DVDs) that therapists can easily search by topic (e.g., assessment and evaluation, low vision, mental health, pediatrics) or keyword (e.g., assessment, cognition, early intervention).

Occupational therapy educational programs are also an excellent resource when exploring and choosing assessments, because they typically have a wide range of assessments for teaching purposes. Members of the faculty are generally willing to assist their students, alumni, and fieldwork educators with clinical issues, including investigating assessments. Additionally, faculty members are usually familiar with the psychometric integrity of the assessments, so they can assist in the interpretation of information. Faculty may also be able to connect therapists who are interested in using the assessments with a network of professional resources.

Reading the assessment manual is paramount to successfully administering and appropriately using the instrument for clinical or research purposes. It is beneficial for therapists to read and reread the assessment manual and relevant literature (i.e., research articles addressing the reliability and validity of the assessment) and to analyze and discuss the information to understand the utility of the instrument for their practice setting. When investigating assessments, therapists should determine the

- Purpose of the assessment (what does the instrument measure?),
- Theoretical approach of the assessment (does it match the theoretical approach of the practice setting and facility?),
- Clinical (or research) utility of the results (how can the results be used?),
- Populations the assessment was developed for (does it match the populations the instrument will be administered to in the clinical or research setting?),
- Reliability of the assessment (how repeatable or consistent is the instrument; to what degree

does it yield the same results or measures the same way each time it is administered under the same condition with the same population?), and
- Validity of the assessment (does the instrument measure the specific concept it is intended to measure; are the conclusions, inferences, or propositions correct?).

Just because an assessment is published and the authors report good psychometric integrity does not necessarily mean that it actually has good psychometric integrity. Therapists should use resources to interpret and better understand the psychometric properties of assessments.

An effective method of learning about the psychometric integrity of assessments is to establish a **journal club** in your practice setting or facility to review publications related to the evaluation process and assessments. The journal club can include staff members and students. It is important to designate specific meetings to address the evaluation process.

For example, if the journal club meets monthly, consider having 4 out of the 12 meetings address evaluation. The articles selected can address the evaluation of particular diagnostic categories (e.g., stroke, brain injury, developmental disabilities) related to your client population, or they could address a particular assessment. Participation in a journal club can build the evidence-based skills of those participating. Participants should not merely read and repeat what the author reports but instead should discuss and interpret the assessments' psychometric properties. Students can be important contributors and facilitators to this process.

Another consideration is the format of the assessment, which ranges from interviews to pencil-and-paper tests, performance-based tasks, and computerized tests. Therapists should consider which format is best for their population and practice setting. Additionally, therapists must consider which format best measures occupational performance and the components that support the client's occupational performance. Although performance-based measures may take therapists more time to administer, these measures yield objective data related to occupational performance. When choosing assessments, therapists should consider both the quality and the quantity of measurable objective data the assessment yields.

Therapists must be knowledgeable of the time it takes to administer the assessment. This factor is particularly important when evaluating younger children or people with low endurance or cognitive limitations. Therapists must also consider the amount of time required to set up and clean up the assessment, as well as the time needed to score and interpret the assessment. Ideally, the assessment selected provides the best objective and most useful information in the shortest amount of time. Other time considerations, include the amount of time required for both formal and informal training, depending on the requirements of the assessment.

Although most occupational therapists commonly use particular assessments in their practice setting, they should go through a thoughtful process to select the most appropriate assessments for their clinical population versus simply using assessments historically used by the facility. It is helpful to have a summary of available assessments.

One effective way of compiling assessment summaries is for therapists to create user-friendly one-page handouts on the best assessments (from the "short list") for their client population. Include the complete reference for the assessment and a brief description of the assessment's format, purpose (what it is intended to measure), populations, length of time for administration, setup and testing criteria, required materials, psychometric properties (reliability and validity), scoring, and helpful hints or considerations for administration. Additionally, a summary chart of the best assessments used to evaluate a specific area (e.g., basic activities of daily living, work, perception, strength, fine motor skills) can guide therapists in the selection of the most appropriate assessments for a specific client (Exhibit 4.4).

Therapists should have the current edition of the assessments they use when evaluating a client. Current editions are particularly important for pediatric assessments that periodically revise normative data for age and skill comparisons. If an outdated version of the assessment is used, the results may not be an accurate measure of the child's skills.

The facility should have an established method for obtaining and maintaining literature and resources relevant to using the assessment. For example, a staff member or pair of staff members can provide a staff development session on updates, revisions, or new evidence related to a specific assessment. An evidence-based library of assessments relevant to the practice of the department can be created and maintained (i.e., updated at least annually). Evidence-based activities are great learning assignments for students during fieldwork experiences.

As a rule, assessments that obtain objective, clearly defined, quantifiable data are most effective to include in the evaluation process for all populations; however, they are essential when the evaluation helps to determine placement decisions (e.g., school-based programs, discharge planning; Exhibit 4.5).

The process of creating an evidence-based library of the assessments used in your clinical practice or at your work site begins by identifying an appropriate organizational structure. The

---

EXHIBIT 4.5. HELPFUL HINTS FOR ASSESSMENTS

- Use your resources
  - Peer-reviewed journals
  - Textbooks
  - Professional organization magazines and forums
  - Educational programs and faculty members.
- Establish a journal club.
- Determine the best assessments for the client population and setting.
- Create user-friendly, 1-page handouts for the best assessments.
- Develop a summary chart of assessments related to the client population.
- Create an evidence-based library.

EXHIBIT 4.4. SAMPLE SUMMARY CHART CATEGORIES

Title	Purpose	Description	Population or Type of Client	Method or Rating	Source or Training

information could be organized by type of assessment (e.g., performance-based, interview, questionnaire), the domain addressed by the assessment (e.g., occupations, performance skills, body functions and body structures, performance patterns, environmental factors), or age group for which the assessment is designed (e.g., 0–3 years, 3–7 years, 7–12 years, adolescent, adult, older adult). Remember to establish a system for adding new evidence related to the evaluation process and assessments to your library.

ENVIRONMENT

Occupational therapists must carefully consider the **environment** when selecting appropriate assessments for their facility and when administering the assessments in their clinical practice. Environment includes both physical and emotional factors. *Physical factors* include space, seating, sound, temperature, people, and tasks; *emotional factors* involve the mood of both the client and the therapist.

Physical Environment

Therapists must consider physical factors such as the size and type of space needed and available for administrating the assessment. Some assessments may require a large space so the client can perform gross motor movements, whereas other assessments may require tasks to be performed in a kitchen or need a table top for administration. Therapists must also take into account the type and amount of objects and materials needed and available.

Additionally, the arrangement of the objects and materials, including seating, is important. Some assessments require specific objects to be positioned in a precise order. Sometimes assessment manuals will state the recommended or required positioning of the therapist and client; for example, the therapist needs to sit across from the client, at a 90° angle, or next to the client. Therapists must know the environmental requirements of the assessment and identify the optimal environment for administering the assessment. Often, the therapist must modify the clinical setting to create the most favorable environment for the administration of the assessment. If the

clinical environment does not match the environmental requirements of the assessment, the therapist needs to determine whether modification is permissible. Therapists must be aware that administering an assessment in an alternative or modified environment may result in skewed data and invalidate the results of the evaluation.

The therapist also must attend to the temperature and sound of the environment. The client's perception, needs, and comfort should be the determining factors in adjusting temperature and monitoring sound. Eliminating excess noise and distractions is optimal for administering most, if not all, assessments, but is essential when conducting an evaluation with a pediatric client or client with a cognitive disability.

The location of the evaluation depends on the type of practice setting. In some practice settings, the evaluation process occurs in a small room, whereas in other settings the therapist administers the evaluations in the client's room or in a clinic area. Ideally, the therapist conducts an evaluation in a private, or at least semiprivate, location to support the client's best performance. The therapist should avoid environments where other people (e.g., practitioners, clients, parents, teachers) are in the area or passing through the area. Therapists often have to be creative in selecting a location for the evaluation. For example, a therapist who works in the school environment may consider using the hallways, cafeteria, gymnasium, playground, auditorium stage, or a classroom not in use. Other clinical environments may have a specified area for conducting evaluations.

The number of people present and their roles can affect the evaluation process and the client's performance. In busy environments, therapists might not obtain the client's best or optimal performance. If a parent or caregiver is present during the evaluation, it may be helpful to ask him or her to leave the room temporarily to observe the client interact with the environment independently. The therapist should consider the use of a two-way mirror, if available, that allows parents (or others) an opportunity to observe the child (or the client) during the evaluation process without creating undue distractions. Unfortunately, this setup is not always available.

An occupational therapist who works in a client's home has special challenges. For example, a therapist who works in early intervention or with older adults often needs to evaluate clients in their homes. If possible, the therapist should request clarification of the evaluation site location before conducting the evaluation. Home environments have many variations that can both positively and negatively affect the evaluation process. Administering assessments in the home requires more spontaneous decision making and flexibility because therapists do not have the opportunity to preplan or familiarize themselves with the environment before the evaluation session.

Therapists must consider the tasks or items required by the assessment and their relationship with the environment. Therapists should ask

- How complex are the tasks?
- Are there time limits and restrictions?
- Are the tasks highly structured or loosely organized?
- Do the tasks require a serious atmosphere or encourage a playful mood?
- Is there a social dimension to the tasks?
- Are the tasks more cooperative or competitive?

Therapists must consider the order in which the assessment tasks or items are administered. First and foremost, the therapist must refer to the assessment manual to determine whether there is a standardized format for the administration of the tasks. If the assessment specifies the order, the occupational therapist must adhere to it so that the results are valid. If the order is flexible, then the therapist must determine the most favorable order of administration for the client while taking into account the environmental constraints (Exhibit 4.6).

EXHIBIT 4.6. HELPFUL HINTS FOR THE PHYSICAL ENVIRONMENT

Refer to the manual of the assessment when considering
- Size and type of space
- Objects and materials, and their arrangement
- Seating and positioning of the therapist and client
- Temperature
- Sound
- People
- Complexity, structure, and order of the tasks.

Emotional Environment

In addition to the physical factors of the environment, a therapist must give special consideration to the environment's emotional factors—the mood of both the client and the occupational therapist. The therapist cannot control the mood of the client; however, a therapist can promote and facilitate desired affective behaviors using effective communication strategies. As health care professionals, occupational therapists may need to modify their natural communication style and learn more effective communication techniques. The challenge is for the therapist to change communication styles on the basis of the needs and styles of the client.

Therapists' clinical effectiveness in the evaluation process is directly related to their communication skills. Therapists can learn communication techniques and incorporate effective techniques into their interpersonal style through ongoing self-evaluation, practice, and feedback. All communication has a nonverbal message (i.e., how the therapist conveys the information) in addition to the verbal message (i.e., the information the therapist gives).

Preparing clients and their family members or significant others for the evaluation process is essential. The initial contact with the client at the start of the evaluation session is key to creating a therapeutic atmosphere that communicates trust and caring. Therapists must make sure to provide a thorough, user-friendly orientation to both occupational therapy services and the evaluation process. A client must understand what the therapist is going to do and what the therapist expects him or her to do. Clients are typically more involved and invested in the process if they understand how the services and evaluation connect with their health goals.

Regardless of the practice setting, occupational therapists have a tendency to use medical and therapy jargon. Therapists should transform their jargon into user-friendly language for clients and their families. For example, therapists working in an educational setting need to define clearly words such as *proprioception, vestibular, sensory integration, sensory processing*, and *kinesthetic* using plain, nonmedical language. Clear, simple language in this situation will ensure that parents and team members (i.e., teachers, school administrators) understand what the therapist says or writes. The therapist needs to accept that preparing the client (including the family and significant other) is an ongoing process and that it is the therapist's responsibility to do so to provide high-quality, individualized services.

The **mood** of the occupational therapist is the other half of the emotional factor of the environment. Mood includes the therapist's temperament, how he or she conveys it, and how it influences communication with the client. Mood can facilitate or hinder desired affective behaviors of the client. Therapists must be aware of their mood, the message they are conveying through their mood, and the effect it has on the therapeutic relationship. Mood is interrelated with communication techniques, and the same ongoing process of self-evaluation, practice, and feedback applies for incorporating effective techniques into one's interpersonal style. See Exhibit 4.7 for helpful hints for improving the emotional environment.

TIME

Occupational therapists need to consider **time-related factors,** including the time requirements for responding to the referral for an evaluation, the time it takes to administer the assessments, and the time needed to become proficient in documenting the evaluation results. In today's practice settings, time demands are great and many, so efficiency is essential.

Occupational therapists must complete the evaluation process in a timely manner. Doing so requires that therapists know the time rules (i.e.,

---

EXHIBIT 4.7. HELPFUL HINTS FOR THE EMOTIONAL ENVIRONMENT

- Consider the mood of the client.
- Be aware of your mood as a therapist and its effect on the therapeutic relationship.
- Modify your communication style to facilitate desired affective behaviors in the client.
- Use self-evaluation, practice, and feedback to improve your communication techniques.
- Prepare the client and their families or significant others for the evaluation process.
- Create an atmosphere of trust and caring.
- Avoid the use of medical and therapy jargon when speaking with clients and their families or significant others.

---

state laws and regulatory codes, facility or setting policies) for evaluations. The timeline for the evaluation process varies by practice setting and facility. The occupational therapist may have 24 hours to respond to and complete the evaluation of a client in an intensive care unit, whereas the timeline for a client in another unit (e.g., acute, skilled, rehabilitation), facility, or practice setting may be within 48 hours, 3 working days, or 1 week. In early intervention (ages birth–2 years), preschool (ages 3–5 years), and school-based (ages 6–21 years) services, there is a 60-calendar-day timeline for all initial evaluations to be completed and for the interdisciplinary team meeting to be held (Jackson, 2008).

A therapist often completes the evaluation in one session; however, it may be acceptable in some practice settings for an evaluation to take more than one session. Facilities may have a policy regarding the time allotted for the completion of the evaluation. The policy of one facility may be for the evaluation to be completed within a 45-minute session, whereas the policy of another facility may allow up to 1.5 hours. Additionally, facilities may have policies regarding the time allotted for the occupational therapist to interpret and document the assessment data, as well as to develop and document objective and measurable goals that address targeted outcomes. The documentation format affects the time needed for documenting the evaluation. The time needed to complete electronic documentation is different from the time needed to complete a written narrative or to dictate the evaluation findings.

There are also time differences within formats. The electronic documentation procedure at one facility may be more or less time intensive than that of another facility. Therapists must include both the hands-on time for administering the assessment and the time for documentation when determining the total time needed for the evaluation. For example, if the hands-on component of a pediatric evaluation takes approximately 1.5 hours, including parental consultation time, followed by documentation time of approximately 1.5 hour, the total time of the evaluation is 3 hours. The more complex the assessment, typically the more time required for administration and documentation—but also typically the greater yield of data regarding the client's occupational performance.

A therapist also needs to know the rules and regulations regarding reevaluation. The time frame for reassessment and reevaluation of the plan may vary from weekly to monthly to every 6 months or annually, depending on the practice setting (e.g., early intervention evaluations are completed yearly, with reviews every 6 months; outpatient reevaluations are typically completed every 2–4 weeks). Occupational therapists must be aware that laws, regulations, and facility policies change, sometimes frequently, so being up-to-date on the rules that affect one's practice is essential. As previously stated, therapists need to have a working knowledge of the current state laws, regulatory requirements, and facility policies relevant to their practice setting. It is important to consider all of these time factors when determining the total time the occupational therapist needs to perform an evaluation, which is necessary information when coordinating the therapist's and departmental schedule (Exhibit 4.8).

TEAMWORK

Therapists must remember they are part of a **team**. Occupational therapists do not work with the client in isolation but are a member of a team of professionals, each contributing unique services but all focusing on maximizing the health and wellness of the client. Team members may include a physician, nurse, physical therapist, speech–language pathologist, audiologist, psychologist, recreational therapist, dietitian, respiratory therapist, neurologist, or other specialized physicians. In the school setting, the team typically includes a teacher, guidance counselor, principal, and director of special education in addition to therapy providers.

Central to the team, and also members of the team, are the client and his or her family (e.g., parent, guardian, spouse, adult child). The communication skills discussed earlier apply not only to interactions with the client and family but also to interactions with all of the team members. Communication among team members may occur in person, in writing, by e-mail, or by phone. Regardless of the format, communication is essential for completion of a comprehensive evaluation. Occupational therapists must ensure that all members of the team understand the unique focus of occupational therapy and its relevance to the client and other services. No matter how indirect or brief the interaction, everyone with whom the occupational therapist comes in contact should understand that the focus of occupational therapy services is on occupations.

Each team member needs to know the unique contributions that the other team members add to the comprehensive evaluation of the client. Occupational therapists must ensure that the evaluation process, including the assessment administered, focuses on the client's occupational performance and the underlying factors that affect performance. The evaluation documentation also needs to reflect the unique focus of occupational therapy. See Exhibit 4.9 for helpful hints for fostering teamwork.

MATERIALS

Occupational therapists need to determine the **materials** needed to complete the evaluation, including general materials and materials specifically required for an assessment. Typically, the assessment manual provides a list of required equipment and supplies. The more occupation-based the assessment, the more likely the materials will reflect real-world

---

EXHIBIT 4.8. HELPFUL HINTS FOR TIME

- Know the time rules (i.e., state laws and regulatory codes, facility or setting policies) for responding to referrals and for completing evaluations and reevaluations.
- The total time needed for an evaluation includes both the hands-on time for administering the assessment and the time for documentation.

EXHIBIT 4.9. HELPFUL HINTS FOR TEAMWORK

- Each member of the team contributes unique services.
- All team members focus on maximizing the health and wellness of the client.
- The client and family are central members of the team.
- Effective communication is essential.
- Know the unique contributions of each team member.
- Ensure that all members of the team understand the unique focus of occupational therapy.

materials (i.e., objects available in people's homes and for purchase in local retail stores). Examples of these materials include dishes, pots and pans, clothing, banking forms, job applications, and medication bottles. Additionally, clients often use their own materials for occupation-based assessments (e.g., hygiene supplies, clothing, medications).

The evaluation process usually involves use of general materials, such as paper, pencil, pen, clipboard, watch or stopwatch, tape measure, and magnifying glass. Materials may also relate to the practice setting. For example, when conducting an evaluation in a pediatric practice setting, the occupational therapist may use a child-size desk and chair, therapy mat, therapy ball, variety of writing implements (i.e., crayons, pencils, markers, colored pencils), pencil grips, sensory items (e.g., Koosh™ balls, sand, rice, dry beans), paper (e.g., construction, lined, unlined), manipulatives (e.g., stress balls, small objects), and scissors (e.g., child sized, right- and left-handed, easy grip).

Therapists should organize evaluation materials for the most efficient access and use. In a setting where several therapists use the same assessments, give careful thought to methods for storing and maintaining assessment materials. As with all equipment and supplies, it is beneficial to establish a system for determining who currently has an assessment and its materials, how the assessment and materials are maintained, and who is responsible for monitoring the system.

Evaluation equipment and materials are often stored in plastic bins, canvas or lightweight portable bags, or rolling upright small suitcases. Therapists working in settings that require them to transport materials from site to site (e.g., home or school settings) often use lightweight portable file boxes to keep files and equipment organized in a car trunk. Some therapists organize supplies alphabetically by the days of the week, whereas other therapists use different colors for each school or program site. Additionally, accordion file folders organized by month, Excel spreadsheets, and book or smart phone calendars are all helpful in keeping track of evaluation due dates and assessment materials. General and organizational supplies and storage containers are available at many retail, sporting goods, discount, and office supply stores. Before starting an evaluation, the therapist needs to make sure that all the necessary materials are available (Exhibit 4.10).

DOCUMENTATION

When therapists provide a skilled service to a client, they must document the services provided. **Documentation** in the form of a well-written and comprehensive evaluation report is essential because it articulates the rationale for providing occupational therapy services and connects the services to the client's targeted outcomes. Occupational therapists need to know and understand the state laws and regulatory requirements of the practice setting and the facility policies regarding documentation. Therapists also need to be mindful of the type of practice setting, service model, and theoretical perspective of the facility or setting when writing evaluation reports. Knowing the focus of the practice setting is important because it directs the focus and language of the report. Hospital-based and outpatient settings are typically more medically driven, whereas community- and school-based settings usually focus on social, family, and educational issues.

The link between documentation and the service model is particularly important in pediatric practice settings. For example, occupational therapists providing early intervention services need to know whether the services in their states are medical based or education based, because the service model varies from state to state. Early intervention services are both family driven and family focused; thus, the family is the primary service model, and the early intervention evaluation focuses on issues that affect both the child and the family (Nanof & Schefkind, 2008).

EXHIBIT 4.10. HELPFUL HINTS FOR MATERIALS

- Determine the materials (general and assessment-specific) needed to complete the evaluation.
- Remember that occupation-based materials usually reflect "real-world" materials.
- Organize evaluation materials for efficient access and use.

Therapists who evaluate preschool children (ages 3–5 years) will generally administer the assessments in a preschool setting, although occasionally they may administer them in the child's home. When services occur in a setting outside of the home, the family is no longer the primary area of concentration but instead is now a secondary service area. The family always remains important, but when writing the evaluation report, therapists must recognize this shift of evaluation and service philosophy because the evaluation content now focuses primarily on educational issues and family issues become secondary.

Another example is the need for therapists evaluating school-age children (ages 6–21 years) to focus their documentation on facilitating educational access to the school environment. An appropriate evaluation in a school setting addresses how the student can successfully access the educational environment (in accordance with the Individuals With Disabilities Education Improvement Act of 2004). Parental input is always important because parents are vital members of the team; however, concentration on school-based issues remains the top priority when providing school-based evaluations. Sometimes therapists provide supplemental school services in addition to education-based programs; however, therapists should get clarification from the school-based work site program supervisor regarding the roles of private outpatient and medical-based services before completing an evaluation.

Recommendations, including frequency and duration of services, are also dependent on the type of practice setting. In a pediatric practice setting, it is helpful to begin by asking the work site supervisor about

- The service philosophy regarding treatment frequency;
- Consultation in addition to direct service;
- Involvement of professionals external to the practice setting;
- Parental involvement;
- Team members and their collaborative roles;
- Potential use of instructional aides; and
- The need for nurses if dealing with a child's medical condition, assistive devices, and supplemental equipment and training needs.

All of these issues are important to understand before writing the evaluation report and providing recommendations. Parents are often confused when they concurrently receive a report from a medical-based outpatient facility and another report from a school-based program. Both sites have differing service philosophies, and billing practices and legal mandates must be explained clearly to the parents and team when determining service needs for the child. Having a clear understanding of the roles and responsibilities of the evaluating occupational therapists before the evaluation is completed helps make the process smoother and more manageable.

The *Guidelines for Documentation of Occupational Therapy* (AOTA, 2013) is a good resource for determining what information to include in an evaluation report. According to the AOTA guidelines, an evaluation report should include client information, the referral source, a description of the client's occupational profile, the assessments used and results, an analysis of occupational performance, interpretation of the findings, and recommendations regarding intervention approaches and types of interventions to be used to achieve the client's targeted outcomes.

Therapists need to consider the people who read their evaluation reports. The readers likely include a range of health professionals on the team (e.g., physician, nurse, physical therapist, speech–language pathologist, audiologist, psychologist, recreational therapist, dietitian, respiratory therapist, neurologist, other specialized physician); in school-based practice, readers also would include numerous education staff (e.g., teacher, guidance counselor, principal, director of special education). Other readers are the client and family. Another important reader in most practice settings is the reimbursement source. Readers review the evaluation report from their perspective, looking for elements relevant to their specific role in the client's services.

Therapists need to make sure the evaluation report addresses the content the readers expect to see in an occupational therapy evaluation. The challenge is to complete the evaluation report in the most efficient yet comprehensive manner. Therapists need to read their documentation through the eyes of those reading it—people who are not occupational therapists. Therapists need to consider how non–occupational therapists interpret the information. Just because the report information seems clear to a therapist and likely clear to other occupational therapists does not mean that the information is understandable to other readers of the report. Similar to when therapists verbally communicate with other team members, when they communicate in writing, they need to use user-friendly language by avoiding or clearly defining medical and educational jargon and acronyms. See Exhibit 4.11 for helpful hints regarding documentation.

ACCOUNTABILITY

Accountability means that each occupational therapist is responsible for the services he or she provides. Accountability includes promoting and maintaining high standards of conduct (AOTA, 2010a). Practical considerations related to accountability apply to a range of professional behaviors, including, but not limited to, truthfulness and honesty, respect, communication, competence, confidentiality, and reimbursement (AOTA, 2010a). An occupational therapist must provide services that are within his or her level of competence and scope of practice.

The occupational therapy evaluation may reveal needs of the client that are not within the scope of occupational therapy practice or the

---

EXHIBIT 4.11. HELPFUL HINTS FOR DOCUMENTATION

- Understand that the evaluation report must articulate the rationale for occupational therapy services and connect the services to the client's targeted outcomes.
- Know the laws and regulatory requirements of the practice setting and facility policies regarding documentation.
- Consider the service model when documenting; this consideration is particularly important in pediatric practice settings.
- Use the *Guidelines for Documentation of Occupational Therapy* (AOTA, 2013), which is a good resource.
- Consider the people who read the evaluation report (e.g., other health professionals on the team, education staff, client, family, reimbursement sources).
- Use user-friendly language (i.e., avoid or clearly define medical and educational jargon and acronyms).

---

expertise of the therapist. If so, and when appropriate, a therapist needs to refer the client to other health care providers. The evaluation report must accurately describe the type and duration of the services provided. Additionally, therapists must inform the client truthfully of the results of the evaluation and the risks and benefits associated with the recommendations.

Effective communication is an important professional behavior. Therapists need to be truthful, candid, and honest in all aspects of communication, including written, verbal, and electronic forms. Effective communication includes honest statements; adherence to applicable laws, guidelines, and regulations; accurate documentation; and avoidance of biased or derogatory language.

Competence includes not only a therapist's current level of skill but also maintaining and increasing competence. Therapists need to take responsibility for maintaining high standards by taking responsible steps through appropriate education and training to ensure their competency when incorporating new assessments into their practice.

Occupational therapists are accountable for ensuring that **confidentiality** and the **right to privacy** are respected and maintained for recipients of their services. Information obtained during or associated with the evaluation process is protected information, and therapists must maintain the confidentiality of the information. Therapists must maintain the confidentiality of all verbal, written, electronic, augmentative, and nonverbal communication as required by the Health Insurance Portability and Accountability Act of 1996 privacy rule and the Family Educational Rights and Privacy Act of 1974, also known as the *Buckley Amendment*.

Therapists working in pediatric settings must be mindful that privacy rules prohibit them from communicating with professionals outside the immediate service agency unless a parent has given specific written permission to allow it. As a rule, therapists should consult with their supervisor or administrator to ensure an understanding of the privacy restrictions related to initiating communication with other professionals.

It is important to maintain the privacy of clients (e.g., keeping names covered on files on a desk in an office or on a table in the clinic). Therapists working in school-, home-, and other community-based practice settings may be required to transport client files in their own car; these confidential files must be protected by being concealed and locked in the vehicle. Additionally, electronic communication must be protected (e.g., using only initials in the subject line of an e-mail rather than the client's full name).

Therapists need to follow their work site's privacy procedures regarding the deleting of electronic files. Privacy rules must be considered when responding to or acknowledging clients both within and outside of the therapy setting. It can be helpful to ask clients how they would like to be recognized during the evaluation session and also how they would like to be recognized (or not recognized) when seen outside of therapy. For example, some older children do not like their therapists to acknowledge them when they are with their peers.

Accountability also includes guaranteeing **fair treatment.** Therapists need to ensure that the evaluation services provided are fair and equitable and the fee for an evaluation is reasonable and commensurate with the service performed. To ensure fair treatment, therapists need to be accountable for their time. Therapists need to keep track of evaluation time, including direct hands-on time and indirect documentation time. Depending on the practice setting, a therapist also may be required to keep track of the time spent in consultation with parents, family, and team members, as well as the travel time associated with an evaluation. Therapists should record their time daily, sometimes in 5- to 15-minute increments, depending on the setting.

Submitting paperwork, including the paperwork associated with billing, is an essential professional task. Paperwork may need to be submitted daily, weekly, or monthly. Regardless of the time requirement, therapists need to submit paperwork on time. There are federal, state, agency, and facility rules regarding the length of time copies of client records, including evaluation reports and associated time and billing reports, must be retained. The typical standard for retaining records is a minimum of 3 years; however, therapists should confirm the appropriate length of time to retain records with their work site supervisor or administrator and follow the procedures accordingly. Although this chapter focuses on the evaluation process, the practical considerations associated with accountability relate to services across the occupational therapy process, not just the evaluation.

In addition to being accountable for the services provided, therapists are also accountable for understanding their employment role. Two basic **reimbursement models** of services are (1) employee and (2) independent contractor. The Internal Revenue Service (2011) has specific rules regarding these two reimbursement models. Essentially, **employees** receive a salary and benefits and work a prescribed number of hours each week, whereas **independent contractors** determine their own schedule. Independent contractors have flexibility regarding their caseload and traditionally receive a higher hourly reimbursement rate than an employee because independent contractors are responsible for their own benefits and tax payments.

In each employment role scenario, it is important that the therapist be clear about how he or she is being reimbursed for services. Therapists must know and understand the implications if being paid by the hour for providing direct and indirect occupational therapy services (which includes evaluations) or if being paid a flat sum for an all-inclusive evaluation session.

Another employment consideration that therapists are accountable for is reimbursement for travel. This issue is important, particularly in pediatric and home-care practice settings. Therapists need to clarify travel reimbursement before they engage in the evaluation process. Typically, an agency does not reimburse therapists travel when they drive to and from their home because this type of travel is considered commuting to and from the work site. However, an agency may reimburse travel time or mileage if a therapist is driving between evaluation sessions on the same day and for the same agency. Therapists in practice settings requiring travel to and from multiple work sites should keep track of travel time by using a paper or electronic travel log.

Therapists who work as independent contractors should consult with a certified public accountant to assist with appropriate tax and expense filing requirements. Independent contractors should also ask their agency supervisor or administrator about the availability and type of assessments available for use, on-site equipment and supplies, evaluation formats and content requirements, mentoring for evaluation education and training, and documentation requirements. Independent contractors may be responsible for purchasing and maintaining their own assessments, whereas for employees, the facility generally provides all the required materials for the evaluation process. Consideration of these issues can assist therapists in determining the most appropriate employment reimbursement model for their needs (Exhibit 4.12).

OCCUPATIONAL THERAPY ASSISTANTS

Occupational therapy assistants are valuable members of the team. An occupational therapist and occupational therapy assistant must know their roles and their contribution to each component of the occupational therapy process, including the evaluation process. AOTA's (2010b) *Standards of Practice for Occupational Therapy* states that

> an occupational therapy assistant contributes to the screening, evaluation, and re-evaluation process by implementing delegated assessments and by providing verbal and written reports of observations and client capacities to the occupational therapist in accordance with federal and state laws, other regulatory and payer requirements, and AOTA documents. (p. S108)

EXHIBIT 4.12. HELPFUL HINTS FOR ACCOUNTABILITY

- Provide services within your level of competence and scope of practice.
- When appropriate, refer clients to other health care providers.
- Reports must accurately describe the type and duration of services provided.
- Be truthful, candid, and honest in all aspects of communication.
- Ensure your competency by seeking out appropriate education and training.
- Ensure the client's confidentiality and right to privacy.
- Guarantee fair treatment to all clients.
- Know the time factors related to the services you provide and keep track of them, as needed.
- Understand your employment role (employee vs. independent contractor).

Occupational therapists and occupational therapy assistants need to know and adhere to the state laws and regulatory requirements of their facility and practice setting, including the rules governing the involvement of occupational therapy assistants in the evaluation process and the supervision requirements for occupational therapy assistants.

PROFESSIONAL DEVELOPMENT

Therapists need to pursue **professional development** activities to ensure their own competency in performance of the evaluation process. Mentorship is a valuable professional development activity, especially for entry-level occupational therapists or therapists new to a practice setting (Gilfoyle, Grady, & Nielson, 2011). A **mentor** can assist a therapist in identifying strategies to obtain education and training in the evaluation process, including the administration of specific assessments. The strategies may include review of specific evaluation guidelines and opportunities to observe the evaluation process. The mentor does not need to have expertise in the administration of a specialized evaluation, such as a sensory processing evaluation, that the therapist wants or needs to learn; however, the mentor can connect the therapist with other occupational therapists with expertise in that area. Mentors also can provide support for managing clients with challenging behaviors during the evaluation process.

A therapist may request mentorship many times throughout his or her career, including when he or she is entry level; when transitioning to a new practice setting, facility, or agency; and when learning a new evaluation process or assessment. Mentoring is an effective professional development activity to enhance a therapist's knowledge and skills. Remember that mentoring is advantageous for both the mentee and the mentor, because both grow professionally.

Being a member of AOTA and a state occupational therapy association can offer a therapist many opportunities for continued professional development and updates on regulations. If one uses the resources provided by these organizations, further professional development can be promoted. Therapists can also attend national and state education events, including annual conferences that typically offer presentations in all practice areas and workshops for specialized content areas. Association members typically receive a reduced registration rate. Additionally, professional associations offer a range of continuing education opportunities, including various publications and online courses. These resources address various practice areas and issues, including topics related to the evaluation process. Therapists can also consider pursuing specialty certifications in a practice area.

Another example is the use of discussion forums related to practice areas on OTConnections (http://otconnectons.aota.org/). Such discussions are a great place to post questions related to the evaluation process and assessments. These forums give therapists the opportunity to receive feedback from therapists across the country and are a great resource for finding a mentor and connecting with experts in the field. See Exhibit 4.13 for helpful hints for maximizing professional development.

SUMMARY

The goal of the occupational therapist is to provide high-quality evaluation services in the most effective and efficient manner. To do so, therapists must be aware of the current laws and regulatory requirements of their practice area and specific facility policies. Therapists also need to seek out and use professional resources to enhance competence in performing evaluations. Therapists with an understanding of the practical aspects associated with the evaluation process will be better able to identify and implement strategies to maximize proficiency in the evaluation process.

EXHIBIT 4.13. HELPFUL HINTS FOR PROFESSIONAL DEVELOPMENT

- Know that you are responsible for your own competency.
- Understand that mentorship is valuable and advantageous for both the mentee and the mentor.
- Be an active member in professional organizations.
- Use your resources, such as attending conferences and continuing education events, reading publications, and participating in a discussion forum.

QUESTIONS

1. Describe what you would do if you had questions regarding a rule or regulation related to a referral for an occupational therapy evaluation.
2. What specific steps would you include in the identification, selection, and analysis of assessments? What resources are available to assist you in identifying, selecting, and analyzing potential assessments for your practice setting?
3. Describe the teaching methods you would use to ensure you are competent in administering, scoring, and documenting the results of a new assessment. Describe the strategies you would implement on an ongoing basis to maintain current knowledge about the assessment.
4. Identify 2 positive features and 2 negative features of the physical environment that affect the evaluation process. How can you improve the physical environment during an evaluation?
5. What can you do to influence positively the emotional environment during the evaluation process?
6. Describe the unique focus of occupational therapy in the evaluation process and its relevance to the services provided in client care. How would your description of the occupational therapy evaluation process change when speaking with a nurse, a physical therapist, a teacher, or a family member?
7. Identify at least 3 readers of your evaluation report and the content each reader expects to see in it. Review an occupational therapy evaluation report through the eyes of those reading it. Identify 2 aspects of the documentation that could be changed to make the information more understandable to the readers of the report.

References

American Occupational Therapy Association. (1997). Statement—Fundamental concepts of occupational therapy: Occupation, purposeful activity, and function. *American Journal of Occupational Therapy, 51,* 864–866. http://dx.doi/10.5014/ajot.51.10.864

American Occupational Therapy Association. (2010a). Occupational therapy code of ethics and ethics standards (2010). *American Journal of Occupational Therapy, 64,* S17–S26. http://dx.doi/10.5014/ajot.2010.64S17

American Occupational Therapy Association. (2010b). Standards of practice for occupational therapy. *American Journal of Occupational Therapy, 64,* S106–S111. http://dx.doi/10.5014/ajot.2010.64S106

American Occupational Therapy Association. (2013). Guidelines for documentation of occupational therapy. *American Journal of Occupational Therapy, 67*(Suppl.), S32–S38. http://dx.doi/10.5014/ajot.2013.67S32

Asher, I. E. (2014). *Asher's occupational therapy assessment tools: An annotated index* (4th ed.). Bethesda, MD: AOTA Press.

Commonwealth of Pennsylvania, Occupational Therapy Practice Act of 1982, Pub. L. 502, No. 140, amended July 5, 2012, Pub. L. 1132, No. 138. Retrieved from http://www.legis.state.pa.us/wu01/li/li/us/htm/2012/0/0138.htm

Family Educational Rights and Privacy Act of 1974, Pub. L. 93–380, 20 U.S.C. § 1232g *et seq.*; 34 C.F.R. § 99.

Gilfoyle, E., Grady, A., & Nielson, C. (2011). *Mentoring leaders: The power of storytelling for building leadership in health care and education.* Bethesda, MD: AOTA Press.

Health Insurance Portability and Accountability Act of 1996, Pub. L. 104–191, 45 C.F.R. § 160, 164.

Individuals With Disabilities Education Improvement Act of 2004, Pub. L. 108–446, 20 U.S.C. § 1400 *et seq.*

Internal Revenue Service. (2011, August). *Determination of worker status for purposes of federal employment taxes and income tax withholding* (Form SS-8). Washington, DC: U.S. Department of Treasury.

Jackson, L. (Ed.). (2008). *The new IDEA: An occupational therapy toolkit* (2nd ed.). Bethesda, MD: AOTA Press.

Law, M., Baum, C., & Dunn, W. (2005). *Measuring occupational performance: Supporting best practice in occupational therapy* (2nd ed.). Thorofare, NJ: Slack.

Mulligan, S. (2013). *Occupational therapy evaluation for children: A pocket guide.* Philadelphia: Lippincott Williams & Wilkins.

Nanof, T., & Schefkind, S. (2008, April). *IDEA overview and early intervention practice.* Paper presented at the AOTA Annual Conference & Expo, Long Beach, CA.

Schell, B. A., Gillen, G., & Scaffa, M. E. (Eds.). (2014). *Willard and Spackman's occupational therapy* (12th ed.). Philadelphia: Lippincott Williams & Wilkins.

Vroman, K. G., & Stewart, E. (2013). *Occupational therapy evaluation for adults: A pocket guide.* Philadelphia: Lippincott Williams & Wilkins.

CHAPTER 5

Evaluation in the Intervention Planning Process

Lou Ann Griswold, PhD, OTR/L, FAOTA

Highlights

- Evaluation process focusing on occupation
- Evaluation leading to intervention planning
- Reassessment throughout the intervention process
- Documentation of evaluation results
- Types of assessments
- Evaluation in context: Pragmatic issues of evaluation
- Learning a new assessment
- Therapeutic use of self during evaluation.

Key Terms

Arena assessment
Compensatory approach
Criterion-referenced assessment
Documentation
Evaluation
Intervention plan
Intervention process
Norm-referenced assessment
Occupational profile

Occupational roles
Performance analysis
Reassessment
Reimbursement
Restorative approach
Review phase
Skill acquisition approach
Standardized assessments
Therapeutic use of self

The occupational therapist strives to enhance a client's occupational performance and participation in activities that are important to him or her. Knowing where to begin and how best to support a client is determined through evaluation. The evaluation process answers many of the questions an occupational therapist has about a client and enables him or her to plan intervention. Evaluation guides the therapist in considering what is important to the client, reflecting client-centered services.

Furthermore, evaluation establishes a baseline for performance against which the therapist can measure the effectiveness of intervention. Occupational therapists emphasize occupation throughout evaluation, highlighting the unique contribution of occupational therapy to improve a client's participation in occupations.

This chapter describes how evaluation informs decision making from the first contact with a client through the intervention process. Specifically, the chapter helps the occupational therapist

- Focus evaluation on occupation,
- Use evaluation results to plan intervention,
- Identify how frames of reference and pragmatic reasoning influence the evaluation process,
- Differentiate types of assessments, and
- Maintain a focus on occupation when documenting evaluation results.

Assessment options are introduced in the context of intervention planning, particularly the purpose of assessments and the intended use of the information gathered. Several case examples illustrate the relationship between evaluation and intervention and allow for examination of the pragmatic issues determined by the context that influence evaluation and intervention. Therapists are then encouraged to continue to update their knowledge and skills in assessments, and a process for learning administration of new assessments is suggested. The chapter concludes with a discussion of therapeutic use of self during evaluation.

EVALUATION PROCESS FOCUSING ON OCCUPATION

An occupational therapist evaluates a client's occupational performance, which centers on the client's capacity and desire to engage in occupations.

Evaluation refers to the process of gathering information about a client. Mulligan (2014) also recognized that evaluation is a thought process. Her point is important because it reflects the occupational therapist's clinical reasoning used throughout the evaluation process.

One might logically assume that evaluation precedes intervention. The *Occupational Therapy Practice Framework: Domain and Process* (3rd ed.; American Occupational Therapy Association [AOTA], 2014; *Framework*) identified evaluation as the first phase in the occupational therapy intervention process. In reality, gathering information about a client continues throughout all phases of the intervention process as the occupational therapist learns more about the client and his or her needs, desires, and abilities, and observes the client's performance and response to intervention (Vroman & Stewart, 2014).

The purpose and timing of the evaluation determine the type of data collected and the assessment instruments or measures used (Ideishi, 2003; Weinstock-Zlotnick & Hinojosa, 2004). When conducted at the beginning of a therapeutic relationship with a client, evaluation provides information to guide decision making regarding occupational therapy services and leads to intervention, beginning with planning and continuing through implementation of intervention and review of the client's progress. Evaluation is also connected clearly to outcomes; during the evaluation process, the client identifies desired outcomes that are then revisited at the conclusion of therapy.

EVALUATION LEADING TO INTERVENTION PLANNING

A therapist synthesizes evaluation findings to develop an intervention plan. The therapist develops a plan by considering evaluation data with information about the client's motivation, prognosis, resources, and personal goals. Evaluation data serve as the groundwork upon which a therapist develops an appropriate evaluation plan.

Getting to Know the Client

Getting to know the client as a person is a critical step in the evaluation process (AOTA, 2014;

Brown, 2009; Fisher & Griswold, 2009; Hocking, 2001; Mulligan, 2014; Trombly Latham, 2008; Vroman & Stewart, 2014). Identifying the activities the client likes to do currently, enjoyed doing in the past, and would like to do in the future enables the therapist to know what is important to the person. Learning the client's history gives the therapist information about patterns of behavior and strengths or interests that might be useful in therapy.

Understanding the client as an occupational being and the occupations that are important to him or her will focus intervention and identify goals that are meaningful to the client (Brown, 2009). Knowing the client as an occupational being also enables a therapist to predict more accurately the outcome of occupational therapy intervention (Simmons, Crepeau, & White, 2000). At times, family members or others (e.g., teachers) provide information to enable the therapist to understand the client, especially when working with children (Mulligan, 2014), but gathering information from others who are close to the client is often used with clients of all ages (Fisher & Griswold, 2009).

During the initial phase of evaluation, an occupational therapist strives to understand the client as a person; the context in which he or she lives, works, and plays; his or her perceived strengths and needs related to occupational performance; and desired goals for occupational engagement.

Learning about the client as a person includes identifying his or her **occupational roles.** Roles often indicate what the client values and suggest possible tasks that are important in supporting the identified roles. The therapist then can explore which tasks are easy and which are difficult for the client to perform. Learning the client's perception of how the environment supports or hinders his or her roles and tasks further enables the therapist to understand more about the person and his or her natural contexts (Fisher, 2009).

While learning about the client from his or her perspective, the occupational therapist helps the client to identify his or her priorities and goals for occupational therapy—what the client would like to do, or do better. The gathered information then guides the occupational therapist to know the focus of the occupational **performance analysis,** the next phase of evaluation, and subsequently leads to intervention planning. Using the identified process helps promote occupation-based practice. Case Example 5.1 illustrates these points as Jean, the occupational therapist, receives a referral from her team members in a community mental health center.

CASE EXAMPLE 5.1. JEAN AND TONYA: OCCUPATION-BASED PRACTICE

Jean, an occupational therapist, worked in a community outpatient mental health center. **Tonya** sought help through the mental health center because she was feeling "depressed and alone."

During an initial occupational therapy interview, Tonya identified her primary role at this time as a mother of 2 toddler-age children. She listed the tasks that supported this role as preparing snacks and meals, cleaning, playing, and supporting and fostering the children's development.

Tonya felt that she was not doing these tasks well; for example, she often started to prepare a meal but then became distracted and changed her plans. She stated that the meals she prepared were not nutritionally complete and that her house was "forever a mess." She stated that she did not feel she really played with the children but rather only watched them.

Tonya had wanted to have children and stay at home with them while they were young, but now she felt isolated. She said that she was not as motivated to keep up with the housework and meal preparation as she would like. Tonya acknowledged that she had little enthusiasm to perform the activities she knew were important to her as a mother. Tonya was married, but her husband was out of town 4 days per week for work. She and her family lived on the outskirts of a small town.

Jean learned that Tonya had been in drama clubs during high school and college and enjoyed that period of her life. Further exploration revealed that Tonya liked not only the acting but also the energy level she felt when in contact with large groups of people. Tonya recalled that in college, her grades improved as the pressures of a theater production increased. Before her children were born, Tonya worked as a kindergarten teacher, where she felt she was able to use her artistic talents in many ways to promote her students' development.

Jean listened as Tonya talked about her past, present, and dreams for the future. Tonya said that she would like to be around other people but did not want to be employed while her children were young. She stated she wanted to feel that she was "doing something worthwhile with her life." She also wanted to do a better job caring for her children's daily needs and to "have fun with them."

Initial Evaluation Phase

During the initial evaluation phase, Jean gathered an occupational profile of Tonya. The *occupational profile* is a summary constructed by the therapist of the client's life, including the set of activities, routines, and roles (AOTA, 2014). Occupational therapists may conduct an informal interview with a client to obtain an occupational profile (as Jean did with Tonya), or they may use assessment protocols to determine how a client spends his or her time, values given occupational roles and routines, engages in interests, and obtains feelings of competence.

Two assessment instruments used to gather such data are the Canadian Occupational Performance Measure (COPM; Law et al., 2005) and the Occupational Performance History Interview (OPHI–II; Kielhofner et al., 2004). The COPM gathers specific information regarding the occupations the client wants or needs to do and his or her perception of his or her performance of and satisfaction with these occupations. The OPHI–II provides a more expansive occupational profile.

Jean used her clinical reasoning and decided that she needed to assess Tonya's performance during daily tasks for which she had reported having difficulty (Fisher, 2009; Gillen, 2013; Trombly Latham, 2008). Observing occupational performance allows the occupational therapist to consider the quality with which the client performs a task and is essential to promote occupation-based evaluation and intervention (Fisher, 2013).

Observing clients engaging in occupations in natural contexts provides the most efficient and valid method of evaluating occupational performance (Gillen, 2013). Jean and Tonya decided that it might be informative to have Jean observe Tonya completing a simple cooking task. Jean could analyze her observations using a nonstandardized analysis or a standardized assessment such as the Assessment of Motor and Process Skills (AMPS; Fisher & Jones, 2012). Jean chose to do a nonstandardized analysis of Tonya as she prepared lunch for her children (Fisher & Griswold, 2014).

After interpretation of the observation of the client's occupational performance, the therapist then determines whether further evaluation is needed to assess specific client factors or environmental contexts (AOTA, 2014; Fisher, 2009; Trombly Latham, 2008). Only the aspects necessary to more thoroughly understand the client's performance need to be assessed.

For some clients, assessing the environmental context of the place of employment might be relevant. For example, visiting a job site would enable the therapist to determine the challenges and supports within that environment. The therapist might consider any physical, social, and cultural aspects of the environment that might be supporting or hindering a client's performance.

In other situations, assessing client factors such as range of motion or strength might help to determine underlying causes of problems in occupational performance (AOTA, 2014). The occupational therapist uses his or her clinical judgment to determine whether the assessment of any of these areas will be helpful in better understanding the client and his or her occupational performance. These areas would be assessed using additional observation or specific assessments or measures as appropriate.

In Tonya's case, Jean determined that she needed more information about how Tonya spent her time each day—the temporal dimension of context. She asked Tonya to keep a log of all activities that she engaged in for a 7-day period, using the Occupational Questionnaire (Smith, Kielhofner, & Watts, 1986). This questionnaire asks the client to indicate the importance, sense of competence, and enjoyment for each activity.

Once all the relevant information has been gathered, the occupational therapist synthesizes and interprets the results of all evaluation data and identifies the client's strengths and weaknesses (AOTA, 2014). The therapist then shares his or her interpretation and hypotheses with the client. Further interpretation of the results may occur with the client, and together the therapist and client then establish goals to lead to the client's desired outcomes.

Jean concluded that Tonya was motivated to carry out her role as a mother. Based on her performance analysis of her observation of Tonya preparing lunch, Jean reported that Tonya had the motor and process skills to do desired tasks of instrumental activities of daily living (IADLs), important for her role as a mother. Motivation and performance skills were Tonya's strengths.

Analyzing Tonya's Occupational Questionnaire, Jean determined that Tonya engaged in many activities throughout the week that she felt she had to do but did not enjoy doing. Jean noted that, in fact, Tonya engaged in very few activities that were enjoyable to her. She hypothesized that the environment in which Tonya lived was not conducive to social contact with others, particularly adults. Jean also hypothesized that Tonya was frustrated by not using her creative talents.

Jean shared her conclusions with Tonya, who agreed with them and said that she would like to have more contact with other adults and to become involved in drama in some way again. These were Tonya's desired outcomes. Jean and Tonya then identified specific goals and a plan that would enable Tonya to reach her desired outcomes.

REASSESSMENT THROUGHOUT THE INTERVENTION PROCESS

The therapist completes a **reassessment** after the initial evaluation to determine whether the intervention is effective or whether an intervention plan needs to be modified. The initial evaluation process ends with setting goals, which establishes the course for intervention. The **intervention process** consists of three steps: (1) planning, (2) implementation, and (3) review (AOTA, 2014). The evaluation process continues throughout intervention as the therapist monitors a client's responses and modifies the intervention as needed. Because of the explicit link between evaluation and intervention, it is helpful to consider how evaluation informs each step of the intervention process.

Planning Phase of Intervention

Evaluation is tied most closely to planning intervention. An *intervention plan* draws on the information gathered during the evaluation phase, particularly the client's desired outcomes of therapy and identified goals for therapy. Intervention planning also includes the approach to be used, and details of service delivery (AOTA, 2014). As illustrated in the example of Tonya and Jean, an occupational therapist bases the intervention plan on the client's desired outcomes and occupational goals to support participation in meaningful life activities (Brown, 2009; Hinojosa, Kramer, Royeen, & Luebben, 2003).

Desired outcomes vary in nature and specificity across clients. Examples of desired outcomes for clients at different ages and with various types of disabilities and needs might include

- Living independently at home,
- Engaging in the activities associated with the role of a grandmother,
- Playing with other children on the playground, or
- Feeling emotionally ready to return to work and interact socially with peers.

Often, the occupational therapist helps the client turn desired outcomes into specific goals that will support what the client would like to do. For example, to live independently at home, a client might need to prepare a simple sandwich and pour a cold beverage into a glass. Playing with others on the playground might include collaborating with others to share playground equipment. The goals are further honed into behavioral objectives based on difficulties that the occupational therapist observed during the occupational performance analysis.

Suppose the occupational therapist observed an older gentleman, who wanted to remain living independently in his home and needed to prepare lunch for himself, to have difficulty choosing the right utensils to make a sandwich and not be able to locate the mustard that he had put into the refrigerator before the assessment began. The occupational therapist can use these observations to write behavioral objectives to support the goal of making a sandwich, contributing to the desired outcome to live independently at home.

Similarly, the occupational therapist would use observation results of the child on the playground to refine the goal of collaborating with others into behavioral objectives. Specifically, the occupational therapist might have observed that the child did not ask questions of her peers or respond to peers' questions or comments, which ultimately resulted in not taking turns during the social interaction that supports playing together. The therapist can use the observations to write behavioral objectives related to asking a peer a question during play activities and responding to peers' questions and comments.

One can see from these two examples presented that observing the quality of occupational performance is necessary to write clear and specific behavioral objectives that emphasize occupation. Because the behavioral objectives are grounded in performance analysis, the intervention plan is occupation focused and client centered. In other words, the intervention plan takes into account what is important to the client and his or her current level of occupational performance.

Occupation-focused evaluation includes

- Gathering information from the client's perspective on desired and challenging occupations,
- Observing occupational performance in natural contexts, and
- Using the analysis of an observation of occupational performance to identify behavioral objectives to support the client's desired occupations.

After the goals and behavioral objectives are determined with the client, the therapist uses his or her clinical reasoning to consider factors that hinder the person from performing at the desired level (Fisher, 2009). Options might include client factors (e.g., motivation, internalized routine, body function), environmental demands (e.g., characteristics of people in the environment, space, available assessments and materials), or task demands (e.g., required steps, required actions).

Based on the occupational therapist's judgment, he or she selects an intervention approach and theoretical perspective or frame of reference to guide the intervention. The occupational therapist decides whether it is more appropriate to take a **skill acquisition approach,** facilitating learning or relearning of skills, such as manipulating small objects or controlling impulsive behaviors (Kaplan, 2010), or a **restorative approach** to establish or restore underlying abilities such as muscle strength or skilled movement (Bass-Haugen, Mathiowetz, & Flinn, 2008). Alternatively, the therapist might choose to take a **compensatory approach** and adapt task demands or modify the environment to promote more successful engagement in desired occupations (Brown, 2009; Fisher, 2009).

The therapist should share his or her knowledge and evidence regarding the different intervention options with the client. In collaboration with the client, the therapist determines the best approach to obtain the identified goals and create a plan for intervention. The therapist uses clinical reasoning, professional experiences, selected theoretical perspective, and evidence-based research to determine reasonable and appropriate methods to reach the desired outcomes.

Implementation Phase of Intervention

As the occupational therapist and occupational therapy assistant work with a client to implement an intervention plan, they engage in ongoing reassessment to ensure that therapy is meaningful and effectively facilitating progress toward the established goals and objectives. As a practitioner implements services, he or she continually seeks new activities to promote the client's progress.

Activities that are relevant and meaningful to the client have been shown to be more effective in helping him or her reach the established goals (Mastos, Miller, Eliasson, & Imms, 2007; Phipps & Richardson, 2007). Monitoring the client's affective response to activities and approaches used during therapy enables a practitioner to determine the meaning they hold for the person (Park, 2008; Price, 2009). Such monitoring and ongoing reassessment keeps the intervention client centered.

Review Phase of Intervention: Monitoring Progress

In addition to the ongoing, informal evaluation throughout intervention, the occupational therapist, with the occupational therapy assistant, formally reevaluates a client's performance and progress throughout intervention to modify the intervention plan (Radomski, 2008; Stewart, 2010). A review of ongoing observations and formal assessment data can redirect a practitioner's decision making and services. A practitioner may observe poor performance during a therapy activity, leading to a change in the intervention approach or additional formal reevaluation that in turn redirects intervention. As the review of progress occurs, the therapist moves into the **review phase** of intervention.

Review time may be built into the intervention plan if allowed by the pragmatic constraints that influence practice. The time frame may be after a certain number of visits or at set intervals (e.g., weekly, monthly), often determined by reimbursement guidelines. During these reviews, the desired outcomes, goals, and behavioral objectives of the occupational therapy intervention plan form the basis for determining the effectiveness of the intervention. The initial assessment measures may be repeated to determine change in occupational performance.

Being aware of how frequently an assessment can be used for reassessment is important for the therapist to consider when choosing the assessments for the initial evaluation. Comparison of assessment data over time enables the therapist and client to objectively measure progress and determine whether therapy should continue or the client should be discharged. Review

of the intervention may also facilitate a referral to another professional colleague.

Case Example 5.2 and Case Example 5.3 illustrate very different types of evaluation approaches that address each client's occupational goals. However, in both examples, the occupational therapists gathered information about each client as a person and observed the quality of occupational performance in relevant tasks. The two cases reflect different types of settings in which the occupational therapists worked, influencing the evaluation process. Finally, the frame of reference each therapist used further influenced her choice of assessments. Consequently, the evaluation process influenced planning intervention, implementing intervention, and reviewing progress.

CASE EXAMPLE 5.2. JOAN AND MR. MUÑIZ: DESIRED OUTCOMES AND INTERESTS

Joan worked as an occupational therapist for a home-based rehabilitation program. She was allowed 4 visits to see her client, **Mr. Muñiz,** including time for evaluation and intervention. Mr. Muñiz had experienced a cerebrovascular accident (CVA) and had already received 2 months of inpatient occupational therapy services.

Joan knew that evaluation was essential to enable her to know what to focus on in intervention; however, she was also very aware that she had limited time to spend with her client and wanted to move into intervention as quickly as possible. She received documentation on Mr. Muñiz from the inpatient rehabilitation setting where he had received services most recently. The documentation Joan received enabled her to quickly establish a therapeutic rapport with Mr. Muñiz. She used the assessment data provided by the previous occupational therapist at the time of discharge and did not need to repeat the same assessments. She also knew the client's interests, concerns, abilities, and needs from this documentation.

Joan built on her existing knowledge of Mr. Muñiz and directed her attention to how he was doing at home, an area not addressed during inpatient rehabilitation. Thus, Joan focused her evaluation on Mr. Muñiz's current needs, which allowed her to begin intervention almost immediately.

Joan spent the first 10 minutes of her home visit talking with Mr. Muñiz and his wife. She quickly learned through her informal interview that Mr. Muñiz wanted to make his own coffee in the morning, tend his rose garden, and grill meat for family meals. Although Mr. Muñiz was not independent in all personal activities of daily living, Mr. and Mrs. Muñiz agreed that the routine they had worked out met his needs, and Mrs. Muñiz felt comfortable assisting him.

Joan determined that she wanted to assess Mr. Muñiz's occupational performance by observing him performing tasks that were important to him. She decided to use the AMPS, a standardized assessment instrument, to determine the effort, efficiency, independence, and safety that Mr. Muñiz exhibited during familiar and desired ADLs. For the assessment, she and Mr. Muñiz chose AMPS tasks that directly related to his desired outcomes. Joan observed him potting a rose plant and making a pot of coffee.

From her assessment, including the discussion with Mr. and Mrs. Muñiz and observing the quality of his occupational performance, Joan gathered a great deal of information about Mr. Muñiz's abilities and needs. She determined that further assessing Mr. Muñiz's specific physical or cognitive skills would not help her plan or implement intervention or review progress. Joan and Mr. Muñiz used his expressed desired outcomes and interests to set goals and plan intervention.

Aware of his abilities and current stage of recovery, Joan decided to use a compensatory approach to support Mr. Muñiz's performance in his desired occupations. At the conclusion of her first visit, Joan began the intervention by making suggestions for modifying Mr. Muñiz's kitchen environment and adapting the task demands in his garden area. Joan efficiently included both evaluation and intervention into the first of her 4 sessions with Mr. Muñiz.

Joan repeated the AMPS at the end of the intervention period to provide a standardized measure of the progress that Mr. Muñiz had made. Another measure of effectiveness of the occupational therapy intervention was Mr. Muñiz's reported improved participation in the 3 occupations that he had identified as being important. By using a client-centered and occupation-based approach, Joan was able to help Mr. Muñiz meet his goals of making his own coffee, tending to his roses, and grilling for his family.

Note. AMPS = Assessment of Motor and Process Skills.

CASE EXAMPLE 5.3. DANIELLE AND PIERRE: BIOMECHANICAL FRAME OF REFERENCE

Danielle, an occupational therapist in an outpatient clinic that specializes in upper-extremity rehabilitation, took a slightly different approach during evaluation than Joan in Case Example 5.2. Danielle was working with **Pierre,** a plumber, as a client. Pierre was eager to return to work after sustaining an on-the-job injury to his left hand. Pierre had a tendon repair and was referred for occupational therapy by his orthopedic surgeon. Because of the nature of the injury, Pierre's insurance preapproved 8 sessions.

Danielle began her first session by interviewing Pierre to get to know his job requirements and leisure interests. She learned about the types of hand movements that Pierre needed to do at work and looked at the tools and materials he used on the job. She also found out that Pierre bowled regularly with friends and built model trains at home. Pierre said that he could still bowl with his right hand but was not able to use his left hand to work on his trains.

Pierre was most concerned about returning to work. Danielle observed Pierre using his plumbing tools; she recognized that limited range of motion and strength in his left hand were the underlying cause of his difficulty with occupational performance. Danielle knew that her intervention approach would be one of remediation of hand function to support Pierre's job performance and enable him to perform other activities that were important to him.

Danielle selected a biomechanical frame of reference to guide Pierre's evaluation and intervention (Flinn, Jackson, McLaughlin Gray, & Zemke, 2008). Further assessment focused on measuring range of motion and grip strength in Pierre's left hand, because these factors would be important in monitoring his progress toward his occupational performance goals supporting his roles as plumber and builder of model trains.

Intervention Planning in the Case Examples

In both case examples, the occupational therapists focused on the occupational interests and desires of the clients. Joan (see Case Example 5.2) had preliminary information about her client, so she did not have to spend as much time collecting information for an occupational profile as Danielle (see Case Example 5.3).

However, Joan did need to do a formal assessment because the focus of her services was different from that of the occupational therapy services her client had received previously. Joan observed Mr. Muñiz as he engaged in occupations that were important to him in his home so that she could determine his occupational ability and plan appropriate intervention. Joan consciously decided not to further assess Mr. Muñiz's abilities around muscle tone, movement, or cognition because information from these types of assessments would not have helped her plan for intervention.

Danielle began her evaluation by gathering information to construct an occupational profile of Pierre. She also observed Pierre performing desired occupations, but did so in the clinic setting, not in his work environment. Her observation allowed her to efficiently determine Pierre's motor abilities and skills. Then, consistent with the biomechanical frame of reference, Danielle focused subsequent assessment on the client factors she knew were the underlying cause of Pierre's inability to engage in work tasks, and such measurements were required by her facility.

These two case examples illustrate that there is no single right way to complete an evaluation. The process varies based on the client, the information available from other sources, and information gathered during the initial steps of the evaluation process. The pragmatics of service delivery (particularly the number of visits allowed by third-party payers) influence what a therapist can do.

In both cases, Joan and Danielle gathered information about their clients as occupational beings and analyzed their clients' occupational performance. Joan was able to move from her performance analysis to intervention. Her intervention plan came directly from the performance analysis that she had done for evaluation and addressed those occupations of concern in therapy sessions to ensure occupation-based intervention.

Because Danielle further assessed components of body function, as was required by her facility, the focus of her assessment at that time was no longer on occupation and she ran the risk of switching her intervention focus to that of body function, specifically range of motion and strength, rather than occupation. Danielle worked hard to remain occupation focused, particularly as she documented her results.

DOCUMENTATION OF EVALUATION RESULTS

The evaluation phase concludes with the **documentation** of results and reporting recommendations. Most importantly, the occupational therapist needs to frame the evaluation results using occupation, discussing the client as an occupational being and reporting the observed quality of occupational performance during desired and necessary tasks. Doing so maintains occupation-centered thinking and emphasizes the unique role of occupational therapy (Fisher, 2013). Documentation should include information that is relevant and important to address the initial referral for evaluation. The purpose of the referral for evaluation may have been clearly stated or may have been vague in nature.

The referral for Pierre (see Case Example 5.3) read "evaluate and treat ROM [range of motion] & strength: post tendon injury and surgical repair." As an occupational therapist, Danielle documented Pierre's performance in occupations that were meaningful to him. Because of the setting's documentation requirements and the referral, she also documented the underlying body functions of range of motion and strength in his hand. To remain occupation focused, Danielle reported on Pierre's occupational performance first, then documented body functions as they related to his occupational performance, as shown in Appendix 5.A.

Occupational therapy evaluation results provide valuable information about the client that will be informative to other professional colleagues, particularly when planning for discharge. Often, the occupational therapist is the professional who is best able to determine how independently and safely a person can perform necessary occupations, information essential in determining discharge readiness and recommendations. Consequently, occupational therapy evaluation reports should be written clearly so that other professionals can easily understand the types of assessment used, the findings, and the interpretation of those findings that relate to occupational performance and subsequent goals and recommendations.

Appendix 5.B provides one example of an evaluation report template based on AOTA's (2013) *Guidelines for Documentation of Occupational Therapy*. The report template leads the occupational therapist through reporting evaluation findings to planning intervention in the recommendations section. Appendix 5.A illustrates using this template for Pierre (see Case Example 5.3 discussed earlier).

Although a facility often determines the format for evaluation reports, most reports conclude with recommendations. The recommendations usually include the broad goals for intervention and a suggested approach to use during therapy and may include details of services to be provided.

For example, Joan (see Case Example 5.2) might recommend that Mr. Muñiz receive three more occupational therapy visits in which the therapist uses a compensatory approach to modify the demands of tasks and Mr. Muñiz's environment to support his safety and independence in performing IADLs at home. The recommendations should be logically based on the evaluation findings reported.

Even if therapy is not warranted, the report should include recommendations (in the form of suggestions) that address the reason for referral. For example, an elementary grade student, Eric, was referred to occupational therapy "to determine if sensory processing difficulties are interfering with his ability to attend in the classroom." If the occupational therapist does not find that Eric has sensory processing difficulties and finds no reason for his difficulty in class that warrants occupational therapy services, the therapist still might offer suggestions that the teacher could implement to enhance Eric's ability to engage in schoolwork tasks. The occupational therapist might suggest moving Eric to a location in the classroom with fewer distractions or suggest that the teacher be sure she has Eric's attention before giving instructions or ensure that Eric has all needed supplies before beginning a schoolwork task.

Suggestions might also include a referral to another professional, for example, to a speech–language pathologist to confirm hearing acuity and processing, which also may influence Eric's schoolwork performance. These suggestions become a form of consultation. The recipients of the evaluation report (in this case, Eric's parents and teachers) receive a written report of not only the evaluation findings but also some guidance regarding how to proceed.

All client information, when written, serves as a permanent record of the client's abilities and progress made during intervention. An evaluation report documents the present performance level and the client's desired outcomes and goals, which can inform others who work with the client in the future.

Such information is especially helpful for clients who are transferred from one facility or type of care to another. In the continuum of health care used in the United States, it is not unusual for a client to receive services in several facilities or different departments within one facility. Information gathered during evaluation often goes into the client's chart for future use by other occupational therapists and professionals in subsequent settings. An occupational therapist at the receiving facility may use and build on previous assessments so that clients do not have to repeat the same assessments and lose valuable intervention time during a limited length of stay.

The therapist should confirm the client's desired outcomes and goals efficiently at the onset of services, helping to establish a therapeutic relationship with the client and keep services client centered. The therapist then can begin intervention almost immediately while continuing to gather more evaluation data throughout intervention. The example of Joan and Mr. Muñiz in Case Example 5.2 illustrates good use of information from another facility.

TYPES OF ASSESSMENTS

Several assessment methods were presented in the three client examples in this chapter. Assessment instruments vary in their specific purpose, procedures for administration and scoring, type of data obtained, and interpretation of results.

It is essential that the occupational therapist consider what each assessment measures and how the results are interpreted to ensure a match with the intended use of the evaluation for a given client (Zur, Johnson, Roy, Laliberte Rudman, & Wells, 2012). Selecting assessments on the basis of the client's situation and needs allows the occupational therapist to maintain client-centered practice. Furthermore, choosing assessments that focus on occupation emphasizes the unique role of occupational therapy (Fisher, 2013). Therapists should not select assessments based just on their own level of comfort or familiarity; learning new assessments is a professional responsibility.

Knowing the purpose of each assessment being considered for use is essential to enable the occupational therapist to choose the most appropriate assessment for a specific client and the questions to be answered. Some assessments gather information about a client's occupational history, interests, or roles. Other assessments provide guidelines for evaluating occupational performance; still others focus on client factors, context, or activity demands.

Standardized assessments should always be scored in a standardized manner. Standardized assessments provide objective data that can help identify or determine a client's level of function and dysfunction. Results from a standardized test may vary in their usefulness in planning an intervention program, depending on the focus of the assessment and its interpretation. Repeating a standardized assessment can document change over time and provide data for evidence-based research (Mulligan, 2014).

Standardized assessments often have specific procedures for administration and scoring that therapists must follow to obtain reliable and valid results. Some standardized assessments require formal training to learn how to administer, score, and interpret, ensuring that the results are reliable.

Many standardized assessments are limited because they often measure behaviors in unnatural conditions, unless occupational performance in a natural environment is a condition of testing. Typically, standardized assessments require the client to perform tasks such as stacking 1-inch cubes, sorting cards or objects, squeezing a dynamometer, or determining correct change in a simulated purchasing task, in a testing room or clinic and therefore outside a meaningful context.

The results may help the therapist understand a client's abilities, but the therapist then needs to transfer the results to a context and relate the findings to occupational performance. As Gillen (2013) pointed out, the transfer of results from an artificial testing environment does not reflect a client's performance in a natural context. Certainly, standardized assessments in which the occupational therapist observes the client perform activities in a natural context provide the most valid way to measure occupational performance. Such assessments directly support intervention planning because the therapist has observed performance in the real context.

Interpreting the assessment results requires the occupational therapist to first refer back to the stated purpose of the assessment used and then to further consider the focus of interpretation stated in the assessment manual. For example, both the ADL-Focused Occupation-Based Neurobehavioral Evaluation (A–ONE; Árnadóttir, 1990, 2011) and AMPS are based on observation of a person performing activities of daily living (ADL) tasks in natural context, making them both occupation-focused assessments.

Interpretation of these two assessments is different: The A–ONE focuses on underlying neurobehavioral impairments that cause decreased ADL performance, and the AMPS evaluates a person's ability to perform ADLs and IADLs, providing a measure of the quality of a person's motor and process abilities when performing ADL tasks. Assessment manuals provide guidelines for interpreting the results.

Using a variety of methods and tools for assessment provides a range of data to inform an evaluation appropriate to the needs of the client. A therapist draws from different quantitative and qualitative methods depending on the questions he or she has about a client.

Case Example 5.4 illustrates an occupational therapist's use of two types of assessments: (1) a standardized, observational, *criterion-referenced assessment* (i.e., designed to provide a measure of performance that is interpretable in terms of clearly defined and delimited criteria) conducted in the natural environment and (2) a *norm-referenced*

CASE EXAMPLE 5.4. LUKE AND CRYSTAL: CRITERION-REFERENCED AND NORM-REFERENCED ASSESSMENTS

Luke, a 10-year-old fifth grader, was referred to occupational therapy by his teacher and the school's special education referral team. Luke had received occupational therapy services as a preschooler for motor skills, particularly fine motor development. Occupational therapy was discontinued when he entered kindergarten because norm-referenced assessments indicated that his motor development was within age range. At the beginning of second grade, Luke was diagnosed with a language-based learning disability and has received speech and language therapy and help with reading since that time.

Luke's fifth-grade teacher is concerned because Luke is not getting his work done in a timely manner. She reported that he frequently does only half of the required writing, with illegible, sloppy handwriting. She wonders if his difficulty with written work is because of fine motor and handwriting issues in addition to his learning disability affecting his spelling. Because of his history of fine motor difficulty in preschool and now handwriting difficulty, the team asked for the occupational therapist to assess his fine motor skills as they related to education.

Crystal, the occupational therapist, talked with Luke's teacher and learned that he had difficulty with all writing tasks but that his problem is more pronounced when he needs to write several paragraphs at one time. Crystal learned that Luke also does not complete most classroom projects in a timely manner and the end product is usually incomplete and sloppily done. Crystal found out that Luke finishes his math work, most of which is done in a math workbook. Crystal's focus was not on how well Luke was performing academically but on Luke's performance while doing his schoolwork tasks—his necessary occupation.

During the conversation with Luke's teacher, Crystal arranged to observe Luke during a science activity in which he, as well as the other students, would be graphing results from an experiment and writing up the results in paragraph form—both tasks that the teacher indicated would be challenging for Luke to finish in a timely and neat manner.

During the observation, Crystal noted that Luke made several trips to gather paper, ruler, and pencils needed to complete the two tasks. His materials were on top of one another within his workspace, making materials difficult for him to locate when he needed them. Luke paused for long periods during each task. He also played with his ruler and pencils, at one point putting a pencil through a hole in the ruler, and spinning the ruler around. Another student sitting near Luke cued him to get back to work. He then worked quickly and wrote without keeping his written work between the lines on the paper.

Crystal noted that Luke held his pencil with a mature grasp and easily manipulated his pencil and other materials in his hands. Crystal concluded that Luke's difficulty in writing was not caused by deficiencies in fine motor skills but by inefficient use of time, space, and materials related to the schoolwork tasks.

(Continued)

**CASE EXAMPLE 5.4. LUKE AND CRYSTAL: CRITERION-REFERENCED
AND NORM-REFERENCED ASSESSMENTS** *(Cont.)*

Crystal was a calibrated rater for the School Assessment of Motor and Process Skills (School AMPS; Fisher, Bryze, Hume, & Grisworld, 2007) and scored her observations using the criteria in the School AMPS manual. She entered the scores into her School AMPS software program to obtain a school motor performance measure of 2.1 logits and a school process performance measure of 0.03 logits.

The motor performance measure indicated that Luke demonstrated a questionable level of effort in using tools and materials. The process performance measure indicated that he demonstrated a mild-to-moderate level of inefficiency when organizing time, space, and materials. Transformation of the 2 performance measures revealed that Luke's motor performance was in the average range when compared with his same-age peers (z score of −1.0), but his process performance was significantly below that of his peers (z score of −2.4). Standardized scores were familiar to other team members and helped them understand Luke's performance in relation to other students of the same age.

Crystal knew that the special education team and Luke's teacher would expect her to have assessed his fine motor and visual–motor skills, factors that support handwriting. Although her clinical reasoning of the observations when using the School AMPS indicated these skills were not issues for Luke, she reasoned that specific assessments in these areas would be relatively quick to do and provide information expected by the team. She also saw combining the 3 assessments as an opportunity to demonstrate to the team the value of a standardized observational assessment over assessments of client factors (Gillen, 2013).

Crystal chose the fine motor control tasks on the Bruininks–Oseretsky Test of Motor Proficiency (BOT2; Bruininks & Bruininks, 2005) and the Beery Visual Motor Integration Test (Beery VMI; Beery & Beery, 2004). Both are standardized assessments of client factors. These two assessments indicated that Luke's fine motor skills and visual–motor integration were in the average range. His performance resulted in a z score of −1.2 as measured by the BOT2 and a standard score of 99, in the 47th percentile, on the Beery VMI. The results from these 2 standardized assessments confirmed the clinical reasoning of Crystal's observation of Luke in his classroom.

Crystal shared her findings with the team and reported that she observed Luke to have difficulty during the schoolwork tasks. However, she clarified that Luke demonstrated no difficulty with the quality of motor performance when writing during the schoolwork project observed and reported that Luke's scores on the standardized assessments of fine motor and visual–motor skills supported her interpretation. Crystal emphasized that Luke had difficulty completing his schoolwork tasks because of inefficiency in gathering materials and organizing time and space, resulting in him rushing to finish his work, compromising the quality of the end product.

Her recommendations to support Luke in the classroom resulted from her observation of his work during schoolwork tasks, the context in which he typically did these tasks. Crystal used her observations and problem solved with the teacher ways to support Luke to gather needed tools and materials. Crystal worked with Luke on strategies to keep his desktop more organized as he works. Luke, his teacher, and Crystal developed a plan to help Luke begin working more quickly and sustain work behaviors throughout a task. Because Crystal was able to use a standardized assessment of her observations using the School AMPS, she will be able to document changes in his performance when she observes him later in the school year.

---

assessment (i.e., designed to provide a measure of performance that is interpretable in terms of clearly defined and delimited criteria) of client factors. The occupational therapist deliberately chose the assessments she used and carefully considered the information they provided. Each type of assessment provided different information to gain an understanding of the client's abilities and challenges. The occupational therapist used her clinical reasoning to interpret all of the findings and to consider intervention.

The example of Luke and Crystal (see Case Example 5.4) enables us to consider the use of a criterion-referenced assessment and norm-referenced assessment. The School AMPS is a standardized criterion-referenced assessment based on observation in a natural context. This particular assessment allowed Crystal to generate a baseline performance measure (i.e., a number) to compare with Luke's future performance. Crystal's observation of Luke in the classroom provided her with a wealth of information to consider while determining Luke's needs and options for occupational therapy services.

The standardized norm-referenced assessments on fine motor and visual–motor skills ruled out difficulty in these areas but did not add any information to help Crystal plan intervention. If Luke had demonstrated difficulty on these two assessments, the results would have informed Crystal of weaknesses in these areas but again would not have helped her know what to do for intervention. Furthermore, if Crystal had limited her evaluation to the assessments of client factors that were conducted outside of the natural classroom environment, the results would have led her to logically conclude that Luke did not need occupational therapy services.

Fortunately, Crystal observed Luke doing tasks that he needed to do in his classroom and she saw difficulties that occupational therapy could address. In Luke's case, occupational therapy played an important role to support his schoolwork performance.

EVALUATION IN CONTEXT: PRAGMATIC ISSUES OF EVALUATION

Although the focus of evaluation is on the client, options are often limited by pragmatic constraints on practice. These constraints include reimbursement implications determined by federal, insurance, or facility policies; facility procedures; resources in the community where the client lives; and the occupational therapist's own attributes (Vroman & Stewart, 2014).

Reimbursement

The time many occupational therapists spend on evaluation is constrained by federal, insurance, or facility policies guiding **reimbursement** (seen in Case Examples 5.2 and 5.3 for Mr. Muñiz and Pierre, respectively). In some cases, an occupational therapist may have only half an hour for evaluation. In other situations, the facility will be reimbursed only if the therapist engages in intervention during the first visit with a client, thus limiting the amount of formal evaluation time, as with Mr. Muñiz (Vroman & Stewart, 2014).

A therapist can blend some direct measures of occupational performance and findings from assessments directly into intervention. Thus, the transition from evaluation to intervention is nearly seamless, leading to time efficiency.

For instance, in the case of Mr. Muñiz, during her interview, Joan discovered that he wanted to tend to his rose garden (occupational profile). Joan observed him pot a plant and scored the observation using the AMPS. Consequently, at the end of the evaluation, Joan had observed

performance in the desired task (i.e., gardening). This observation led her to know how to help Mr. Muñiz participate in his desired occupation. Joan used the entire evaluation process to guide intervention immediately.

When evaluation time is limited, a therapist may also rely on screening techniques. Screening is a preliminary assessment process used to determine whether a problem exists. Results of a screening are not sufficient for intervention planning but may indicate the need for more extensive evaluation (Vroman & Stewart, 2014; Radomski, 2008). Screening can include observation of the client, review of a client's medical records, or administration of a standardized assessment designed as a screening instrument (Mulligan, 2014).

Because of reimbursement constraints, it is imperative that the occupational therapist is clear about the purpose of evaluation and the usefulness of the information gathered for decision making. The therapist needs to ensure that he or she is gathering information that is useful and relevant to the desired purpose. Knowing the potential use of evaluation data and the type of information that is relevant to address a client's needs will enable therapists to gather the essential information more efficiently.

In Case Examples 5.2 and 5.3, the therapists began their evaluations by getting to know the clients as people and learning what was important to them so that further evaluation focused on the clients' goals and supported their occupational interests and performance of desired tasks. In these examples, both therapists quickly determined what other assessment data would enable them to plan and monitor intervention. Both therapists chose assessments with a specific purpose in mind.

Facility Procedures

Each facility has its own way of conducting business. Professionals work together in a variety of ways to gather evaluation information and provide services to clients. The working relationship, or structure of teamwork, to which the facility subscribes influences how the occupational therapist works with colleagues who are simultaneously gathering evaluation data. Teams might be multi-disciplinary, interdisciplinary, or transdisciplinary in nature.

Coordinating efforts always proves to be efficient, informative, and cost-effective. Clearly identifying each professional's domain of focus and services may help to determine the purpose of their respective evaluations, regardless of the type of team used in a facility. Some evaluation information may be universally desired, and team members can determine who is in the best position to gather that information and share it with the team. Having one professional gather information for the rest of the team reflects client-centered thinking, because the client has to give information or perform similar assessment tasks only once.

The type of setting and the mission and philosophy of the facility, the composition of professionals, and the complexity of clients' needs often determine how professionals coordinate their efforts for evaluation and intervention. In medical settings and frequently in mental health practice, each professional on a multidisciplinary team typically gathers his or her own assessment data and then shares results with other team members (Falk-Kessler, 2014). This team model may result in an overlap of assessments performed.

In some rehabilitation settings and in many pediatric settings, professionals work as an interdisciplinary team, collaborating in the assessment process. Team members determine the type of assessment data needed and how each member will contribute to the process. They share their respective evaluation results and develop an integrated intervention plan (Falk-Kessler, 2014; Mulligan, 2014).

When a team has worked together in a facility over time, each professional knows the team expectations and focuses on discipline-specific information. An occupational therapist usually gathers information to complete an occupational profile and focuses on how a disability affects the client's occupational performance; other team members may gather specific client-factor information. When team members coordinate their evaluation efforts they avoid duplication for the client and reduce costs.

Transdisciplinary teams are commonly seen in early intervention programs for infants and young children (Mulligan, 2014), but they also may be used in other areas of practice. In this model, team members have a stable relationship from working together over time and have shared knowledge and skills, enabling them to observe and record assessment results for one another. With a transdisciplinary team, professional boundaries are blurred and expertise is shared so that assessment and intervention services are integrated and often done by one person (Mulligan, 2014). Transdisciplinary teams may use an **arena assessment** to conduct an evaluation; one person presents assessment tasks, and each professional gathers respective information (Mulligan, 2014).

Community Resources

Communities vary greatly in the options and natural supports available to residents. Natural community supports include health care options, religious supports, employment and volunteer opportunities, and leisure and social networks. Communities with senior citizen centers may have a cadre of volunteers who provide supports to older adults to enable them to live longer in their homes.

Knowing the availability of natural supports for all community members helps a therapist ensure that clients are at the right level of independence and, before discharge, have access to supports to help ensure their safety and well-being. Knowing the community options for discharge helps a therapist anticipate goals for clients and make decisions regarding assessment foci. For example, knowing that Meals On Wheels is available for a client might enable the therapist to focus on other aspects of IADLs. When a therapist evaluates a client living in a community that is unfamiliar to the therapist, an environmental assessment might be helpful to identify the broader community resources.

Therapist Attributes

Pragmatically, a therapist's own knowledge and experience naturally limit what he or she does during an evaluation. Staying abreast of new models of practice and frames of reference, as well as the implications of new perspectives for evaluation and intervention, enables therapists to reflect current professional thinking. Reviewing and critiquing evidence related to how to best evaluate or enhance occupational performance informs therapists of the best practices known to date (Baker & Tickle-Degnen, 2014). In addition, knowing a range of assessment instruments enables a therapist to practice in a client-centered manner; learning new assessment instruments should be part of a therapist's ongoing professional competence objectives.

LEARNING A NEW ASSESSMENT

Learning is a process that requires time and practice, and learning a new assessment procedure or instrument is no exception. Some assessments require specific education and certification processes. For example, the Sensory Integration and Praxis Tests (Ayres, 1989) and the AMPS both require that therapists take a course, practice using the assessment, and then demonstrate standardized use or calibration of scoring. Other assessments, such as the Sensory Profile (Dunn, 1999), the OPHI–II, and the COPM require the therapist to study the administration manual and practice the assessment according to described procedures to competently administer, score, and interpret the results.

In all cases, an occupational therapist learning a new assessment instrument should know the purpose of the assessment and the type of information it will provide. He or she should have read the manual and know, before using it with a client, how to administer, score, and interpret the results. Practice administering the assessment is essential to acquiring competence in its use.

Some assessments require standardized administration, meaning that the therapist must use very specific directions and responses during administration. Giving too much or too little information or doing the assessment tasks wrong, including not giving instructions as described in the assessment manual, can influence the client's response and invalidate the results. Some assessments do not require specific wording in directions given to the client, but the manual provides parameters for client instructions.

When learning a new assessment, a single reading of a manual is never sufficient, even for experienced therapists. Tests that have standardized administration may require the therapist to create note cards or other prompts as reminders of what to do next or what to observe while assessing. The therapist needs to imagine using the assessment instrument, then practice using it, possibly without another person present, before giving the assessment to another person who is not a client. Some instruments have objects to present to a client, such as blocks, small toys, or pegs and a pegboard. Therapists may need to know which side of the client to sit on, because it may affect test administration.

Once the therapist is comfortable with the assessment instrument's items, their order of presentation, and the scoring of a person's performance, he or she should practice giving the instrument to another person with the same characteristics as the population for whom the assessment was intended. This practice person may be a friend or colleague, but therapists learning a new assessment must anticipate a response from someone who might be less able.

Therapists should be prepared to provide certain types of support as appropriate. For example, the assessment manual may have specific guidelines to follow when a person makes an error; therapists need to know in advance what constitutes an error as well as how to respond. Some assessments end after a person has made a certain number of errors, so therapists should know when to end the assessment.

Learning a new instrument can be daunting. However, the rewards of learning and using a new assessment protocol are worth every minute of preparation. Further, it increases the accuracy of the assessment findings and ensures that the therapist is competent in administering and interpreting the assessment. The end result is a valid, ethical, fair evaluation process leading to increased confidence when reporting the results and using them to plan intervention.

New assessments will continue to be developed as the profession evolves. The influence of the *Framework* (AOTA, 2014) and the focus on observing occupational performance will generate new protocols that highlight what occupational therapists do best—evaluate and promote occupational performance and engagement in occupation. Therapists will have many opportunities to learn new assessments throughout their careers, to stay current in practice, and to provide the quality of services that they want to offer to clients.

THERAPEUTIC USE OF SELF DURING EVALUATION

Regardless of the type of assessment used or the constraints on evaluation and practice, the occupational therapist should always consider how he or she is influencing the evaluation process. The value of establishing a positive working relationship with clients has been important to occupational therapists throughout the profession's history (Peloquin, 2003). Use of one's own personal and professional attributes, termed *therapeutic use of self*, promotes collaboration with a client.

A therapist uses therapeutic use of self continually throughout the evaluation process as he or she and the client determine what occupation is of greatest concern and what tasks the therapist might observe the client perform. If the task is difficult for the client to perform successfully, the experience will likely trigger frustration, sadness, anger, or despair. The therapist must be ready to support the client as appropriate. Poor performance may lead to a goal and motivation for therapy; it also may be the point at which the therapist needs to help the client consider other options in his or her life and find meaning in new activities.

Using one's self in this way, as a medium of therapy, is considered the "art of therapy" and is just as important as the theoretical and technical knowledge and skills that therapists possess (Peloquin, 2003).

SUMMARY

Evaluation provides the foundational information on which occupational therapy services are built. The process begins by getting to know the client as a person and understanding the occupations that are important to him or her. The occupational therapist examines the client's occupational performance in tasks that are relevant, important, and challenging to the client. The therapist may determine that further assessment of client factors, context, or task demands would provide greater understanding of

a client's strengths and limitations. The evaluation process is as long or short as necessary to enable the therapist to plan and implement appropriate occupational therapy services.

Many methods can provide information that might be interesting; however, a longer evaluation is not necessarily a better one. The therapist must determine the salient information to answer the questions posed by the referral and support the client's desire and need to participate in meaningful life experiences. A sound evaluation process leads to informed planning and intervention services.

QUESTIONS

1. The author describes how evaluation leads to intervention planning in Case Example 5.1. What other assessments might you have used with Tonya?
2. Can you think of some additional types of interventions that Jean might have developed for Tonya based on the information provided? Are there other areas on which you would have focused?
3. Reflect on a case with which you are familiar. When reviewing interventions to consider making changes, what kind of information would have made you consider changing the intervention plan? Identify specific data that you wanted to gather before changing the plan with the client in the case you chose.
4. In Case Example 5.2, how might the evaluation (and possibly the intervention) have been different if the number of visits had not been limited?
5. Think about a case with which you are familiar. What were the critical elements that needed to be included in the documentation to justify occupational therapy intervention in that setting?
6. In Case Example 5.1, what strategies might Jean have used to develop a therapeutic rapport with Tonya that supported occupational therapy intervention?
7. Consider a case of your own. What other type of evaluation questions might you ask to enhance the focus of evaluation and intervention on occupation? What assessments or methods would help you glean the desired information?

References

American Occupational Therapy Association. (2013). Guidelines for documentation of occupational therapy. *American Journal of Occupational Therapy, 67*(Suppl.), S32–S38. http://dx.doi.org/10.5014/ajot.2013.67S32

American Occupational Therapy Association. (2014). Occupational therapy practice framework: Domain and process (3rd ed.). *American Journal of Occupational Therapy, 68*(Suppl. 1), S1–S48. http://dx.doi.org/10.5014/ajot.2014.682006

Árnadóttir, G. (1990). *The brain and behavior: Assessing cortical dysfunction through activities of daily living.* St. Louis: Mosby.

Árnadóttir, G. (2011). Impact of neurobehavioral deficits on activities of daily living. In G. Gillen (Ed.), *Stroke rehabilitation: A function-based approach* (3rd ed., pp. 456–500). St. Louis: Mosby.

Ayres, A. J. (1989). *Sensory Integration and Praxis Tests.* Los Angeles: Western Psychological Services.

Baker, N., & Tickle-Degnen, L. (2014). Evidence-based practice. In B. A. B. Schell, G. Gillen, & M. E. Scaffa (Eds.). *Willard and Spackman's occupational therapy* (12th ed., pp. 398–412). Philadelphia: Lippincott Williams & Wilkins.

Bass-Haugen, J., Mathiowetz, V., & Flinn, N. (2008). Optimizing motor behavior using the occupational therapy task-oriented approach. In M. V. Radomski & C. A. Trombly (Eds.), *Occupational therapy for physical dysfunction* (6th ed., pp. 598–617). Philadelphia: Lippincott Williams & Wilkins.

Beery, K. E., & Beery, N. A. (2004). *The Beery–Buktenica Developmental Test of Visual–Motor Integration* (5th ed.). Minneapolis: NCS Pearson.

Brown, C. (2009). Functional assessment and intervention in occupational therapy. *Psychiatric Rehabilitation Journal, 32,* 162–170. http://dx.doi.org/10.2975/32.3.2009.162-170

Bruininks, R. H., & Bruininks, B. D. (2005). *Bruininks–Oseretsky Test of Motor Proficiency* (2nd ed.). Circle Pines, MN: AGS Publishing.

Dunn, W. (1999). *Sensory Profile: User's manual.* San Antonio: Psychological Corporation.

Falk-Kessler, J. (2014). Professionalism, communication, and teamwork. In B. Schell, G. Gillen, & M. Scaffa (Eds.), *Willard and Spackman's occupational therapy* (12th ed., pp. 452–465). Philadelphia: Lippincott Williams & Wilkins.

Fisher, A. G. (2009). *Occupational therapy intervention process model: A model for planning and implementing top–down, client-centered, and occupation-based interventions.* Fort Collins, CO: Three Star Press.

Fisher, A. G. (2013). Occupation-centred, occupation-based, occupation-focused: Same, same or different. *Scandinavian Journal of Occupational Therapy, 20,* 162–173. http://dx.doi.org/doi:10.3109/11038128.2012.754492

Fisher, A. G., Bryze, K., Hume, V., & Griswold, L. A. (2007). *School Assessment of Motor and Process Skills.* Fort Collins, CO: Three Star Press.

Fisher, A. G., & Griswold, L. A. (2009). *Evaluation of social interaction.* Fort Collins, CO: Three Star Press.

Fisher, A. G., & Griswold, L. A. (2014). Performance skills: Implementing performance analyses to evaluate the quality of occupational performance. In B. Schell, G. Gillen, & M. Scaffa (Eds.), *Willard and Spackman's occupational therapy* (12th ed., pp. 249–264). Philadelphia: Lippincott Williams & Wilkins.

Fisher, A. G., & Jones, K. B. (2012). *Assessment of Motor and Process Skills* (7th ed., rev.). Fort Collins, CO: Three Star Press.

Flinn, N. A., Jackson, J., McLaughlin Gray, J., & Zemke, R. (2008). Optimizing abilities and capacities: Range of motion, strength, and endurance. In M. V. Radomski & C. A. Trombly (Eds.). *Occupational therapy for physical dysfunction* (6th ed., pp. 573–597). Philadelphia: Lippincott Williams & Wilkins.

Gillen, G. (2013). A fork in the road: An occupational hazard. *American Journal of Occupational Therapy, 67,* 641–652. http://dx.doi.org/doi:10.5014/ajot.2013.676002

Hinojosa, J., Kramer, P., Royeen, C. B., & Luebben, A. (2003). Core concept of occupation. In P. Kramer, J. Hinojosa, & C. B. Royeen (Eds.), *Perspectives in human occupation: Participation in life* (pp. 1–17). Philadelphia: Lippincott Williams & Wilkins.

Hocking, C. (2001). Implementing occupation-based assessment. *American Journal of Occupational Therapy, 55,* 463–469. http://dx.doi.org/10.5014/ajot.55.4.463

Ideishi, R. I. (2003). Influence of occupation on assessment and treatment. In P. Kramer, J. Hinojosa, & C. B. Royeen (Eds.), *Perspectives in human occupation: Participation in life* (pp. 278–296). Philadelphia: Lippincott Williams & Wilkins.

Kaplan, M. (2010). A frame of reference for motor acquisition. In P. Kramer & J. Hinojosa (Eds.), *Frames of reference for pediatric occupational therapy* (3rd ed., pp. 390–424). Philadelphia: Lippincott Williams & Wilkins.

Kielhofner, G., Mallinson, T., Crawford, C., Nowak, M., Rigby, M., Henry, A., . . . Walens, D. (2004). *A user's guide to the Occupational Performance History Interview–II* (OPHI–II; version 2.1). Chicago: Model of Human Occupation Clearinghouse, Department of Occupational Therapy, University of Illinois.

Law, M., Baptiste, S., Carswell, A., McColl, M. A., Polatajko, H., & Pollock, N. (2005). *Canadian Occupational Performance Measure* (4th ed.). Toronto: CAOT Publications ACE.

Mastos, M., Miller, K., Eliasson, A. C., & Imms, C. (2007). Goal-directed training: Linking theories of treatment to clinical practice for improved functional activities in daily life. *Clinical Rehabilitation, 21,* 47–55. http://dx.doi.org/10.1177/0269215506073494

Mulligan, S. (2014). *Occupational therapy evaluation for children: A pocket guide* (2nd ed.). Philadelphia: Lippincott Williams & Wilkins.

Park, M. (2008). Making scenes: Imaginative practices of a child with autism in a sensory integration-based therapy session. *Medical Anthropology Quarterly, 22,* 234–256. http://dx.doi.org/10.1111/j.1548-1387.2008.00024.x

Peloquin, S. M. (2003). The therapeutic relationship: Manifestations and challenges in occupational therapy. In E. B. Crepeau, E. S. Cohn, & B. A. B. Schell (Eds.), *Willard and Spackman's occupational therapy* (10th ed., pp. 157–170). Philadelphia: Lippincott Williams & Wilkins.

Phipps, S., & Richardson, P. (2007). Occupational therapy outcomes for clients with traumatic brain injury and stroke using the Canadian Occupational Performance Measure. *American Journal of Occupational Therapy, 61,* 328–334. http://dx.doi.org/10.5014/ajot.61.3.328

Price, P. (2009). The therapeutic relationship. In E. B. Crepeau, E. S. Cohn, & B. A. B. Schell (Eds.), *Willard and Spackman's occupational therapy* (11th ed., pp. 328–341). Philadelphia: Lippincott Williams & Wilkins.

Radomski, M. V. (2008). Planning, guiding, and documenting practice. In M. V. Radomski & C. A. Trombly Latham (Eds.), *Occupational therapy for physical dysfunction* (6th ed., pp. 40–64). Philadelphia: Lippincott Williams & Wilkins.

Simmons, D. C., Crepeau, E. B., & White, B. P. (2000). The predictive power of narrative data in occupational therapy evaluation. *American Journal of Occupational Therapy, 54,* 471–476. http://dx.doi.org/10.5014/ajot.54.5.471

Smith, N. R., Kielhofner, G., & Watts, J. H. (1986). The relationships between volition, activity pattern, and life satisfaction in the elderly. *American Journal of Occupational Therapy, 40,* 278–283. http://dx.doi.org/10.5014/ajot.40.4.278

Stewart, K. B. (2010). Purposes, processes, and methods of evaluation. In J. Case-Smith & J. C. O'Brien (Eds.), *Occupational therapy for children* (6th ed., pp. 193–211). St. Louis: Mosby/Elsevier.

Trombly Latham, C. A. (2008). Conceptual framework for practice. In C. A. Trombly Latham & M. V. Radomski (Eds.), *Occupational therapy for physical dysfunction* (6th ed., pp. 1–20). Philadelphia: Lippincott Williams & Wilkins.

Vroman, K., & Stewart, E. (2014). *Occupational therapy evaluation for adults: A pocket guide* (2nd ed.). Philadelphia: Lippincott Williams & Wilkins.

Weinstock-Zlotnick, G., & Hinojosa, J. (2004). Bottom-up or top-down evaluation: Is one better than the other? *American Journal of Occupational Therapy, 58,* 594–599. http://dx.doi.org/10.5014/ajot.58.5.594

Zur, B., Johnson, A., Roy, E., Laliberte Rudman, D., & Wells, J. (2012). Beyond traditional notions of validity: Selecting appropriate measures for occupational therapy practice. *Australian Occupational Therapy Journal, 59,* 243–246. http://dx.doi.org/10.1111/j.1440-1630.2012.01007.x

APPENDIX 5.A. SAMPLE OCCUPATIONAL THERAPY EVALUATION REPORT

Facility/Agency Name
Occupational Therapy Evaluation Report

Name: Pierre Sample
Date of Birth: November 25, 1990
ID #: 77007
Date of Evaluation: January 31, 2014
Age: 23 years
Primary Diagnosis: Limited function postinjury and postsurgery of flexor pollicis longus

Reason for Referral

Pierre was referred by A–1 Hand Surgery, Inc., 5 weeks' post–surgical repair of flexor pollicis longus in his left hand, surgical restrictions removed. The injury was sustained on the job when equipment crushed his hand while he was working as a plumber. Presenting problems include an inability to use his left hand for work-related tasks as well as leisure activities and some ADLs. Evaluation included gathering information from Pierre regarding difficulties in task performance, observation of his performance during tasks he reported he needed for his job, and goniometric measurements, as well as evaluation of grip strength required for hand use.

Occupational Profile

Pierre reported that he lives with his girlfriend, who does most of the meal preparation and is willing to do household chores that he typically does until his hand function returns. Pierre works for a local plumbing company where he primarily installs pipes and heating systems in new home construction. He described his primary job tasks to be drilling holes, cutting and fitting pipes, and soldering. He usually works with one other plumber when he goes out to a job site. Pierre enjoys his job and is working toward advancing his status. He said that his boss is holding his job for him. In addition to work, Pierre reported that he is an avid bowler and bowls 2–3 times a week for a social

outlet. Pierre stated that he can continue bowling because he bowls with his uninjured right hand. He also builds model trains, which he began doing with his father when he was a young boy. Building model trains has become a large part of Pierre's identity; his trains have been shown in many public events, particularly around the holidays. Pierre expressed concern regarding his inability to pinch the tiny train parts with his left hand. He reported that after experiences recovering from past sports injuries in high school, he knows he needs to do his exercises and is eager to begin therapy. His goals are to return to work and to building model trains.

Assessments Used and Evaluation Results

When observed cutting and soldering pipes, Pierre was unable to grip and stabilize the pipes and fittings with his left hand, resulting in his inability to do routinely performed work tasks. Functionally, he was unable to pick up objects smaller than 3 inches in diameter. Evaluation of left thumb ROM indicated moderate limitation. AROM for thumb MP was 30° and thumb IP 55°. Secondary to prolonged immobility, lumbrical strength for digits 2 through 4 was MMT score of 3, limiting grasp and pinch. Evaluation of strength for flexor pollicis longus was MMT score of 2. Dynamometer results indicated a left grasp of 70 pounds. Secondary to AROM limitation, pinch strength was not evaluated. Sensory evaluation noted no deficits in sensory functioning.

Analysis of Occupational Performance

At the time of the initial evaluation, Pierre demonstrated limited left-hand function that is hindering his return to work as a plumber because he needs his left hand to grasp and support copper pipe of 1-inch diameter. An important leisure activity of building trains is also compromised. He is able to perform personal ADLs with adaptation, and he is independent with necessary IADLs.

(continued)

Pierre had limited ROM and strength in left-hand flexors and thumb adduction and opposition. He was unable to oppose and achieve forceful thumb flexion to pinch and pick up objects less than 3 inches in diameter and had functional issues with grasp.

Summary and Analysis

Pierre's goals of returning to work and engaging in all leisure activities are realistic. He is motivated to participate in occupational therapy to achieve his goals.

Recommendations

Outpatient occupational therapy services are recommended to address left-hand function, postsurgical repair of flexor pollicis longus and intrinsic muscle weakness, to meet the goal of grasping and manipulating tools and materials, as required to return to work. Services include 8 sessions over a 4-week period of time and a home exercise program. Adapted handles on work tools will enable return to work before obtaining full ROM and strength.

Danielle Exemplar, MS, OTR/L
Occupational Therapist

Note. ADLs = activities of daily living; AROM = active range of motion; IADLs = instrumental activities of daily living; IP = interphalangeal; MMT = manual muscle testing; MP = metacarpophalangeal; ROM = range of motion.

APPENDIX 5.B. OCCUPATIONAL THERAPY EVALUATION REPORT TEMPLATE

Facility/Agency Name
Occupational Therapy Evaluation Report

Name: (Client's Full Name)
Date of Birth:
ID #: (given by facility/agency)
Date of Evaluation:
Age:
Primary Diagnosis: (if known)

Reason for Referral

Include the referral source, reason for referral, and the presenting primary concerns. Identify the evaluation procedures and assessments used and a brief notation regarding the purpose of each.

Occupational Profile

Include information about the client's current living situation, employment status, and leisure activities. For each relevant occupation (e.g., work, education, leisure, ADLs), discuss the tasks necessary, context (social and physical environment), and satisfaction level. Discuss the client's occupational history if it provides information about the client's ability to adapt to the presenting situation. Identify the client's self-identified strengths, limitations, desired outcomes or goals, and priorities.

Assessments Used and Evaluation Results

Results may be organized in a variety of formats. Often the information in this section is organized by the evaluation procedure used, by areas of occupation, or the assessment. To promote occupation-focused reporting, begin with a description of the quality of the client's observed occupational performance. Specific numeric findings or results often are included in an appendix.

Analysis of Occupational Performance

Provide a synthesis of the evaluation results reported above, specifically as they relate to occupational performance. The interpretation may be what busy colleagues read first (or solely), so it should provide a complete overview of the evaluation findings and lead into summary and analysis and recommendations in the following sections.

Summary and Analysis

Begin by noting problems in occupational performance to help clarify the occupation-centered nature of occupational therapy, as unique from other professions. Summarize the data as it relates to the concerns stated in the referral, and summarize interpretation of that data as it relates to the occupational profile.

Recommendations

Recommendations for occupational therapy services, if warranted, should include suggestions for the focus of intervention, intervention approach, and service delivery model, often with suggested frequency and duration of services. The recommendations should address the reason for referral and reflect the client's occupational goals and priorities noted earlier in the report.

Note. ADLs = activities of daily living.

CHAPTER 6

Administration of Evaluation and Assessments

Jim Hinojosa, PhD, OT, BCP, FAOTA
Paula Kramer, PhD, OTR, FAOTA

Highlights

- Categories of assessments with standardized protocols
- Assessment techniques
- Considerations in administration of assessments
- Developing competence in use of assessments
- Evaluator and situational issues
- Types of error in assessment
- Implications for intervention.

Key Terms

Activity configuration
Assessment environment
Capacity
Classical test theory
Criterion-referenced assessments
Errors
Interviews
Ipsative assessment
Item bias
Item response theory
Nonstandardized assessments
Normative assessment
Normed sample

Observation
Open-ended interviews
Performance
Performance assessments
Proxy
Questionnaire
Rater bias
Reliability
Standardized assessments
Structured interviews
Test-taker variables
Therapeutic relationship
Validity

This chapter discusses the key issues that occupational therapists need to consider when administering and interpreting an assessment. We begin by detailing concerns regarding specific categories of assessments, followed by a discussion of general principles that guide the administration of standardized and nonstandardized assessments, including environmental considerations and sources of error in testing. We conclude with a brief description of how the findings from assessments influence the development of an intervention plan and determine the effectiveness of the intervention.

CATEGORIES OF ASSESSMENTS WITH STANDARDIZED PROTOCOLS

The purpose of an evaluation is to obtain useful information about the client and his or her life situation. Occupational therapists use data from assessments to identify a client's strengths and limitations and develop an appropriate intervention plan. The first step in the evaluation process is selecting the most appropriate assessment. Best practice requires therapists to use **standardized assessments** whenever possible. Standardized assessments, when administered in the recommended manner, provide reliable and valid data. In many situations, laws governing practice and reimbursement, including the Individuals With Disabilities Education Improvement Act of 2004 and the Outcomes and Assessment Information Set–C (Centers for Medicare and Medicaid Services, 2013), require the use of standardized assessments.

Many standardized assessments are appropriate for reevaluation because therapists can compare the retest scores, performance measures, or behavioral indicators to identify changes in a client's performance. Occupational therapists should read the literature regarding the specific standardized assessment they are using or planning to use to increase their knowledge about the assessment, including its advantages and limitations. Moreover, knowledge about the specific assessment and its standardization determines whether therapists can use the assessment as part of a reevaluation. In situations in which a standardized assessment is not designed for reevaluation, therapists should look for another standardized assessment that addresses

the same domain or area of concern to obtain comparison data.

Standardized assessments have specific set procedures or protocols. When therapists follow these set procedures, it ensures that all clients who undergo evaluation using a particular assessment have consistent testing experiences. Following standardized procedures when administering the assessments is necessary to obtain reportable, valid results. Many standardized assessments have specific processes for data analysis.

There are three types of standardized assessments:

1. *Normative assessments* compare data obtained against a normed sample.
2. *Criterion-referenced assessments* determine a set score for mastery and compare data obtained against the set score.
3. *Ipsative assessments* have standardized procedures and are individualized so that the same domain can be compared over time.

Normative Assessments

The developer of a test designs a **normative assessment** from data using research conducted on a specific sample of people (i.e., the normative group). Often, the normative group is the "normal" population, or **normed sample**. Data from a normed sample forms a probability distribution shaped like a bell curve, with the scores of a majority of the people clustered in the center.

When therapists obtain data about a client from a normative assessment, they can compare the client's performance against the normed sample. When the standardization sample is a group of people who are normal, therapists compare the client's scores, behaviors, or performance against the group's scores, behaviors, or performance. When a test developer designs an assessment for a group with a specific disability, the standardization often describes how the person with a disability performs relative both to the normed sample and to other people with the specific disability. It is critical that therapists understand to whom the client is being compared and explicitly state this information in the evaluation summary report.

Therapists must consider the psychometric integrity and potential limitations of a standardized assessment when interpreting data. Psychometrics includes the reliability and validity of the assessment, the sample size and demographics of the normed sample, and the standard error of measurement. All of these factors are important for judging how valuable the data from the assessment will be in understanding the client's abilities and limitations.

Reliability measures the consistency of the results an assessment provides, whereas *validity* measures how true the measure is to the underlying theory and concepts. Reliability is necessary but not sufficient to determine psychometric integrity. A measure can be reliable but not valid, but a valid measure will provide reliable information. A reliable measure is relatively free of measurement error. Reliability estimates can range from 0 to 1.00. Generally, a score of ≥0.70 indicates that a measure is reliable (Fleiss, Levin, & Paik, 2003; Nunnally & Bernstein, 1994). Scores of >0.80 have excellent reliability. There is no single score or system to determine an assessment's validity; therefore, therapists do not have one score of value they can use to determine validity. In reality, many of the assessments occupational therapists use do not meet these standards. However, the assessment selected may be the only available instrument or the best instrument available for the purpose. See Chapter 10, "Standardized Testing: Scoring and Interpretation of Results," for a more complete discussion of psychometric concepts.

Therapists should always seek assessments with the most psychometric integrity. When selecting an assessment, if that assessment's psychometric integrity is relatively low, therapists need to consider whether other assessments are available for the population of interest. If there is a better assessment, they should explore using it.

Sometimes, however, therapists decide on a particular assessment with lower psychometric integrity for a particular reason. When therapists make this decision, they should be clear about why they have made this choice. Greater familiarity with an assessment is not a good justification for choosing an assessment with less psychometric integrity. Sometimes the only assessment available for testing a specific factor has weak psychometric integrity; in such cases, therapists should report the limitations of the assessment in the evaluation summary.

Some normative assessments frequently used by occupational therapists are the Mini-Mental State Exam (Folstein, Folstein, McHugh, & Fanjiang, 2001), the Sensory Integration and Praxis Tests (Ayres, 1989), the Lowenstein Occupational Therapy Cognitive Assessment (Itzkovich, Elazar, Averbuch, & Katz, 2000), the Assessment of Motor and Process Skills (AMPS; Fisher & Jones, 2012), and the School Version of the Assessment of Motor and Process Skills (School AMPS; Fisher, Bryze, Hume, & Griswold, 2007).

Criterion-Referenced Assessments

Criterion-referenced assessments measure how well a person performs against a set of criteria rather than against another person. The developer of a criterion-referenced assessment selects items that reflect mastery of the area of concern or content. For example, if the area of concern is reading, a teacher might develop an assessment on the basis of the components required to demonstrate mastery of reading. The development of an assessment on the basis of a particular criterion begins with the construction of a table of specifications that lists the indicators associated with each component specification. For example, if an assessment developer wanted to assess the ability to dress oneself, he or she would begin by identifying the component aspects of dressing (e.g., selecting clothes, putting on a shirt, putting on pants or a skirt, putting on socks, putting on shoes).

Generally, a criterion-referenced assessment provides an established score that reflects mastery. A person's performance on a criterion-referenced assessment is how well the person performs against the set score for mastery. A criterion-based assessment does not compare scores, behaviors, or performances to a norm; instead, the focus is on the mastery of the area of interest.

Sometimes a test developer selects criteria for a criterion-referenced assessment for which normative information is available. When using a criterion-referenced assessment, therapists cannot use information about the normal range of the criteria as a basis for comparing the client's performance against the known norm. Comparing criterion-referenced data with normative-referenced data is like comparing apples to oranges.

Criterion-referenced data are based on mastery; normative-referenced data are based on performance as it relates to a normative sample, as described earlier. A criterion-referenced assessment cannot become a normative assessment just because normative data are available. Driving tests, course exams, and the National Board for Certification in Occupational Therapy examination are all criterion-referenced assessments.

Some criterion-referenced assessments that occupational therapists might use with a client are the School Function Assessment (Coster, Deeney, Haltiwanger, & Haley, 1998), the Klein–Bell Activities of Daily Living Scale (Klein & Bell, 1979), the Kohlman Evaluation of Living Skills (Kohlman-Thompson, 1992), and the Árnadóttir OT–ADL (Occupational Therapy–Activities of Daily Living) Neurobehavioral Evaluation (Árnadóttir, 1990).

Just as with normative assessments, the psychometric integrity of criterion-referenced assessments and other limitations identified in the test manual must be examined. Again, therapists must determine which assessment is the most appropriate one to use.

Ipsative Assessments

An *ipsative assessment* has standardized procedures and is individualized so that the person compares himself or herself in the same domain across time. Frequently, the person contrasts present performance against the prior performance in a specific domain. Two common forms—interview-based and observation-based assessments—do not have specific expected outcomes. Ipsative assessments use a standardized method of collecting data so that a therapist can obtain information from different clients under consistent conditions.

The ipsative assessment developer outlines the specific procedures, the order in which they are to be followed, and sometimes the conditions that are most appropriate for administering the specific assessment. A common ipsative assessment that has standardized (although not published) procedures is an *activity configuration* (Cynkin & Robinson, 1990; Mosey, 1986), which consists of a series of questions that the therapist asks a client during the initial interview.

The activity configuration begins with the therapist asking the client to describe a typical weekday in detail. During the interview, the therapist asks follow-up questions about specific activities and the amount of time spent in each activity. After outlining a weekday, the therapist asks the client to describe a typical weekend day. Again, the therapist asks follow-up questions about the specific amount of time spent in each activity. Using the client's descriptions, the therapist forms a rough understanding of the client's activities. At this point, the therapist asks the client to indicate which activities he or she enjoys, dislikes, or finds dissatisfying. The therapist may also ask about difficult activities and responsibilities.

A standardized order of questions provides a clear and detailed understanding of the client's daily life. A change in the procedures (e.g., a change in the order of the questions) would result in less thorough information about the client's life.

Other ipsative assessments used by occupational therapists are the Canadian Occupational Performance Measure (Law et al., 2005), the Pediatric Volitional Questionnaire (Geist, Kielhofner, Basu, & Kafkes, 2002), the Pediatric Interest Profiles (Henry, 2000), the Occupational Performance History Interview (Kielhofner et al., 1998), and the *Occupational Therapy Practice Framework: Domain and Process* (3rd ed.; American Occupational Therapy Association [AOTA], 2014).

ASSESSMENT TECHNIQUES

One method of grouping assessments is by the techniques used for gathering information. These categories can be labeled *watching* (observation), *measuring* (observation using instruments for performance measures), *listening* (interviews), and *asking* (written questionnaires). The most basic techniques are observation and interviewing.

Observation involves therapists directly perceiving the actions of a client and then recording what they see. Observation can be aided (by the use of an assessment) or unaided. Many assessments of activities of daily living (ADLs) and instrumental ADLs originated with unaided observation of activities and behaviors that led to the development of standardized observational assessments. The FIM™ (Uniform Data System for Medical Rehabilitation [UDSMR], 1997), one of the most widely used rehabilitation assessments, was developed from a standardized method of directly observing and rating ADLs.

Observation has advantages over interviews and questionnaires. First, observation allows occupational therapists to witness directly how a client performs in a given situation, without the rationalization or explanation therapists might interject during an interview and without the bias inherent in a self-report or proxy-report questionnaire. Second, observational assessment does not rely on the client's interpretation of questions or memory of events or activities.

One disadvantage of observation is that for an observational assessment to be accurate and consistent, therapists must be unbiased and experienced. Some observational assessments require certification, which means the evaluator must receive advanced training. Another disadvantage of observational assessment is the extensive time required to gather the information. An assessment using the FIM™ can take a therapist an hour or more to perform and interpret, whereas a therapist can complete the self-report FIM™ in less than 30 minutes (Cohen & Marino, 2000).

Occupational therapists often select **performance assessments** to measure functional limitations. For example, therapists can assess reaching, lifting, and standing balance with the Berg Balance Scale (Berg, Wood-Dauphinee, Williams, & Gayton, 1989) and walking speed with the Timed Get-Up-and-Go Test (Wall, Bell, Campbell, & Davis, 2000). Unlike ADL observations, performance assessments often focus on a specific bodily function and its associated impairment. Performance assessments often rely on calibrated instruments for measurement. Therefore, they are independent of individual judgment and not as susceptible to influence from the client or rater bias as are observations, interviews, and questionnaires.

However, because performance assessments focus on the function of a particular body part, they usually ignore the environment and the person as a whole. A study comparing performance assessments to self-reported ADL ability noted cultural differences that could be due to sociocultural and environmental factors not accounted for in performance assessments (van den Brink et al., 2003). Performance assessments may also assess cognitive functioning. These assessments require the client to perform a cognitive task, such as telling time from an analog clock or spelling or reading given

words. These examples of cognitive assessments are not standardized; therefore, it is difficult to interpret the results of such assessments.

Interviews are another common means of gathering information. The interview technique involves a conversation between the therapist and the client or a proxy. Optimally, an observation assessment should involve direct interaction with the client. When direct interaction is not possible, a therapist, with the client's permission, can conduct an interview with a *proxy,* or someone who has sufficient knowledge of the client's situation to act on his or her behalf (e.g., spouse, parent, significant other, or caregiver). A proxy may also be used if the client is a minor or is legally incapable of being interviewed. Whenever possible, therapists should conduct an interview in person to observe the respondent's reactions and behaviors. When an in-person interview is impossible, therapists can interview someone by telephone or through a computer.

Interviews range from structured to open-ended. *Structured interviews* contain specific questions that therapists ask in a specific order. When an interview is highly structured, the information obtained is more likely to be consistent across interviewees. *Open-ended interviews* allow the interviewee to tell his or her story in the manner that is most comfortable, sharing his or her lived experience.

Interview information can be recorded using written notes, audiotaping, or videotaping for later review. Audiotaped interviews allow independent raters to score the data, which can ensure verification of the interpretation. Whenever a person is audio- or videotaped, the therapist must obtain written consent from the participants. This written consent should identify who will have access to the data and what the therapist will do with the audio- or videotapes after the evaluation is completed.

Structured interviews, when conducted in person, provide information that is more consistent and require less training for therapists. One of the most widely used health status assessments, the SF–36 Health Survey (Ware, Snow, Kosinski, & Gandek, 1993), initially developed as an interview assessment, is now extensively used as a self-report questionnaire. Less structured and open-ended interviews require more effort to organize and analyze the information obtained. An advantage of these less structured and open-ended interviews is that they provide therapists with an opportunity to probe for more or clarifying information. Probing is more likely to be used in these types of interviews. When a therapist asks clarifying questions, the client can explain answers to difficult-to-comprehend questions.

Whenever interpreting data from an interview, the therapist must consider the method of data collection (face-to-face vs. remote, structured vs. open-ended) because it can affect the credibility of the information obtained. One challenge for therapists during an interview is to establish rapport with the client or proxy so that he or she shares information truthfully. Therapists conducting open-ended interviews need advanced training on how to engage the client in a guided conversation to solicit appropriate information from the client. It is important that therapists realize that an open-ended interview is not a give-and-take conversation with the interviewee but a guided exchange designed to elicit specific information.

The two major advantages of a **questionnaire** are (1) the ease of administration and (2) low cost. The client or proxy can complete questionnaires, like interviews. A highly structured questionnaire in which the client answers multiple-choice or true–false questions (called *forced-choice responses*) provides highly reliable information. A client can complete a self-report questionnaire at his or her convenience and can be interrupted or stopped easily.

Although easy for therapists to administer, questionnaires have many disadvantages. Questionnaires with highly structured and clearly worded questions provide valid and reliable information, but those with vague or difficult-to-interpret questions provide questionable information. Moreover, the information obtained using questionnaires may be less accurate than information obtained from direct observations or interviews.

For example, when completing a questionnaire, a client can easily misinterpret a question. Should a client misunderstand a question asked during an interview, a therapist has a chance to probe for clarification or additional information. A client can be less accurate when reporting his or her own behavior than when a therapist is directly observing it. In addition, a client may be unable to judge his or her own abilities accurately or may answer a question with personal bias. Again, unlike during an interview or observation, the therapist does not have an opportunity to seek clarification or probe for more in-depth understanding. However, a well-designed questionnaire provides therapists with ways to detect untruths and biases through questions designed to test the veracity of the client's answers.

Finally, the client's ability to complete a questionnaire depends on his or her understanding of the language as well as reading and cognitive abilities. In cases in which therapists are unsure of the client's ability to complete the questionnaire independently, they should read the questionnaire to the client and help him or her complete it.

CONSIDERATIONS IN ADMINISTRATION OF ASSESSMENTS

Occupational therapists must consider various issues when determining the best assessments to use for specific conditions and specific needs of clients. To address client needs, therapists select assessments on the basis of the purpose of the evaluation, therapists' skills, the amount of time available to administer the assessment, and the assessment's requirements (e.g., equipment, space, expertise). Typically, therapists conduct an initial screening in an informal manner, obtaining general information about the client. Screening often includes a review of referral information; general observations; or other information that the client, significant others, or other professionals provide. Depending on the situation and availability, screening can involve the administration of a standardized screening assessment.

On the basis of screening data, therapists may decide to proceed with a full evaluation. They must then decide which assessments to administer and develop a plan to conduct the evaluation. The evaluation plan must be realistic and created in such a manner that therapists can appropriately carry it out under real circumstances, sensitive to the client's situation. Sometimes space, equipment, resources, or expertise limits the choice of available assessments.

Because professionals in many disciplines use the same assessments, occupational therapists may revise the evaluation plan based on which assessments others in the practice setting are using. If the assessment administered by another professional provides information needed to complete the occupational therapy evaluation, the occupational therapist should obtain and use that information in preparing his or her final evaluation summary. When using information from another professional's report, the therapist should always reference the other professional's report and the specific assessments the professional used.

Once occupational therapists have developed an evaluation plan, they inform the client about the process and what the client will be expected to do during the evaluation. It is important to tell the client how long the evaluation will take and what exactly it will involve. Clients have the right to be informed about the purpose of each assessment and how the results will be used.

Moreover, each client has the absolute right to refuse an evaluation or a specific assessment, without consequences. When the client is a child, the family should be involved during the explanation process and also has the right to refuse an evaluation. If the client is an adult but not capable of understanding the rationale for an assessment, therapists should inform the designated health proxy about the focus and purpose of the selected assessments.

> The Health Insurance Portability and Accountability Act of 1996 states that only those persons who have been formally designated by the client or hold a health proxy for the client can be informed about the evaluation plan and process.

In the past, it was customary to discuss such issues with family members and significant others. However, since passage of the Health Insurance Portability and Accountability Act of 1996, only persons who have been formally designated by the client or hold a health proxy for the client can be involved throughout this process. A client's refusal should not affect the outcome of the evaluation. Therapists are responsible for explaining the evaluation process in a manner that is appropriate for the client.

DEVELOPING COMPETENCE IN USE OF ASSESSMENTS

Standardized assessments are generally multifaceted; often, they are not easy for therapists to master. Some assessments require extensive training and certification before use. Using new or unfamiliar assessments requires study and rehearsal on the part of therapists before administration to a client. First, therapists must carefully read the assessment manual. This thorough reading provides an understanding of the scope and purpose of the assessment. Most manuals discuss the administration procedures, identify limitations of the assessment, and present facts about the psychometric integrity. The manual also explains what therapists will learn about the client from the assessment. For example, the manual might explain that therapists will learn about a client's strengths, limitations, performance skills, personal characteristics, roles, and values. At times, this information is not as readily available as one would like.

It is helpful for therapists to examine published literature about the assessment. Research and clinical narratives provide important information about an assessment and its efficacy in a practice situation. Research in journals and reference books using the specific assessment can provide valuable information about the assessment and its usefulness. Additionally, the *Mental Measurement Yearbook* website (www.unl.edu/buros), the Educational Testing Service website (http://ets.org/tests/), and the Health and Psychosocial Instruments (HAPI) database (published by Behavioral Measurement Database Services; http://www.bmdshapi.com/mission.html) provide up-to-date and relevant information. These sources can give therapists a broader understanding of an assessment and its appropriate use. If there is little published information about the assessment, it would be wise for the therapist to seek out someone with more experience in evaluating people similar to the therapist's client to identify whether more appropriate assessments are available.

Once a therapist decides that a standardized assessment is appropriate and will provide useful data, he or she must develop competence in administering the assessment efficiently (Exhibit 6.1). The therapist should practice administering the assessment until he or she is competent in the mechanics of giving directions and manipulating materials. The therapist should also practice administering the assessment to several age-appropriate people without disabilities.

Occupational therapists must develop competence in interpreting the data appropriately by practicing scoring and interpreting the data. Administering and interpreting the assessment data for people without disabilities provide insight into the range and variety of responses for any test item.

EXHIBIT 6.1. DEVELOPING COMPETENCE IN ADMINISTERING AN EVALUATION

- Read the assessment manual thoroughly.
- Review published literature about the assessment.
- Become competent in administration of the assessment.
- Get feedback on your administration of the assessment from an experienced therapist.
- Have an experienced therapist review your interpretation of an assessment.
- Use a combination of standardized and nonstandardized assessments to get a complete picture of the client.
- Write an accurate report, including strengths and areas of concern.

Optimally, once a therapist has obtained basic competence in administering an assessment, he or she should have someone with experience observe him or her administering the assessment and provide feedback to help the therapist refine skills and confirm that the data collected are reliable and accurate.

Therapists often use a combination of standardized and **nonstandardized assessments** (e.g., observation, checklist, interviewing, screening) to identify a client's overall strengths and limitations. Reports from nonstandardized instruments and clinical observations should include comprehensive descriptions of specific behaviors or performance. Data from nonstandardized instruments can establish the client's baseline occupational performance. As with standardized assessments, therapists must establish competence in the administration and interpretation of nonstandardized assessments. Therapists can practice administering nonstandardized assessments by observing and interviewing people without disabilities and then interpreting the data to enhance skill development and competence.

After mastering administration of the assessment, occupational therapists need to become competent in writing up the results in a clear, concise summary. In this written summary, therapists present evidence and provide clear baseline data to either support the need for occupational therapy or illustrate that the client has adequate occupational performance. The written summary should give an overall perspective of the client's ability to function and participate in occupations. All written reports must be accurate and portray data honestly. Therapists should state accurately actual scores and resulting interpretations. Therapists should not overinterpret scores or make conclusions not supported by the data.

PREPARING THE ASSESSMENT ENVIRONMENT

Occupational therapists need to consider the **assessment environment**—both the physical environment and the psychological environment—when administering an assessment. Therapists are part of the environment, and they play an important role in ensuring that the environment is optimal for obtaining the appropriate data. The assessment environment should be conducive to eliciting real performance skills and abilities from the client. The environments needed for standardized and nonstandardized assessments, as discussed in the following sections, are often distinctly different. The type of assessment, and the occupational performance that therapists are trying to elicit, will determine the appropriate environmental setting for the assessment. The realities of the setting and the reimbursement system in which therapists work may also influence the assessment environment.

> Assessment environments can affect a client's test performance. Therapists must be aware that standardized assessments may have prescribed environments for the assessment. Such assessments performed in a controlled clinical environment can yield optimal performance.

Appropriate environments for nonstandardized assessments

Most nonstandardized assessments do not specify the characteristics of the testing environment. Although occupational therapists may take many different approaches, they can gain the most trustworthy information when they conduct the assessment in a natural environment. Therapists can tell more about a child's attention skills in the classroom if they observe the child's performance in the classroom rather than in a clinical environment. Similarly, therapists can gather more information about the home maintenance skills of a woman recovering from a cerebrovascular accident by observing her as she navigates her kitchen at home than by observing her performance in the adapted kitchen in the hospital. Therapists obtain more accurate and realistic information about the client's true occupational performance skills when they use the natural environment for a nonstandardized assessment. Similarly, clients are more likely to provide more information during an interview when they are in a comfortable, familiar setting. When therapists collect data in a more natural, comfortable environment, the data tend to be more trustworthy.

It is often not realistic for occupational therapists to administer an assessment in the natural environment. In these situations, therapists must be creative and develop an appropriate simulated situation to obtain valid information about clients' skills and abilities. An effective simulated environment should have similar characteristics to the natural environment. For example, to assess cooking skills, therapists would use an appropriate setting that has a stove, pots, and pans. To evaluate bathroom transfer skills, therapists should choose a setting as close as possible to the environment in the client's home. In addition, simulated environments may be helpful in increasing the client's comfort with the assessment process.

Sometimes therapists cannot create a simulated environment to match the natural environment. In this situation, they might strive for creating a simulated environment that is ergonomically correct for both them and the client to increase the comfort of both. Therapists should provide the client with a proper setting, appropriate table height, a footrest for the client's feet, and adherence to safety precautions. Proper ergonomics will increase the potential for optimal performance and comfort during the assessment.

Appropriate environments for standardized assessments

Standardized assessments compare the performance of a person against normative or criterion-referenced data. Some standardized assessments prescribe the type of testing environment. If such a prescription exists, therapists must follow it to achieve valid results. If the assessment manual provides no description of the assessment environment, therapists should create an environment that fosters the optimal performance of the client. In most situations, the natural environment may not be the best setting for standardized assessments, because it tends to have distractions that may impede optimal performance. Optimal assessment environments should be comfortable, private, well lit, distraction free, and quiet.

When choosing the environment, therapists must consider the requirements of the assessment. Some assessments require specific equipment; others require a large amount of space. Therapists should make sure that the environment and equipment for a particular assessment are available before administering the assessment so that the results are not compromised. When therapists administer a standardized assessment in a controlled clinical setting, it is assumed that the client will demonstrate optimal performance. If therapists administer a standardized assessment in a noisy room with distractions, the results would not be valid and the client may not demonstrate his or her optimal performance.

Psychological environment for assessment

From a psychological perspective, therapists should try to help the client become an active participant in the assessment process. Establishing rapport with the client increases the client's level of comfort, which is critical because a person tends to perform better when he or she is comfortable than when anxious. Therapists should start the evaluation of the client by introducing themselves. At this point, it is important to find out how the client would like to be addressed. Many older clients prefer to be called by their surnames and are offended when called by their first names, especially by someone who is younger. It is essential to build a rapport and not offend the client before the start of the evaluation.

Therapists should explain the assessment to the client and answer any questions that the client may have. This communication relieves anxiety and creates a more client-centered atmosphere. In addition, when the client knows the rationale for the assessment and what is expected of him or her while completing the assessment, the client is likely to be a more active participant in the process.

Therapists should also consider the client's personality and timetable when scheduling the assessment. Whenever possible, therapists should administer the assessment when the client is most alert and responsive. Therapists will obtain the best results when the client is alert and calm; however, they have to work within the constraints of the system and should recognize that a client's mood and frame of mind will affect the quality of information obtained from the assessment.

The Therapeutic Relationship

The **therapeutic relationship** often begins with the therapist evaluating the client. In most situations, building rapport with the client assists the evaluation process. In the developing relationship between the therapist and the client, the client is in a vulnerable position. The client depends on the therapist to explain the nature of the evaluation and the intervention process. In most cases, the client relates to this information not from a position of knowledge but from one of trust. The client needs to trust the therapist and to believe that the information the therapist provides is accurate and honest.

Additionally, the client needs to trust that the therapist has the required expertise to carry out the evaluation and intervention. Typically, people are more comfortable with those whom they feel they know. Rapport building between therapist and client helps to build comfort, and a basis for communication (Taylor, 2008) can help the client develop that trust. Once the client and therapist have established a relationship of trust, the therapist must fulfill his or her ethical responsibility to not abuse this trust and to provide expert care to the best of his or her capabilities.

Once the client develops trust in the therapist, the client may feel more able to reveal important aspects of his or her life, fears, and concerns. As the client reveals information that is more personal, the client becomes more aware of his or her own thoughts and feelings, enabling him or her to come to terms with personal reactions to illness, injury, or disability. Strong rapport between the client and therapist also can empower the client to feel comfortable enough to ask awkward or difficult questions that he or she might not have otherwise asked. Strong rapport also allows the client to reveal his or

her strengths and abilities. The information gained from this relationship helps the therapist to choose assessments that will meet the client's needs.

Ultimately, this information helps the therapist construct a client-centered evaluation and then a client-centered intervention. Throughout this process, the best interests of the client have to be the primary concern of the therapist. Thus, the therapist must be careful that the nature of the evaluation does not impede the establishment of rapport.

EVALUATOR AND SITUATIONAL ISSUES

Each therapist has specific strengths and limitations that influence his or her selection and use of assessments. Therapists' knowledge, manipulative motor skills, and analytic reasoning all influence how they select and use assessments. Most commonly, therapists gravitate toward assessments that they know better and are more comfortable with, or that are readily available, rather than researching the best assessment to use. Thus, an awareness of the factors that influence their choice of assessments can be useful for therapists as a reflective professional. Reflection on assessment practices may lead to a willingness to explore new or alternative assessments rather than repeatedly using one assessment. Therapists should choose assessments that are most appropriate for the client and his or her needs rather than one that they like and feel comfortable administering.

The therapists' mindset or attitude at the time of the assessment may influence the administration of an assessment. For example, a therapist who is not feeling well or is having a bad day may have difficulty attending to the tasks at hand. Therapists must maintain heightened awareness to prevent personal situations from influencing the evaluation. Thus, when administering and interpreting evaluation data, therapists must consider themselves as a possible intervening variable.

The environment in which occupational therapists administer the assessment also influences the data collected. Physical space, time of day, and distractions influence both the evaluator's and the client's performance and behaviors. When therapists administer an assessment in an environment that is less than ideal (e.g., that has distractions or inadequate space), they should consider how this environment might influence the resulting data from the assessment. If a therapist believes that the environment affected the data, then this information should be reflected in the evaluation summary.

Therapists must consider the whole evaluation experience. During an evaluation, the therapist and client form an exclusive relationship within a shared lived experience. Although the primary focus is on the client, the therapist has the responsibility of analyzing the data to develop an appropriate intervention plan for the client. The knowledge that the therapist gains about the client during the evaluation; the rapport that is established; and the feelings, both emotional and intuitive, of the therapist toward the client make the evaluation experience richer. When interpreting data, therapists should consider other factors about themselves as evaluator. Any recommendations for the intervention plan must reflect both what has been learned from the total evaluation and the shared experience.

The results of the evaluation can have an effect on the client's life. For example, when a child is evaluated in a school system, the results of the data may lead to a classification (e.g., class placement) that may follow that child for many years. In older adult clients, assessment data and the subsequent evaluation summary may determine whether the client is capable of living alone or must be in a supervised placement. Therapists must be certain of the integrity of the assessments and the accuracy of their data when writing evaluation summaries that may result in high-stakes decision making (Plake, 2002).

TYPES OF ERROR IN ASSESSMENT

Therapists make important decisions, such as intervention protocols and disposition, based on assessment data. Therefore, it is critical that evaluators try to minimize errors in the assessment process. **Errors** occur from the assessment itself in the form of item bias or are made by the rater who scores the test or the client's behavior or performance. Therapists should control for error in assessing a client for areas of strength and weakness to ensure that the data are an accurate reflection of the client's abilities. Choosing the best assessment available for the purpose, ensuring that therapists are competent in the administration of the assessment, and adequately

preparing the client for the tasks he or she needs to perform can keep errors to a minimum.

Item Bias

Item bias occurs when people of similar abilities perform differently on a given assessment or test item because of age, gender, ethnicity, cultural, socioeconomic, or other group differences. Items can be biased when they contain content or language that is unfamiliar to, or interpreted differently by, different groups (see Chapter 13, "Evaluating Special Populations").

When choosing an assessment, occupational therapists should know the group of people for whom the instrument was originally designed and whether it was validated on other specific groups of interest. For example, the SF–36 (Ware et al., 1993), one of the most widely used measures of quality-of-life health status, was originally designed as a generic health status measure and validated against large groups of people with various health problems. Because none of these groups contained people whose primary means of mobility was a wheelchair, the developers wrote questions about mobility for people who could walk. To make this instrument unbiased for people who use wheelchairs, the word *walk* was replaced with the word *go*. Item bias introduces errors into an assessment; people with equal abilities should be able to attain the same score. Therapists should research the populations used for standardization in the assessment manual or other literature about the assessment.

Therapists should always consider the psychometric properties of an instrument. **Classical test theory** relies on the psychometric concepts of reliability, validity, and responsiveness. This theory divides total scores into two components: (1) the true score and (2) a margin for error. This approach cannot separate individual ability from item difficulty.

Item response theory, frequently associated with educational and psychological assessments, has become more important to occupational therapy. Item response theory is sometimes referred to as *latent* (or *underlying*) *trait theory*. This theory, developed in the 1960s as a means of separating item difficulty from underlying individual abilities (respondent traits), involves a series of statistical procedures. This approach can also be used to evaluate whether items have equivalent meanings for different groups of respondents and whether items within a scale have the same response format (difficulty). A variant of item response theory, Rasch analysis, was used extensively in evaluating the underlying response format of the FIM™ (UDSMR, 1997). These analyses have shown that the FIM™ has three underlying scales: (1) self-care, (2) motor, and (3) cognitive functions (Cohen & Marino, 2000).

Although further discussion of psychometrics is beyond the scope of this chapter, the differences between classical test theory and item response theory and their implications for health care are discussed in detail in several publications (Chang & Reeve, 2005; Hays, Morales, & Reise, 2000; Schwartz & Rapkin, 2004). Item response theory analyses can also be used to determine whether raters are using the same standards of measurement and can assess whether physical functioning, as assessed by a particular measure, is based on the person's response, the properties of the questions asked, or the severity of a rater's observation.

Evaluator Variables

Rater bias or observer bias, another source of error in assessments, occurs when different evaluators disagree in their assessment of the same person (i.e., *interrater reliability*) or when the same evaluator scores the same person differently on repeated testing (i.e., *intrarater reliability*). If different therapists assessing the same person use different standards of measurement (i.e., if some are more lenient than others), results are not comparable across therapists. Therapists need special training and testing against a standard to eliminate this possibility. For this reason, some assessments, such as the AMPS, require that therapists being trained in usage are calibrated to ensure reliability of ratings.

A more subtle rater bias takes the form of coaching a client (Victor & Abeles, 2004). A therapist may coach, or "push," a client to perform beyond his or her normal capacity. Sometimes this situation occurs because the therapist believes that the client has more skills than he or she is showing during the evaluation. At other times, it occurs because the therapist and client have developed a rapport so that the therapist views that particular client with a subtle bias.

Other therapist factors also contribute to the validity of the assessment results. The therapeutic relationship, for example, contributes to the quality of a client's performance. A therapist facilitates the client's optimal performance when the client trusts the therapist and feels that the therapist is concerned about him or her.

Additionally, the amount of experience that a therapist has in administering and interpreting a specific assessment can influence the results. As therapists have more experience administering an assessment, they become more comfortable and skilled. When therapists first learn to administer an assessment, they usually focus on the mechanics of administering the test, giving less attention to the client's behaviors and performance. Practice and experience allow therapists to become skilled in the mechanics involved in administering an assessment.

Likewise, multiple experiences provide therapists with pragmatic knowledge about when to give breaks; therapists are sensitive to clients' moods and manipulate the environment to ensure best performance within the standardized procedures. A skilled therapist uses the evaluation process to establish a solid therapeutic relationship with the client and his or her significant others.

Test-Taker Variables

Many **test-taker variables** can affect an assessment. Coaching, tolerance for pain or discomfort, and fatigue can influence a client's scores on an assessment. In addition, the process of being evaluated may stress a client. A client realizes that the occupational therapist will make decisions about him or her using the data collected. The client is also conscious of the fact that information gathered using an assessment may determine the services he or she receives or the level of independence with which he or she will live. Even very young children seem to realize that they are being observed and judged during an evaluation.

Anxiety and stress are always important concerns. A moderate amount of anxiety can enhance performance in a testing situation; however, too little or too much anxiety can result in poor performance. Therefore, therapists should try to make clients at ease in the testing situation. Therapists should inform the client about what the assessment involves and what he or she will be asked to do. Moreover, therapists should outline the procedures the assessment will entail; this knowledge of the process can reduce client anxiety. Questioning a client about prior experiences with testing and his or her views on testing can provide information that will promote rapport and provide therapists with some insights about the client.

Additionally, anxiety, stress, depression, or paranoia may be concerns during the evaluation process. Should anxiety, stress, depression, or paranoia appear to interfere with the client's ability to complete the assessment, the therapist may have to adjust the evaluation plan. The therapist must continually reaffirm the purpose and goal of the occupational therapy evaluation.

Sometimes a client's beliefs and views about testing influence his or her behavior or performance. A client who does not care about the results or who does not understand the purpose of the assessment may put little effort into the process of evaluation. A client may not be motivated to perform well on an assessment when he or she believes that assessment scores will not reflect real abilities. When a client's beliefs or views about testing appear to be interfering with the collection of valid assessment data, the therapist needs to adjust the evaluation plan. The therapist may decide to report the limited data collected or may decide to explore other options with the client.

Clients' physical status can interfere with their ability to complete an assessment. During the administration of an assessment, the therapist might observe that the client has limited energy, activity tolerance, or physical stamina. The therapist should modify the evaluation plan to match the client's physical capacity to complete the assessment. Sometimes a therapist needs to postpone the assessment until the client has sufficient physical capacity.

Influence of Previous Testing Activities

A comprehensive evaluation usually involves several assessments, and the order in which they are administered needs to be planned. The activities involved in one assessment may influence performance on another assessment. Some testing demands may lead to fatigue or inability to attend to a task. Some assessments involve tasks that may excite a specific

client, and other assessments contain questions that may upset a client, so it is critical that therapists consider the order in which they administer specific assessments. Therapists must consider what they have learned about the client from the screening. The evaluation plan takes into account the demands that each assessment will put on the client.

At times, facility policies and third-party payers determine which evaluations are used and how they are administered. Therapists may have to adhere to these policies. However, in either situation, therapists should make the experience as comfortable as possible for the client and should indicate any demands that the evaluation is placing on the client in the ensuing report. Therapists have a dual responsibility, to both the client and the facility.

Performance vs. Capacity

Two components of a comprehensive evaluation are the client's performance and capacity. **Performance** is what a person can and does do in the real world, whereas **capacity** is what a person can do in a hypothetical or optimal situation (Spilker, 1990; Weingarden & Martin, 1989). Performance—what a person actually does in a given situation—provides a true picture of the person's functional status. Performance better reflects the assistance a person may need to function in the home environment, whereas capacity may be a better measure for determining the course and type of therapeutic intervention. Personal factors such as motivation and personality can influence performance. Coaching may influence capacity. During the administration of the assessment and when writing the report, occupational therapists need to consider what they have learned about the client's performance and capacity.

IMPLICATIONS FOR INTERVENTION

The evaluation process necessitates that occupational therapists obtain trustworthy data. To do so requires the accurate administration of assessments and candid observations of the client's performance and behaviors. Therapists derive a complete picture of the client through data from reliable and valid assessments, including observations and interviews with the client. The data are tempered by the therapists' judgment and clinical reasoning skills, often gained through experience. A thorough evaluation, combined with consultation with the client whenever possible, is a complex process, providing the foundation for the development of a sound intervention plan. An intervention plan developed from inadequate data or data that were not gathered in an organized and standardized manner is like a house built on an inadequate foundation. Just as a house may not stand without the proper infrastructure, the intervention plan may not be adequate or successful without a basis in strong evaluative data.

> It is impossible to analyze outcome data from interventions without reliable and valid evaluation data to serve as a baseline.

Identifying clear outcomes for the client requires the administration of a comprehensive and sound evaluation that provides clear baseline data. If clear baseline data do not exist, it is difficult to determine the extent of the client's progress. Therapists often are able to identify tasks that clients are able to do after a course of intervention, but without clear baseline data, it is often hard to determine exactly what has changed to account for the improved performance.

SUMMARY

Administering and interpreting an assessment require competence and skills. The role of an evaluator is one of the more daunting roles that occupational therapists undertake. Evaluation serves as the basis for understanding the client, determining his or her needs, and developing a plan for intervention. Performing an assessment requires skill and competence. Therapists must become familiar and competent in administering various assessments. They need to understand the psychometric data and protocols used in standardized tests and the nature of the various assessments. Moreover, therapists must consider the complexities of the assessments, the environment, and the potential variables that might affect the outcome of the assessments. Organizing and understanding all the necessary information for performing a comprehensive evaluation is like managing a three-ring circus—one must be aware of many factors at the same time to ensure a comprehensive and accurate evaluation.

QUESTIONS

1. Describe the process that an occupational therapist would use to develop skills in administering a standardized assessment. Why is such an extensive process necessary?
2. Select a criterion-referenced assessment. Review the manual and identify the elements used to determine mastery.
3. Select a norm-referenced assessment. Review the manual and identify the specific components used for the normative data.
4. Select an ipsative assessment. Review the manual and identify the specific components used to develop the test.
5. How would the environment influence the administration of a developmental assessment for a young child?
6. Consider your own life and self-observations. Can you identify any factors that would influence your ability to administer a standardized assessment? How?
7. Do you think it would be easier for you to administer a standardized assessment to a child or an adult? Why?

References

American Occupational Therapy Association. (2014). Occupational therapy practice framework: Domain and process (3rd ed.). *American Journal of Occupational Therapy, 68*(Suppl. 1), S1–S48. http://dx.doi.org/10.5014/ajot.2014.682006

Árnadóttir, G. (1990). *The brain and behavior: Assessing cortical dysfunction through tasks of daily living.* St. Louis: Mosby.

Ayres, A. J. (1989). *Sensory Integration and Praxis Tests.* Los Angeles: Western Psychological Services.

Berg, K., Wood-Dauphinee, S., Williams, J. I., & Gayton, D. (1989). Measuring balance in the elderly: Preliminary development of an instrument. *Physiotherapy Canada, 41*, 304–311.

Centers for Medicare and Medicaid Services. (2013). *Outcome and Assessment Information Set–C (OASIS–C).* Retrieved from http://www.cms.gov/Medicare/Quality-Initiatives-Patient-Assessment-Instruments/HomeHealthQualityInits/OASISC.html

Chang, C.-H., & Reeve, B. B. (2005). Item response theory and its applications to patient-reported outcomes measurement. *Evaluation and the Health Professions, 28,* 264–282.

Cohen, M. E., & Marino, R. J. (2000). The tools of disability outcomes research functional status measures. *Archives of Physical Medicine and Rehabilitation, 81*(Suppl. 2), S21–S29.

Coster, W., Deeney, T., Haltiwanger, J., & Haley, S. (1998). *School function assessment.* San Antonio: Psychological Corporation.

Cynkin, S., & Robinson, A. M. (1990). *Occupational therapy and activities health: Toward health through activities.* Boston: Little, Brown.

Fisher, A. G., Bryze, K., Hume, V., & Griswold, L. A. (2007). *School AMPS: School version of the assessment of motor and process skills* (2nd ed.). Ft. Collins, CO: Three Star Press.

Fisher, A. G., & Jones, K. B. (2012). *Assessment of motor and process skills* (7th ed., rev.). Ft. Collins, CO: Three Star Press.

Fleiss, J. L., Levin, B. A., & Paik, M. C. (2003). *Statistical methods for rates and proportions* (3rd ed.). Hoboken, NJ: Wiley.

Folstein, M. F., Folstein, S. E., McHugh, P. R., & Fanjiang, G. (2001). *Mini-mental state exam.* Odessa, FL: Psychological Assessment Resources.

Geist, R., Kielhofner, G., Basu, S., & Kafkes, A. (2002). *The Pediatric Volitional Questionnaire (PVQ), Version 2.0.* Chicago: University of Illinois at Chicago, Model of Human Occupation Clearinghouse, Department of Occupational Therapy.

Hays, R. D., Morales, L. S., & Reise, S. P. (2000). Item response theory and health outcomes measurement in the 21st century. *Medical Care, 38*(Suppl.), II28–II42.

Health Insurance Portability and Accountability Act of 1996, Pub. L. 104–191, 45 C.F.R. § 160, 164. Retrieved from http://www.hhs.gov/ocr/hipaa

Henry, A. D. (2000). *The Pediatric Interest Profiles: Surveys of play for children and adolescents.* San Antonio, TX: Therapy Skill Builders.

Individuals With Disabilities Education Improvement Act of 2004, Pub. L. 108–446, 20 U.S.C. § 1400 *et seq.*

Itzkovich, M., Elazar, B., Averbuch, S., & Katz, N. (2000). *Lowenstein Occupational Therapy Cognitive Assessment (LOTCA) battery manual* (2nd ed.). Pequannock, NJ: Maddak.

Kielhofner, G., Mallinson, T., Crawford, C., Nowak, M., Rigby, M., . . . Walens, D. (1998). *The Occupational Performance History Interview (OPHI–II), Version 2.0.* Chicago: University of Illinois at Chicago, Model of Human Occupation Clearinghouse, Department of Occupational Therapy.

Klein, R. M., & Bell, B. (1979). *The Klein–Bell ADL Scale manual.* Seattle: University of Washington, Educational Resources.

Kohlman-Thompson, L. (1992). *Kohlman evaluation of living skills* (3rd ed.). Rockville, MD: American Occupational Therapy Association.

Law, M., Baptiste, S., Carswell, A., McColl, M. A., Polatajko, H., & Pollock, N. (2005). *Canadian occupational performance measure* (4th ed.). Ottawa: CAOT Publications.

Mosey, A. C. (1986). *Psychosocial components of occupational therapy.* New York: Raven Press.

Nunnally, J. C., & Bernstein, I. H. (1994). *Psychometric theory* (3rd ed.). New York: McGraw-Hill.

Plake, B. S. (2002). Evaluating the technical quality of educational tests used for high-stakes decisions. *Measurement and Evaluation in Counseling and Development, 35,* 144–152.

Schwartz, C. E., & Rapkin, B. D. (2004). Reconsidering the psychometrics of quality of life assessment in light of response shift and appraisal. *Health and Quality of Life Outcomes, 2,* 16–26.

Spilker, B. (Ed.). (1990). *Quality of life assessments in clinical trials.* New York: Raven Press.

Taylor, R. (2008). *The intentional relationship: Occupational therapy and use of self.* Philadelphia: F. A. Davis.

Uniform Data System for Medical Rehabilitation. (1997). *Guide for the uniform data set for medical rehabilitation (Adult FIM™), Version 5.1.* Buffalo: State University of New York.

van den Brink, C. L., Tijhuis, M., Kalmijn, S., Klazinga, N. S., Nissinen, A., Giampaoli, S., . . . van den Bos, G. A. (2003). Self-reported disability and its association with performance-based limitation in elderly men: A comparison of three European countries. *Journal of the American Geriatrics Society, 51,* 782–788. http://dx.doi.org/10.1046/j.1365-2389.2003.51258.x

Victor, T. L., & Abeles, N. (2004). Coaching clients to take psychological and neuropsychological tests: A clash of ethical obligations. *Professional Psychology, Research and Practice, 35,* 373–379. http://dx.doi.org/10.1037/0735-7028.35.4.373

Wall, J. C., Bell, C., Campbell, S., & Davis, J. (2000). The Timed Get-Up-and-Go Test revisited: Measurement of the component tasks. *Journal of Rehabilitation and Development, 37,* 109–113.

Ware, J. E., Jr., Snow, K. K., Kosinski, M., & Gandek, B. (1993). *SF–36 Health survey: Manual and interpretation guide.* Boston: Health Institute.

Weingarden, S. I., & Martin, C. (1989). Independent dressing after spinal cord injury: A functional time evaluation. *Archives of Physical Medicine and Rehabilitation, 70,* 518–519.

CHAPTER 7

Contextual Evaluation to Support Participation

Kristie Patten Koenig, PhD, OTR/L, FAOTA

Highlights

- Influence of context on evaluation
- Evaluating a client's context
- Supporting participation through evaluation
- Contextual evaluation to support participation
- Client-centered, occupation-based evaluation
- Strengths-based approach to evaluation.

Key Words

Activity Card Sort
Bottom-up approach
Client-centeredness
Community Integration Questionnaire
Context
Craig Handicap Assessment and Reporting
    Technique
Function
Nonstandardized assessment of context
Participation

Personal context
Poles of function
School Function Assessment
Social context
Standardized assessment of context
Strengths-based assessment
Temporal context
Top-down approach
Virtual environment
Work Environment Impact Scale

The occupational therapist's assessment provides an understanding of the person as an occupational being and identifies his or her participation in life roles. A unique skill of the occupational therapist is to evaluate the whole client within his or her context. During an assessment, the therapist learns about the client's ability to engage and participate in home, school, workplace, and community life, which is done in part by looking at the client's functioning in occupations.

Evaluation must consider factors that empower and make possible clients' engagement and participation in positive health-promoting occupations (Wilcock & Townsend, 2008). According to the American Occupational Therapy Association's (AOTA; 2014) *Occupational Therapy Practice Framework: Domain and Process* (3rd ed.; *Framework*), the **context** includes a person's cultural, personal, temporal, virtual, physical, and social aspects. When considering these factors, therapists examine the variety of interrelated conditions within and surrounding the clients that influence their occupational performance.

Doucet and Gutman (2013) talk about two **poles of function.** In the **top-down approach,** *function* should be "defined and measured by the client's performance of life roles and meaningful activities that are a part of that role" (p. 7). The other pole would be considered a **bottom-up approach** to evaluation and looks at "specific discrete body impairments that affect larger daily life activities" (p. 7). The authors argue that function is defined by both poles. An evaluation that examines a client's context must use information from both poles to understand the influence of context and the environment on the client's participation.

> Actual occupational performance can be assessed only by examining the influence of a person's physical, cultural, personal, temporal, and social contexts on his or her personal and social environments.

INFLUENCE OF CONTEXT ON EVALUATION

When a therapist conducts an evaluation, context matters. *Context* refers to a variety of interrelated conditions that are within and surrounding the client and includes the client's external physical and social environments. It is within these surrounding environments that a client's daily life occupations occur (AOTA, 2014). Contexts are broadly and comprehensively defined in the *Framework* as cultural, personal, temporal, virtual, physical, and social. Table 7.1 defines these areas and, because the client is not limited to the individual level, outlines examples of context for the person, groups, and populations.

Some contexts are external to clients (e.g., virtual), some are internal to clients (e.g., personal), and some may have both external features and internalized beliefs and values (e.g., cultural). A client who has difficulty performing effectively in one context may be successful when the context is changed. The context within which the client engages in his or her occupations is unique for each client. A client's actual occupational performance can only be assessed when the therapist examines the influence of the physical, cultural, personal, temporal, and social contexts as well as personal and social environments. Further, a client's extent, amount, and quality of participation may be influenced by the context in which the occupational therapist administers the assessment (AOTA, 2014).

EVALUATING A CLIENT'S CONTEXT

Frequently, the assessment of context involves both standardized and nonstandardized assessments. Using both types of assessments provides a broad perspective of the client's lived world and is useful in understanding the client's strengths and the challenges the client may be facing. When deciding which assessments to use, the therapist must consider what kind of information would be most helpful in planning an occupation-based intervention.

Standardized assessments, when administered following established procedures, provide valid and reliable results. When using a **standardized assessment of context,** it is critically important that the therapist select an assessment that was standardized on an appropriate population with the same demographics and disabilities as the client being assessed. In occupational therapy, only a few standardized assessments exist that specifically address the context of a client. These assessments address personal context, temporal context, and the environment and will be discussed in the next sections, after which nonstandardized assessments are discussed.

Table 7.1. Contexts and Environments

Context and Environment	Definition	Example
Cultural	Cultural context includes customs, beliefs, activity patterns, behavioral standards, and expectations accepted by the society of which a client is a member. These beliefs and behavioral standards influence the client's identity and activity choices.	*Person:* A person delivering Thanksgiving meals to home-bound people *Group:* Employees marking the end of the work week with casual dress on Friday *Population:* People engaging in an afternoon siesta or high tea
Personal	"Features of the individual that are not part of a health condition or health status" (WHO, 2001, p. 17). Personal context includes age, gender, socioeconomic status, and educational status. Can also include group levels (e.g., volunteers, employees) and population levels (e.g., members of society).	*Person:* A 25-year-old unemployed man with a high school diploma *Group:* Volunteers working in a homeless shelter *Population:* Older drivers learning about community mobility options
Temporal	The experience of time as shaped by engagement in occupations. The temporal aspects of occupation that "contribute to the patterns of daily occupations" are "the rhythm . . . tempo . . . synchronization . . . duration . . . and sequence" (Larson & Zemke, 2004, p. 82; Zemke, 2004, p. 610). Includes stages of life, time of day or year, duration, rhythm of activity, or history.	*Person:* A person retired from work for 10 years *Group:* Annual fundraising campaign *Population:* People celebrating Independence Day on July 4
Virtual	Environment in which communication occurs by means of airwaves or computers and an absence of physical contact. Includes simulated or real-time or near-time existence of an environment via chat rooms, email, videoconferencing, or radio transmissions; remote monitoring via wireless sensors; or computer-based data collection.	*Person:* Friends who text message each other *Group:* Members who participate in a video conference, a telephone conference call, instant messaging, or interactive board use *Population:* Virtual community of gamers
Physical	Natural and built nonhuman environment and the objects in them. Natural environment includes geographic terrain, sensory qualities of environment, plants, and animals. Built environment and objects include buildings, furniture, tools, or devices.	*Person:* A person's house or apartment *Group:* Office building or factory *Population:* Transportation system

(Continued)

Table 7.1. Contexts and Environments *(Cont.)*

Context and Environment	Definition	Example
Social	Is constructed by presence, relationships, and expectations of persons, groups, or populations. Availability and expectations of significant persons, such as spouse, friends, and caregivers. Relationships with persons, groups, or populations. Relationships with systems (e.g., political, legal, economic, institutional) that are influential in establishing norms, role expectations, and social routines.	*Person:* Friends, colleagues *Group:* Occupational therapy students conducting a class get-together *Population:* People influenced by a city government

Note. WHO = World Health Organization.

From "Occupational Therapy Practice Framework: Domain and Process," 3rd Edition, by American Occupational Therapy Association, 2014, *American Journal of Occupational Therapy, 68*(Suppl. 1), p. S28. Copyright © 2014 by the American Occupational Therapy Association. Used with permission.

Standardized Assessments

Standardized assessments that evaluate context focus on a client's personal context, temporal context, and the environment.

Standardized assessments of the personal context

Personal context refers to demographic features of the person, such as age, gender, socioeconomic status, and educational level that are not part of a health condition (World Health Organization [WHO], 2001). The personal context has a direct influence on assessment results. For example, age, educational status, and gender can affect performance, which interacts with the health condition. This interaction is illustrated in a study by Law and colleagues (2006), who assessed participation of 427 children with health and developmental problems, approximately half of whom had cerebral palsy. This large survey showed that children with physical disabilities participated extensively in informal activities, particularly recreational, social, and self-improvement activities. Their participation in formal activities, such as sport teams or choir, was lower and less intense. They also participated less in active physical activities.

For standardized assessments, validity studies are often associated with the personal context to establish discriminative validity. One example is the study by Davies, Soon, Young, and Clausen-Yamaki (2004) that compared students with three types of disabilities (autism, learning disabilities, and traumatic brain injury) on the **School Function Assessment (SFA;** Coster, Deeney, Haltiwanger, & Haley, 1998). Scores on the SFA differed for students with autism and learning disabilities. Students with autism scored much lower on cognitive and behavioral tasks than students with learning disabilities or traumatic brain injury, and the cognitive and behavioral scale was the most accurate predictor of disability across the different groups of students.

Known groups differ on adult measures as well. The **Activity Card Sort (ACS;** Baum & Edwards, 2008) is a standardized assessment that evaluates an adult's amount and level of involvement in various activities, including instrumental activities, low-demand leisure activities, high-demand leisure activities, and social activities.

Another validity study conducted in Israel of healthy adults, healthy older adults, spouses or caregivers of people with Alzheimer's disease, people with multiple sclerosis, and stroke survivors found that the ACS differentiated among these groups (Katz, Karpin, Lak, Furman, & Hartman-Maeir, 2003). Groups differed greatly for activity level and individual activity areas. In healthy adults, participation changed with aging in social–cultural and high physical leisure areas. For caregivers of people with Alzheimer's disease, participation became restricted in leisure areas. For persons with multiple sclerosis, the changes were manifested in instrumental activities of daily living (IADLs) and high physical leisure activities; for persons with stroke, all activity areas were affected. These are all powerful examples of how context impacts assessment.

According to the *Framework,* the personal context includes gender (AOTA, 2014). Gender differences are seen in the **Community Integration Questionnaire (CIQ;** Willer, Ottenbacher, & Coad, 1994) that was developed as an outcome measure for persons with brain injury. CIQ results revealed some interesting relationships among client factors, context, occupations, and community integration in clients with head injury. For example, after rehabilitation, women tend to have greater home integration, and men tend to have higher productivity.

Age also matters. Young clients with spinal cord injury tend to be more integrated in terms of social and productivity dimensions, whereas older clients have more limited community integration (Dijkers, 1997; Ritchie, Wright-St. Clair, Keogh, & Gray, 2014).

Standardized assessments of the temporal context

Temporal context includes stages of life, time of day or year, duration, rhythm of activity, or history. Depending on the stage of life one is in, results with assessments will vary and may even measure different constructs. In a factor analysis study of the first edition of the ACS (Baum & Edwards, 2001), Sachs and Josman (2003) confirmed the original factors with slight variation for older adults and young adults (students). The ACS items for the older adults clustered into four categories: (1) IADLs, (2) leisure, (3) demanding leisure, and (4) maintenance activities. For the young adults, the items clustered into five categories: (1) IADLs, (2) leisure, (3) demanding leisure, (4) maintenance, and (5) social recreational activities. This analysis of construct validity suggests that the ACS measures slightly different constructs based on personal characteristics of the client.

The **Craig Handicap Assessment and Reporting Technique (CHART;** Whiteneck, Charlifue, Gerhart, Overholser, & Richardson, 1992) was originally developed to assess community participation in people with spinal cord injury and was expanded to include people with cognitive impairment. It has been demonstrated that CHART scores are affected by contextual factors such as age, race or ethnicity, education, and occupation at the time of evaluation (Hall, Kijkers, Whiteneck, Brooks, & Krause, 1998). Approximately one-third to one-half of the variance in CHART subscale scores is accounted for by age. Scores decrease with increasing age on all subscales except for the Economic Self-Sufficiency subscale. Although the CHART's scores are based on normative data and it only measures objective aspects of participation, the CHART is a well-established measure of community integration in people with disabilities.

Context clearly affects the performance on an assessment. The environment where occupations occur and how the client interacts with the personal and social environments also have a substantial effect on the evaluation process and individual assessments.

Standardized assessments of the environment

Assessments of the environment relevant to the occupational therapist are examinations of the interaction between person and environment that enables accomplishment of occupations. The goal of most environmental measures is to determine whether the environment constrains or supports a person's occupational performance and what can be adapted or changed to enhance that person's performance. These assessments give the occupational therapist information about what environmental elements enable or interfere with a person's participation in life activities as the therapist determines what services the client may need. For example, a parental report of environmental barriers to participation may highlight the importance of home-based occupational therapy intervention to optimize participation (Law et al., 2013). By modifying or adapting the environment, an occupational therapist can improve a client's participation and decrease levels of caregiver assistance.

Contextual assessments for a child often emphasize the role of the physical and social environments in promoting skill development. The goal of many assessments of a child's contexts is to determine the transactions between the environment and child. These assessments emphasize the elements of the context known to promote development (e.g., parent support and responsiveness, availability of toys and learning materials). Positive data from assessments of a child's context are often predictive of the child's future performance (Bradley, Corwyn, McAdoo, & Coll, 2001).

In contrast, adult assessments emphasize the safety and accessibility of the physical environment, workplace supports, or social supports within a community context. In much of occupational therapy practice, contexts are informally assessed, with a focus on understanding the supports and constraints available within the environment. Few assessments of the environment have been developed, perhaps because environments are dynamic and complex, and change rapidly over time and space. It often is difficult to determine how a person will move through environments and how contexts will change over time.

The environmental assessments that have been developed tend to focus on one environment (e.g., home, work) and tend to focus on a single problem (e.g., physical access, fall prevention, social participation). Assessments of the home environment have focused on barriers to function, particularly for persons using wheelchairs or mobility devices, and safety for older adults who are at risk for falling or other injuries. These assessments often identify barriers and problems that need to be modified to promote optimal function and safety (Wahl, Fänge, Oswald, Gitlin, & Iwarsson, 2009).

Measures of a person's work environment have been developed to identify potential environmental modifications that can increase safety, access, and optimal function. They assess the worker's perception of the social environment, including peer and supervisor support. Research has shown that a supportive work environment is predictive of employee productivity and well-being (Billings & Moos, 1982; Dorman, 2009). The social environment is highlighted in this research and shows how important it is to consider both physical and social environments.

For example, the **Work Environment Impact Scale** (Corner, Kielhofner, & Lin, 1997) assesses the experience of persons with disabilities in their workplace. Both physical and social factors are considered, including transportation, safety, lighting, time, equipment, tools, sound, and architecture. In addition, social environment is assessed, including attitudes, social climate, social support, communication, and expectations. Table 7.2 presents examples of contextual assessments that consider the physical and social environments.

Nonstandardized Assessments of a Client's Contexts

To develop a client's comprehensive occupational profile, the therapist will use nonstandardized assessment strategies to learn about the client's personal lived experience and the context of his or her life. Using observation, interviews, photographs, and engagement in an art activity to conduct a **nonstandardized assessment of context** can provide the therapist rich, insightful information about the client's life. Observations offer the opportunity to see the client interact with others in context. Interviews allow the client to express his or her perceptions and feelings about life. Viewing photographs offers a glimpse into the client's current and past life. Finally, drawing or painting a picture can facilitate the client's expression of his or her context. For example, a child's picture of his or her family or home can provide the therapist useful information that the child is unable to express verbally.

Although the occupational profile typically is used to identify those occupations that are meaningful to the person, it can also be used to explore context. The therapist can ask the client how the environment of his or her life supports or hinders those occupations. Further, the therapist can explore the client's social context and obtain the client's view about the role social context plays in his or her life. It is up to the therapist to creatively ask questions in a nonthreatening manner to determine the role of context in the client's life and learn how it may support active participation. Nonstandardized assessments that evaluate context focus on the personal context, environment, cultural context, social context, and virtual environment.

Nonstandardized assessment of the personal context

In the *Framework*, personal context includes qualities that are not part of the client's health condition or health status (AOTA, 2014). During an interview or from the chart, the therapist can get information about the client's age and socioeconomic

Table 7.2. Sample Assessments of Context

Child Assessments	Purpose	Context
Home Observation for the Measurement of the Environment (Bradley & Caldwell, 1984; Caldwell & Bradley, 1984)	Four versions assess home context of infants, young children, school-aged children, and adolescents	*Physical:* Lighting, safety, equipment, and toys *Social:* Interpersonal relationships, social support, family organization, community life, and use of services
Test of Environmental Supportiveness (Bundy, 1999; Skard & Bundy, 2008)	Assesses supportiveness of the environment for play for children 18 months to 15 years	*Physical:* Safety, objects, accessible space *Social:* Caregiver support, availability and competence of peers

Adult Assessments	Purpose	Context
Housing Enabler (Iwarsson & Slaug, 2001)	Measures physical or architectural barriers with a primary focus on home accessibility of older persons	*Physical:* Indoor and outdoor housing barriers that would be a safety concern *Social:* Not assessed
Safety Assessment of Function and the Environment for Rehabilitation–Health Outcome Measurement and Evaluation (Chiu, Oliver, Marshall, & Letts, 2001)	Assesses a person's ability to function safely in the home with 14 safety domains	*Physical:* Safety hazards, mobility, ADLs, and IADLs *Social:* Living situation, communication, family support
Westmead Home Safety (Clemson, 1997)	Identifies fall hazards in the home environment of older adults	*Physical:* Fall hazards *Social:* Not assessed
Work Environment Impact Scale (Corner, Kielhofner, & Lin, 1997)	Measures the fit between the client and aspects of the environment	*Physical:* Accessibility, arrangement, design, comfort, or sensory qualities *Social:* Time and productivity demands, work schedules, coworker interactions, supervisor communication, and client and customer interactions
Work Environment Scale (Moos, 1994)	Measures worker's perceptions of a workplace's social environment and its impact on morale	*Physical:* Not assessed *Social:* Interpersonal interaction, social communication exchanges, cohesion among workers, friendship and support provided by coworkers and management

Note. ADLs = activities of daily living; IADLs = instrumental activities of daily living.

status. Information about the client's gender identity is more difficult to obtain. Although observation may be a beginning point, information about gender identification is best obtained through a guided conversation with the client. Although some questions can be answered straightforwardly, others may require the therapist to probe gently into the client's self-identity. The therapist must be open to ideas, practices, and preferences that are different from his or her own. The therapist must conduct the interview in a sensitive and nonjudgmental manner to get accurate information.

Nonstandardized assessment of the environment

Obviously, the best way to understand a client's environment is to observe the physical environment and the objects within it. If this is not possible, the therapist can obtain this information by having the client describe his or her nonhuman world. When interviewing clients, it is critical that the therapist ask them to describe their world, including the geographic terrain, plants, and animals (AOTA, 2014). The therapist can also ask clients to share photographs, if available, of their lives. With clients' permission, the therapist can also ask significant others in the clients' lives to share photographs.

Nonstandardized assessment of the cultural context

A client's culture is unique to that person and how he or she practices the customs, beliefs, standards, and expectations of the culture with which he or she identifies. Although a client may describe himself or herself as a member of a specific culture, the practices of the client may be unique to his or her situation. Again, observation is a good beginning point. However, the therapist needs to be careful not to make generalizations based on observation alone. As with personal context, the most effective method of obtaining information is directly from the client. During the interview, the therapist should let the client describe his or her cultural practices. The therapist can sensitively probe for information that is important for developing an appropriate intervention plan. Again, the therapist must be open to ideas, practices, and preferences that are different from his or her own.

Nonstandardized assessment of the social context

A person's social context consists of people with whom the client interacts. The **social context** is constructed around the significant others and important activities in the person's life. If possible, observing the client's interactions with significant others (e.g., spouse, friends, caregivers) provides insightful information about the client's social life. It is also helpful to ask about important occupations that may be done in the social context of groups or clubs.

Nonstandardized assessment of the virtual environment

The **virtual environment** is becoming increasingly important in people's lives. The virtual environment includes communication by means of airwaves or computers with no physical contact with another person (AOTA, 2014). Some examples of these interactions are emails, social networking sites, chat rooms, and videoconferencing. When interviewing the client, the therapist can obtain useful information about the client's participation. Further, the therapist can explore how important participation in the virtual environment is to the client.

> A comprehensive occupational profile includes information obtained from nonstandardized assessments about a client's personal, cultural, social, and virtual contexts. Nonstandardized assessments help the therapist understand the client's personal lived experience and the context of his or her life.

SUPPORTING PARTICIPATION THROUGH EVALUATION

There is an adage in most testing that what we evaluate or assess is what we will treat or, in education, what students will study. If the occupational therapy evaluation does not address participation in life through engagement in occupations but only focuses on the bottom-up pole at the impairment level, chances are that impairment is what the occupational therapy intervention will address. Participation must be central to the evaluation process to successfully fulfill occupational therapy's charge to facilitate engagement and participation in occupations in context.

Participation means sharing with others, taking part in an activity, or being involved in a life situation. Participation in life's activities is an important aspect of health and quality of life. Law (2002) described its importance: "Through participation, we acquire skills and competencies, connect with others and our communities, and find purpose and meaning in life" (p. 640). Participation in occupations is a central concept to occupational therapists and defines an essential goal of intervention.

WHO (2001) defines *participation* as involvement in a life situation and considers it to be a key indicator of health. WHO recognizes the complexity of participation by stressing the interrelationships among body function and structure, activity, personal factors, and environment characteristics. A person's participation does not occur in isolation and must be considered in relation to his or her abilities and the environment in which he or she lives. It can be assessed only by considering the contexts in which people live, work, and play.

Participation implies engagement in a life situation or life activity, but it does not always mean performing the activity. For example, a person can meaningfully participate in an activity by observing that activity, partially performing it, performing it in an adapted way, or directing others to perform it. All of these types of performing imply "engaged involvement," which is the essence of participation. Key aspects of participation that relate to health are that the person can make decisions about participating, finds the activity to be meaningful, and participates in opportunities that are consistent with his or her life goals.

By definition, assessments of participation consider the contexts of a person's activities, recognizing that the physical, social, temporal, and cultural context can support or constrain participation. When participation is measured, the concept of environment is dynamic, varying across time and space and changing with activities and roles. The environment has an essential role in determining the quality, frequency, and level of a person's participation in life activities.

Because the environment can contribute to disability, comprehensive evaluation to understand the basis for disability and to plan intervention includes assessment of the environment. In the *International Classification of Functioning, Disability and Health (ICF*; WHO, 2001), *environment* is broadly defined to include physical, social, cultural, economic, and organizational components. In the *Framework* (AOTA, 2014), environment and its various components are recognized under the broad term of *context.*

A majority of occupational therapy measures assess the client's occupational performance (i.e., how a person completes an activity or task). Measures of participation are challenging to conceptualize, given the dynamic and evolving nature of participation. Scholars (e.g., Law, 2002; Law, Dunn, & Baum, 2005) have discussed the difficulty

of measuring participation. It is not only a broad concept but also a multidimensional and complex one. Participation measures need to consider not only the person, environment, and occupation but also the interactions of these variables. Rather than defining specific attributes of the person, his or her occupations, and relevant environments, participation assessments have to examine the transaction of these variables.

It can be argued that measures of participation have certain characteristics. Scholars have attempted to define the characteristics of this broad, multidimensional concept and have made assumptions about how to measure it. The field has yet to reach consensus on how to measure participation (Coster & Khetani, 2008; Law, 2002; Law et al., 2005); nevertheless, in recent years, several participation measures have been published, and sample measures are presented in Table 7.3.

Defining characteristics of existing participation measures include that they

- Use self-report or caregiver report,
- Focus on a person's everyday occupations or common occupations,
- Consider a person's natural environment or multiple environments,
- Focus on activities that are goal-directed, and
- Assess the perceived importance of participation and associated feelings of well-being or satisfaction.

Self-Report or Caregiver Report

Measures of participation are most often self-reported scales that define participation across environments and time. Coster and Khetani (2008) discussed the temporal and spatial aspects of participation that are inherent in the meaning of the term. Through self-report or caregiver report, participation is assessed as a personal and individualized experience. By using self-report, the evaluator gains a perspective on the opportunities and environmental supports available to the client and how he or she participates in those opportunities.

A variety of methods have been developed to elicit self-report. Many instruments, such as the Life Habits Assessment (Fougeyrollas et al., 1998) and the

Table 7.3. Sample Measures of Participation

Child Assessment	Purpose	How Does It Measure Participation?
Children's Assessment of Participation and Enjoyment/ Preferences for Activities of Children (CAPE/PAC; King et al., 2004)	Measures how a child (with or without disabilities) participates in everyday activities outside of schoolwork or home chores in the context of the natural environment (CAPE) and their preference for doing activities (PAC)	Examines how a child participates, including diversity (i.e., number of activities done), intensity (i.e., frequency of participation), and enjoyment of activities. The CAPE reflects participation in the following areas: • Formal and informal activities • Recreation • Active physical • Social • Skill-based • Self-improvement.
School Function Assessment (Coster, Deeney, Haltiwanger, & Haley, 1998)	Measures a child's participation in academic and social school-related activities	Assesses participation, assistance and adaptations to perform tasks, and school-related performance in physical, cognitive, and behavioral tasks. Includes sections on level of participation in the following school activity settings: • General or special education classroom • Playground • Transportation to and from school • Bathroom • Transition to and from class • Mealtimes.
Participation and Environment Measure in Children and Youth (Coster, Law, & Bedell, 2010)	Examines environmental impact on children's participation within home, school, and community settings for 5- to 17-year-olds with and without disabilities	Identifies numbers of activities done, frequency, level of involvement, number of activities in which change is desired, and two summary scores of environmental barriers and supports on participation in the following settings: • Home • School • Community.
Adult Assessment	**Purpose**	**How Does It Measure Participation?**
Activity Card Sort (Baum & Edwards, 2008)	Identifies levels of occupation and activity participation to develop intervention goals and measure outcome of intervention	Evaluates an adult's amount and level of involvement in various activities, including • Instrumental activities • Low-demand leisure activities • High-demand leisure activities • Social activities.

(Continued)

Table 7.3. Sample Measures of Participation *(Cont.)*

Child Assessment	Purpose	How Does It Measure Participation?
Craig Handicap Assessment and Reporting Technique (Whiteneck, Charlifue, Gerhart, Overholser, & Richardson, 1992)	Assesses community participation in people with spinal cord injury as well as people with cognitive impairments, including persons with traumatic brain injury, stroke, and multiple sclerosis	Asks the client to indicate time spent performing each task in the following domains or roles: • Physical independence • Mobility • Occupation • Social integration • Economic self-sufficiency.
Late-Life Function and Disability Instrument (Haley et al., 2002; Jette et al., 2002)	Assesses of physical function and disability of community-dwelling older adults, measuring functional limitations (i.e., inability to perform activities encountered in daily routines) and disability (i.e., inability to participate in major life tasks and social roles)	Function Scale assesses participation in 32 physical activities, and Disability Scale evaluates self-reported limitations in and frequency of performing 16 major life tasks. The client reports how limited he or she feels in doing a particular task and how often he or she does that task.
Life Habits Assessment (Fougeyrollas et al., 1998)	Measures social participation, life habits, and daily activities of people with disabilities	Appraises the quality of social participation by judging the difficulty of carrying out life habits in the following areas: • Daily activities • Nutrition • Fitness • Personal care • Communication • Housing • Mobility • Social roles • Responsibility • Interpersonal relationships • Community life • Education • Employment • Recreation.
London Handicap Scale (Jenkinson, Mant, Carter, Wade, & Winner, 2000)	Measures global function and disability in adults with chronic, multiple, or progressive diseases	Rates a person's perception of independence from no disadvantage to extreme disadvantage in the areas of • Physical independence • Social integration • Economic self-sufficiency.
Community Integration Questionnaire (Willer, Ottenbacher, & Coad, 1994)	Rates home, work, and community activities that require both physical and cognitive performance to measure intervention outcome for persons with brain injury	Examines frequency of the activities performed and whether done jointly in the following areas: • Home integration • Social integration • Productivity in work, school, and volunteer activities.

Late Life Function and Disability Instrument (Haley et al., 2002; Jette et al., 2002), use a questionnaire that can be administered as an interview or in pencil-and-paper format. Other measures (e.g., ACS) use a card-sort activity in which the client identifies the amount and level of involvement in activities as depicted on the cards. Measures tend to be organized by activities, occupations, or roles and rate the frequency of participation, the supports necessary to participate, how well a person performs in that role or occupation, satisfaction with participation, and restrictions or limitations.

Everyday Occupations and Roles

Occupational therapy has traditionally categorized occupations as activities of daily living (ADLs), IADLs, rest and sleep, education, work, play, leisure, and social participation (AOTA, 2014). As noted by Coster and Khetani (2008), measures of child participation are often organized by role or life situations. Examples of life situations defined in the *ICF* (WHO, 2001) include recreation and leisure, engagement in play, education, self-care, and work. The occupational therapist also recognizes the importance of assessing the subjective experience embedded in these occupations and roles.

The meaning that a person gives to an occupation is essential to determining how it matches his or her life roles. For example, cooking may be leisure to one person, work to another, and an IADL to a third person. In evaluating participation, perception of the experience can be as important as actual performance. For example, a family may rate a child's performance as independent when it is actually supported by equipment, adapted methods, and physical assistance. When these adapted methods are integrated into a family's everyday life, they often consider them as natural and routine and would not consider the child's dependence on supports to be a lack of independence.

Natural Contexts and Multiple Environments

The context is of particular interest when evaluating participation because different environments can support, enhance, or restrict participation. When an assessment does not specify the context, the occupational therapist should consider multiple environments to rate assessment items because performance can change in different environments.

Child measures of participation will often include home, school, and community sections, with the realization that occupational performance and participation may differ by setting. A client who has difficulty performing effectively in one context may be very successful when the context is changed (AOTA, 2014).

Adult participation is assessed by examining how a person functions in his or her natural context, with emphasis on essential daily living activities, including ADLs, social participation, and mobility. Attempting to assess in the natural context makes an accurate indication of participation more likely. Simulated task performance in a clinic kitchen or hospital bathroom may not be indicative of performance in the natural context.

Goal-Directed Activities

Because participation in life activities is goal directed and purposeful, participation measures consider the purpose of activity to the person. A person's goal in a specific activity (e.g., swimming, work) determines both the meaning of participation and the intervention plan. For example, if the goal of going to the movies is to be with friends, then independent mobility in the theater or understanding the movie's plot may not be important aspects of participating in this activity. Activities such as housekeeping are perceived to be work to some people or leisure to those who derive great pleasure from maintaining a clean home. A child's learning in school can be work and lead to a career, but it is also social activity that enables learning about society and culture unrelated to work as an adult.

The meaning a person assigns to an activity may determine whether that activity is a desired or appropriate focus for a rehabilitation program. For example, when a mother with multiple sclerosis finds that baking cookies with her 10-year-old daughter has become difficult, it is important to know whether baking is valued as a leisure pursuit or as a time for the mother–daughter relationship. If baking is an important and desired activity, the

> The occupational therapist inquires about, rather than assumes, a client's goals or purposes in desired activities to fully interpret their meaning and value to the client.

therapist can adapt the techniques to bake; if mother–daughter interaction is most important, the therapist can recommend a substitute joint activity.

Well-Being and Satisfaction

Participation in meaningful occupations has a direct and substantial effect on health and quality of life (Coster & Khetani, 2008; Law, 2002; Wilcock, 1998). Most measures of participation include personal satisfaction, similar to measures of quality of life. The key difference between measures of quality of life and of participation is that most scales that rate quality of life do not specify certain occupations or human functions. In contrast, participation measures link satisfaction and well-being to a client's involvement in specific activities.

CONTEXTUAL EVALUATION TO SUPPORT PARTICIPATION

Occupational performance is defined by Forsyth et al. (2014) as doing a task related to participation, so how can contextual evaluation be used to assess participation? How does the occupational therapist evaluate the varied contexts and understand their effects on occupations? More importantly, how can a contextual evaluation support participation by revealing what the barriers and supports are in the environment?

By adopting a client-centered, strength-based, and occupation-based approach to evaluation and choosing assessments that consider the contextual factors that support or hinder participation, the occupational therapist can develop a more informed understanding of the conditions that are necessary for the client to "achieve health, well-being, and participation in life through engagement in occupation" (AOTA, 2014, p. S4). This stance cannot be an afterthought to the evaluation process. Including participation in baseline measures during the evaluation process can help the occupational therapist focus on this unique area of practice (Kessler & Egan, 2012).

CLIENT-CENTERED, OCCUPATION-BASED EVALUATION

Client-centeredness is a defining principle of occupational therapy practice. This principle guides how an occupational therapist evaluates performance strengths and concerns, selects goals, plans interventions, and evaluates the effects of an intervention program. This principle has been a defining construct of occupational therapy over time (Yerxa, 1967), across international borders (AOTA, 2014; Canadian Association of Occupational Therapists [CAOT], 1997; Wilcock, 1998), and across areas of practice (Law & Mills, 1998). Elements of a client-centered approach include demonstrating respect for clients, involving clients in decision making, advocating with and for clients in meeting their needs, and recognizing clients' experience and knowledge (CAOT, 1997).

In a client-centered evaluation, the occupational therapist assesses the client's ability to engage in meaningful occupations and the interplay among performance, activity demands, and context (Rogers & Holm, 2009).

> A comprehensive occupational therapy evaluation consists of an occupational profile and analysis of occupational performance. The occupational profile is a critical part of the client-centered evaluation to fully understand the client. Client-centered evaluation that evaluates strengths and challenges is the first step of a contextual evaluation.

A primary goal of evaluation is to understand the person as an occupational being. Through evaluation of a client's participation in work, school, leisure, and play in natural physical, social, and cultural contexts, the therapist develops an occupational profile to use in establishing goals and in framing and interpreting further analysis of performance. Based on data from the occupational profile and other assessments, the occupational therapist develops intervention goals and strategies that enhance the client's participation in the occupations most important to him or her (Law, 2002).

Occupation-based intervention is a highly individualized process because it incorporates the unique perspective of the client, the client's occupational performance problems, and the performance context (Rogers & Holm, 2009). These principles—the use of a client-centered approach, the understanding of a person as an occupational being, and the focus on the client's participation in life roles—have important implications for the evaluation process, the types of assessments selected, the methods used to assess clients, and the interpretation of evaluation results.

A client-centered approach recognizes that the client's perspective is the most important one in the intervention process. Almost always, the client and his or her caregivers have the most accurate understanding of his or her strengths, limitations, and priorities. Client-centered evaluation includes the client's perceptions and concerns about performance, roles, interests, goals, and priorities.

A client-centered approach counters the traditional medical model, in which an expert determines a diagnosis and prescribes a treatment based on that diagnosis. In the traditional medical model, the client is the recipient of the treatment but is not actively involved in making treatment decisions. On the basis of the client's diagnosis and performance deficits, professionals determine the treatment approach. In such an approach, it becomes unlikely that treatment goals meet the client's interests and concerns. Because the traditional medical approach promotes passivity and dependency, it contradicts the goal of the occupational therapist that clients actively engage and fully participate in work, daily living, and leisure roles.

In a client-centered evaluation, the occupational therapist helps the client identify and prioritize the occupations and activities that become the focus of intervention. By determining with the client what occupations are most relevant to him or her, the therapist can design meaningful interventions. When the therapist facilitates the client's self-direction and values the importance of the client's self-identified goals, the client becomes invested in the intervention program and is motivated to achieve the outcomes. As a result, outcomes are likely to be more satisfying and important to the client. In addition, the probability that outcomes are successfully achieved increases (Law, 1998).

A client-centered approach supports the client's perception that he or she can make decisions about intervention and can problem solve how to adapt activities to enhance participation. This approach encourages the client's sense of self-determinism and promotes his or her confidence in making decisions and directing therapy services toward his or her own goals. The three main psychological needs that are at the core of self-determination theory—(1) autonomy,

(2) competence, and (3) relatedness (Ryan & Deci, 2000)—can be fostered in a client-centered, strength-based approach to evaluation. Many clients who receive occupational therapy have disabilities that endure throughout their lifetimes; therefore, promoting and respecting clients' self-determinism can encourage them to independently manage services and direct the personal assistance they need.

STRENGTHS-BASED APPROACH TO EVALUATION

An evaluation of a client's context must examine client's strengths, motives, habits, and skills. These assessments are by nature strength based, but a **strengths-based assessment** goes a step further and looks at what about the disability experience can help shape occupations. As Dunn et al. (2013) stated,

> It is even more important to consider a strengths approach when people have obvious challenges. Complexities are just another feature of a person's overall characteristics; for example, having severe spasticity likely means a person moves slowly and without precision; it might also mean that the person can sit quietly and pay attention to what is going on in the room. When we point out what is helpful about a person's characteristics, we acknowledge that the disabilities do not define them as human beings. We might describe a person as "intellectually disabled" or as "working best with structure and routines in place." By stating what the person can do, we set the stage for fostering participation on that person's terms. (p. 1)

A person's spasticity is irrelevant when sitting quietly to watch TV but may become a challenge when the person tries to change the channel. The context and how it can support participation are the crux of a strength-based approach. Evaluation and interventions can focus on adaptations to support this preferred activity. Knowing the impact of the person's spasticity on his or her performance provides the basis for designing an adaptation for channel changing. Therefore, in a strengths-based approach, spasticity is a feature to understand and focus on the client's abilities, rather than the "deficit." This innovative approach requires a more intensive look at how context can support participation.

A contextual evaluation must take into account the strengths of the person, which are often neglected in favor of focusing on the barriers to participation. During the assessment, the therapist must actively listen to the priorities and goals of the client. Many of us acquired our professional skills at a time when the focus of assessment and consequently intervention was identifying what was wrong with a person and then attempting to fix it (Dunn et al., 2013). The traditional medical model led to people with disabilities being acted on by professional experts who defined them in terms of their impairments and then sought to remediate those impairments.

For example, autobiographical narratives and interviews with self-advocates with autism spectrum disorder (ASD) suggest that although remediation may be needed at times, they have not built their lives on remediated weaknesses. Rather, they seek assistance in modifying and adapting their environments and in building on their strengths and unique interests to engage in meaningful occupations that foster participation (Kotler & Koenig, 2012). As one self-advocate noted, "The autism spectrum is inclusive of more than a series of impairments; many of the traits we possess can be, in the proper contexts, strengths or at least neutral attributes" (Ne'eman, 2010).

Occupational therapists are in a unique position to offer innovative services that embrace a client-centered occupation- and strengths-based practice for adolescents and adults with autism. By being a central agent of change in this paradigm shift, occupational therapists can be at the forefront of using restricted interests as meaningful occupation rather than impairments with people who have ASD.

Specifically, much of the current literature on autism has negatively referred to the interests of persons diagnosed with ASD as perseverative, restrictive, and obsessive. Historically, the focus of intervention has been on the need to extinguish these interests to "normalize" the person. An innovative strengths-based practice emphasizes the need to recognize these interests as part of the person. This innovation has to start with the contextual evaluation. The occupational profile must answer two questions for a contextual evaluation:

1. What aspects of the environments or contexts are seen by the client as supporting engagement in desired occupations?
2. What aspects of the environments or contexts are seen by the client as inhibiting engagement?

Completing a strength-based, client-centered, and occupation-based occupational profile allows the therapist to answer these questions to inform interventions that support engagement and participation and enables the therapist to explore how context affects occupational performance, engagement, and participation.

SUMMARY

Context is an important part of a client's life, yet ways of exploring context have been limited. This chapter reviews the importance of context to a client as a support or deterrence to participation in occupations. It outlines both the standardized and nonstandardized ways that context can be evaluated.

An important nonstandardized way for assessing context is through the occupational profile, which provides the basis for the occupational therapist and client to identify priority goals and essential outcomes that become the focus of intervention. By evaluating the client's participation in life roles, the occupational therapist can construct an occupational profile that explores the client's natural contexts. Participation assessments often use self-report or interview with the client, consider the client's everyday occupations and natural environments, and evaluate goal-directed activities. Participation assessments also may assess the client's satisfaction with participation and his or her perception of barriers. This chapter includes discussion of participation assessments that give insight into the client and his or her contextual life.

Assessment of the client's environment is included in holistic evaluation of his or her occupations and participation. Assessments of a child's environments often focus on contextual factors that promote development of specific skills, such as play. Assessments of an adult's environments tend to measure safety, accessibility, comfort, and social supports. The strengths-based assessment can ensure the performance of a contextual evaluation that supports participation. The measures described in this chapter are part of the occupational therapist's evaluation toolbox and enable a comprehensive understanding of a client's occupations, the constraints and supports in the client's environment, and the ability of the client to participate in different environments.

QUESTIONS

1. What role does context play in a client's life?
2. Discuss how the occupational profile can be used to explore context.
3. How can a participation assessment tell the therapist about the client's context?
4. Identify 3 standardized assessments that can be used to explore context. What aspect of context can be identified through each?
5. Why is an occupation-based evaluation important to an occupational therapist's evaluation process? How does it complement observational assessments of performance?
6. What is a strengths-based approach? How would it change the focus of evaluation?

References

American Occupational Therapy Association. (2014). Occupational therapy practice framework: Domain and process (3rd ed.). *American Journal of Occupational Therapy, 68*(Suppl. 1), S1–S48. http://dx.doi.org/10.5014/ajot.2014.682006

Baum, C. M., & Edwards, D. (2001). *Activity Card Sort*. St. Louis: Washington University School of Medicine.

Baum, C. M., & Edwards, D. (2008). *Activity Card Sort* (2nd ed.). Bethesda, MD: AOTA Press.

Billings, A. G., & Moos, R. H. (1982). Social support and functioning among community and clinical groups: A panel model. *Journal of Behavioral Medicine, 5,* 295–311. http://dx.doi.org/10.1007/BF00846157

Bradley, R. H., & Caldwell, B. M. (1984). The HOME inventory and family demographics. *Developmental Psychology, 20,* 315–320. http://dx.doi.org/10.1037/0012-1649.20.2.315

Bradley, R. H., Corwyn, R. F., McAdoo, H. P., & Coll, C. G. (2001). The home environments of children in the United States Part I: Variations by age, ethnicity, and poverty status. *Child Development, 72,* 1844–1867. http://dx.doi.org/10.1111/1467-8624.t01-1-00382

Bundy, A. (1999). *Test of Environmental Supportiveness.* Ft. Collins: Colorado State University.

Caldwell, B., & Bradley, R. (1984). *Home Observation for Measurement of the Environment.* Little Rock: University of Arkansas at Little Rock.

Canadian Association of Occupational Therapists. (1997). *Enabling occupation: An occupation therapy perspective.* Ottawa: CAOT Publications.

Chiu, T., Oliver, R., Marshall, L., & Letts, L. (2001). *Safety Assessment of Function and the Environment for Rehabilitation (SAFER) tool manual.* Toronto: COTA Comprehensive Rehabilitation and Mental Health Services.

Clemson, L. (1997). *Home fall hazards: A guide to identifying fall hazards in the homes of elderly people and an accompaniment to the assessment tool, the Westmead Home Safety Assessment (WeHSA).* West Brunswick, Victoria: Co-ordinates Publications.

Corner, R. A., Kielhofner, G., & Lin, F.-L. (1997). Construct validity of a work environment impact scale. *Work, 9,* 21–24.

Coster, W., Deeney, T., Haltiwanger, I., & Haley, S. (1998). *School Function Assessment.* San Antonio, TX: Psychological Corporation.

Coster, W., & Khetani, M. A. (2008). Measuring participation of children with disabilities: Issues and challenges. *Disability and Rehabilitation, 30,* 639–648. http://dx.doi.org/10.1080/09638280701400375

Coster, W., Law, M., & Bedell, G. (2010). *The Participation and Environment Measure in Children and Youth (PEM–CY).* Boston: Boston University.

Davies, P. L., Soon, P. L., Young, M., & Clausen-Yamaki, A. (2004). Validity and reliability of the school function assessment in elementary school students with disabilities. *Physical and Occupational Therapy in Pediatrics, 24,* 23–43. http://dx.doi.org/10.1300/J006v24n03_03

Dijkers, M. (1997). Quality of life after spinal cord injury: A meta analysis of the effects of disablement components. *Spinal Cord, 35,* 829–840. http://dx.doi.org/10.1038/sj.sc.3100571

Dorman, J. P. (2009). Statistical tests conducted with school environment data: The effect of teachers being clustered in schools. *Learning Environments Research, 12,* 85–99. http://dx.doi.org/10.1007/s10984-009-9054-y

Doucet, B. M., & Gutman, S. A. (2013). Quantifying function: The rest of the measurement story. *American Journal of Occupational Therapy, 67,* 7–9. http://dx.doi.org/10.5014/ajot.2013.007096

Dunn, W., Koenig, K. P., Cox, J., Sabata, D., Pope, E., Foster, L., & Blackwell, A. (2013). Harnessing strengths: Daring to celebrate everyone's unique contributions, Part 2. *Developmental Disabilities Special Interest Section Quarterly Newsletter, 36,* 1–4.

Forsyth, K., Taylor, R. R., Kramer, J. H., Prior, S., Richie, L., Whitehead, J., . . . Melton, J. (2014). The Model of Human Occupation. In B. A. B. Schell & M. E. Scaffa (Eds.), *Willard and Spackman's occupational therapy* (12th ed., pp. 505–526). Baltimore: Lippincott Williams & Wilkins.

Fougeyrollas, P., Noreau, L., Bergeron, H., Cloutier, R., Dion, S. A., & St-Michel, G. (1998). Social consequences of long term impairments and disabilities: Conceptual approach and assessment of handicap. *International Journal of Rehabilitation Research, 21,* 127–141. http://dx.doi.org/10.1097/00004356-199806000-00002

Haley, S. M., Jette, A. M., Coster, W. J., Kooyoomjian, J. T., Levenson, S., Heeren, T., & Ashba, J. (2002). Late Life Function and Disability Instrument: II. Development and evaluation of the function component. *Journals of Gerontology, Series A: Biological Sciences and Medical Sciences, 57,* M217–M222. http://dx.doi.org/10.1093/gerona/57.4.M217

Hall, K., Kijkers, M., Whiteneck, G., Brooks, C. A., & Krause, J. S. (1998). The Craig Handicap Assessment and Reporting Technique (CHART): Metric properties and scoring. *Topics in Spinal Cord Injury Rehabilitation, 4,* 16–30. http://dx.doi.org/10.1310/v5ru-frfe-50e6-e2na

Iwarsson, S., & Slaug, B. (2001). *The Housing Enabler. An instrument for assessing and analysing accessibility problems in housing.* Nävlinge and Staffanstorp, Sweden: Veten & Skapen HB & Slaug Data Management.

Jenkinson, C., Mant, J., Carter, J., Wade, D., & Winner, S. (2000). The London Handicap Scale: A re-evaluation of its validity using standard scoring and simple summation. *Journal of Neurology, Neurosurgery, and Psychiatry, 68,* 365–367. http://dx.doi.org/10.1136/jnnp.68.3.365

Jette, A. M., Haley, S. M., Coster, W. J., Kooyoomjian, J. T., Levenson, S., Heeren, T., & Ashba, J. (2002). Late Life Function and Disability Instrument: I. Development and evaluation of the disability component. *Journals of Gerontology, Series A: Biological Sciences and Medical Sciences, 57,* M209–M216. http://dx.doi.org/10.1093/gerona/57.4.M209

Katz, N., Karpin, H., Lak, A., Furman, T., & Hartman-Maeir. (2003). Participation in occupational performance: Reliability and validity of the Activity Card Sort. *OTJR: Occupation, Participation and Health, 23,* 10–17.

Kessler, D., & Egan, M. (2012). A review of measures to evaluate participation outcomes. *British Journal of Occupational Therapy, 75,* 403–411. http://dx.doi.org/10.4276/030802212X13470263980757

King, G., Law, M., King, S., Hurley, P., Hanna, S., Kertoy, M., & Young, N. (2004). *Children's Assessment of Participation and Enjoyment (CAPE) and Preferences for Activities of Children (PAC).* San Antonio, TX: Harcourt Assessment.

Kotler, P. D., & Koenig, K. P. (2012). Authentic partnerships with adults with autism: Shifting the focus to strengths. *OT Practice, 17,* 6–9.

Larson, E., & Zemke, R. (2004). Shaping the temporal patterns of our lives: The social coordination of occupation. *Journal of Occupational Science, 10,* 80–89. http://dx.doi.org/10.1080/14427591.2003.9686514

Law, M. (1998). Does client-centered practice make a difference? In M. Law (Ed.), *Client-centered occupational therapy* (pp. 19–29). Thorofare, NJ: Slack.

Law, M. (2002). Participation in the occupations of everyday life. *American Journal of Occupational Therapy, 56,* 640–649. http://dx.doi.org/10.5014/ajot.56.6.640

Law, M., Anaby, D., Teplicky, R., Khetani, M. A., Coster, W., & Bedell, G. (2013). Participation in the home environment among children and youth with and without disabilities. *British Journal of Occupational Therapy, 76,* 58–66. http://dx.doi.org/10.4276/030802213X13603244419112

Law, M., Dunn, W., & Baum, C. (2005). Measuring participation. In M. Law, C. Baum, & W. Dunn (Eds.), *Measuring occupational performance: Supporting best practice in occupational therapy* (2nd ed., pp. 107–128). Thorofare, NJ: Slack.

Law, M., King, G., King, S., Kertoy, M., Hurley, P., Rosenbaum, P., & Hanna, S. (2006). Patterns of participation in recreational and leisure activities among children with complex physical disabilities. *Developmental Medicine and Child Neurology, 48,* 337–342. http://dx.doi.org/10.1017/S0012162206000740

Law, M., & Mills, J. (1998). Client-centered occupational therapy. In M. Law (Ed.), *Client-centered occupational therapy* (pp. 1–18). Thorofare, NJ: Slack.

Moos, R. (1994). *Work Environment Scale manual* (3rd ed.). Palo Alto, CA: Consulting Psychologists Press.

Ne'eman, A. (2010). The future (and the past) of autism advocacy, or why the ASA's magazine, *The Advocate,* wouldn't publish this piece. *Disability Studies Quarterly, 30*(1). Retrieved from http://dsq-sds.org/article/view/1059/1244

Ritchie, L., Wright-St. Clair, V. A., Keogh, J., & Gray, M. (2014). Community integration after traumatic brain injury: A systematic review of the clinical implications of measurement and service provision for older adults. *Archives of Physical Medicine and Rehabilitation, 95*(1), 163–174. http://dx.doi.org/10.1016/j.apmr.2013.08.237

Rogers, J., & Holm, M. (2009). The occupational therapy process. In E. B. Crepeau, E. S. Cohn, & B. A. B. Schell (Eds.), *Willard and Spackman's occupational therapy* (11th ed., pp. 428–434). Philadelphia: Wolters Kluwer/Lippincott Williams & Wilkins.

Ryan, R. M., & Deci, E. L. (2000). Self-determination theory and the facilitation of intrinsic motivation, social development, and well-being. *American Psychologist, 55,* 68–78. http://dx.doi.org/10.1037/0003-066X.55.1.68

Sachs, D., & Josman, N. (2003). The Activity Card Sort: A factor analysis. *OTJR: Occupation, Participation and Health, 23,* 165–176.

Skard, G., & Bundy, A. C. (2008). Test of Playfulness. In L. D. Parham & L. S. Fazio (Eds.), *Play in occupational therapy for children* (2nd ed., pp. 71–94). St. Louis: Mosby/Elsevier.

Wahl, H. W., Fänge, A., Oswald, F., Gitlin, L. N., & Iwarsson, S. (2009). The home environment and disability-related outcomes in aging individuals: What is the empirical evidence? *Gerontologist, 49,* 355–367. http://dx.doi.org/10.1093/geront/gnp056

Whiteneck, G. G., Charlifue, S. W., Gerhart, K. A., Overholser, J. D., & Richardson, G. N. (1992). Quantifying handicap: A new measure of long-term rehabilitation outcomes. *Archives of Physical Medicine and Rehabilitation, 73,* 519–526.

Wilcock, A. A. (1998). Reflections on doing, being, and becoming. *Canadian Journal of Occupational Therapy, 65*(5), 148–157. http://dx.doi.org/10.1177/000841749806500501

Wilcock, A. A., & Townsend, E. A. (2008). Occupational justice. In E. B. Crepeau, E. S. Cohn, & B. B. Schell (Eds.), *Willard and Spackman's occupational* therapy (11th ed., pp. 192–199). Philadelphia: Lippincott Williams & Wilkins.

Willer, B., Ottenbacher, K. J., & Coad, M. L. (1994). The community integration questionnaire. A comparative examination. *American Journal of Physical Medicine and Rehabilitation, 73,* 103–111. http://dx.doi.org/10.1097/00002060-199404000-00006

World Health Organization. (2001). *International classification of functioning, disability and health.* Geneva: Author.

Yerxa, E. J. (1967). Authentic occupational therapy [Eleanor Clarke Slagle Lecture]. *American Journal of Occupational Therapy, 21,* 1–9.

Zemke, R. (2004). Time, space, and the kaleidoscopes of occupation [Eleanor Clarke Slagle Lecture]. *American Journal of Occupational Therapy, 58,* 608–620. http://dc.doi.org/10.5014/ajot.58.6.60

CHAPTER 8

Nonstandardized Assessments

Charlotte Brasic Royeen, PhD, OTR, FAOTA
Lenin C. Grajo, EdM, OTR
Aimee J. Luebben, EdD, OTR, FAOTA

Highlights

- Standardized vs. nonstandardized testing
- Why use nonstandardized testing?
- When to use nonstandardized testing
- Occupational profile as a guide to choosing additional assessments
- Using nonstandardized assessments.

Key Terms

Class evidence
Conditional processing
Criterion-referenced assessment
Duration recording
Elements of nonstandardized assessments
Event recording
Interactive reasoning
Interview
Ipsative-referenced assessment
Narrative reasoning
Norm-referenced assessment
Observation
Occupational performance assessments

Occupational profile
Operations of nonstandardized assessments
Outcomes of nonstandardized assessments
Questionnaires
Rate recording
Research Pyramid
Screening
Standardized assessment
Structured assessments
Testing bias
Time sampling
Unstructured assessments

This chapter begins with an introduction to nonstandardized testing as a method of information gathering, including a discussion of how it relates to standardized assessments. It then presents why, when, and how occupational therapists use nonstandardized assessments. The remainder of the chapter reviews nonstandardized assessment methods in four major categories: (1) observation, (2) interview, (3) questionnaire, and (4) performance.

STANDARDIZED VS. NONSTANDARDIZED TESTING

What makes an assessment standardized? According to Anastasi and Urbina (1997), "*Standardization*, implies uniformity of procedure in administering and scoring the test" (p. 6, italics added). Standardization means that each time an occupational therapist administers a standardized assessment, the therapist administers the instrument and scores it in the same manner. Standardization also means that the environmental conditions under which the

assessment is administered are prescribed. Standardized assessments have psychometric data regarding their reliability and validity.

In addition, most standardized assessments are categorized as either criterion referenced or norm referenced. A *criterion-referenced assessment* allows comparison of clients' results to a specified criterion. A *norm-referenced assessment* allows comparison of the results for an individual with those of a group of people, often people with similar characteristics or conditions. When a therapist administers a standardized assessment and does not follow the prescribed procedures in the manual, it is no longer considered standardized. Characteristics of nonstandardized and standardized assessment instruments are compared in Table 8.1.

Nonstandardized assessments may not be uniform in administration or scoring. In addition, full and complete psychometric data about the assessment may not exist. Because nonstandardized testing is not built on prescribed processes of administration and scoring, it allows for flexibility and individualization. Just as standardized

Table 8.1. Comparison of Nonstandardized and Standardized Assessment Characteristics

Characteristic	Nonstandardized Assessment	Standardized Assessment
Focus	Ipsative-referenced	Norm referenced Criterion referenced
	Individual, system	Standard, groups
	Individualized, self	Others
Personal	Intrapersonal	Interpersonal
Setting	Naturalistic	Laboratory controlled, prescribed
Type of evidence	Individuated	Class
Examples	• DNA • Fingerprints • Performance observation • Ethnographic observation	• Blood type • Percentile rank • Standard score • Derived score
Data generated	Qualitative and quantitative	Primarily quantitative
Procedures	Less formal	Formal
Structure	Less structured	More structured
Clinical reasoning	Requires strong clinical reasoning for assessment and interpretation	Less dependent on clinical reasoning for administration and interpretation
Validity	Strong internal validity	Strong external validity

assessments are norm-referenced or criterion-referenced, nonstandardized tests are individualized. Individualized assessments can also be called ***ipsative-referenced assessments*** (ipsitive is an alternative spelling); the word *ipsative* is Latin for herself, himself, or itself. Anastasi and Urbina (1997) stated,

> While the ipsative frame of reference may be the most suitable for intraindividual comparisons, such as those needed in the assessment of interests and other preferences, normative reference data are necessary for the sort of interindividual comparisons used, for example, in the assessment of abnormality. (p. 370)

Nonstandardized assessments using an ipsative reference provide unique opportunities for occupational therapists to delve deeply into the individual or a group within the natural environment. Just as research methods evolve to meet a particular field's need, methods of assessment develop in response to a discipline's need. For occupational therapy evaluation, ipsative-referenced nonstandardized assessments are becoming more recognized and useful as individualized assessment instruments. In fact, Donnelly and Carswell (2002) reviewed the literature to report on individualized outcome measures that are client centered.

WHY USE NONSTANDARDIZED TESTING?

Nonstandardized testing results in the collection of individuated information that can be traced to a single entity. Individuated evidence (e.g., fingerprints; DNA; a well-written, detailed performance observation) provides strong internal validity; the information collected is indicative of a person's uniqueness. Such ipsative information is considered an *intrapersonal,* or "within-the-person," comparison.

If *interpersonal* (i.e., between persons) comparisons are the goal, then occupational therapists need to use standardized assessments that have strong external validity. A **standardized assessment** allows comparison of a person's ability, behavior, performance, and so on to a standard (i.e., criterion referenced) or a group (i.e., norm referenced). The resulting information from many standardized assessments, however, is considered **class evidence:** classification within a category (e.g., blood type, perceptual–motor percentile). Class evidence does not offer the corresponding intrapersonal uniqueness that individuated evidence or ipsative reference provides, which is an *intrapersonal,* or within-the-person, comparison.

Nonstandardized Testing in Occupational Therapy

In the history of occupational therapy, perspectives on assessments and intervention have evolved across different periods in the profession. For many years, the profession has tried to move away from traditional medical models of practice to focus on understanding the individualized, unique perspectives of occupation (i.e., an ipsative reference point); the dynamic systems of the person engaging and participating in occupations; and the environments where the person performs the occupations. Many aspects of occupational therapy service delivery, however, particularly assessments, still focus on static protocols. Hinojosa (2007) pointed out that "occupational therapy practice has become less individualized and more routine, and that therapy becomes all about protocols, techniques and procedures" (p. 634).

To be faithful to the principles and philosophy of occupational therapy, the profession emphasizes theory-driven and occupation-based practice, which may include more ipsative-referenced assessments. In her Eleanor Clarke Slagle Lecture focused on measurement challenges in practice, Coster (2008) stated, "instruments provide a way to extract pattern from the performance of an individual for some purpose" (p. 748).

Therapists have used various assessments in everyday practice to justify reimbursement practices rather than looking at client's individual and specific needs. Using specific examples in cognitive assessments, Gillen (2013) asserted in his Slagle Lecture that many of our assessments are "originally and primarily adopted from other disciplines, not occupation based, contrived, novel, and two dimensional in a three-dimensional world" (p. 647). He further added that our assessments must theoretically resemble everyday demands and not be dominated by artificially controlled, unnatural testing environments.

Many paradigms in occupational therapy practice support the use of both standardized and nonstandardized assessments. Models and theories predict what occurs within the person and in his or her performance of occupations. Further, most describe how the environment influences occupational performance. Each of these models or theories then lends itself to the use of nonstandardized forms of assessments (Table 8.2).

Kielhofner (2008), in the Model of Human Occupation (MOHO), used terminology different from the conventional *standardized* and *unstandardized* terms to describe assessments that support his conceptual model, using the terms *structured* and *unstructured* instead. **Structured assessments** have fixed procedures, specified guidelines for use, standardized administration procedures, and evidence of reliability and validity. **Unstructured assessments** use natural circumstances that arise for learning about a client.

Do not get confused. Many occupational therapy assessments (e.g., those based on MOHO) have specific protocols, guidelines for administration, and established reliability and validity properties. Nevertheless, these assessments are ipsative referenced and therefore are nonstandardized assessments.

Kielhofner (2008) recommended routinely using unstructured assessments in practice. To ensure dependability of unstructured forms of assessments, Kielhofner emphasized the importance of evaluating the contexts of occupational performance, triangulating or comparing gathered data with other sources, and performing validity checks through proper and reasoned interpretation of data. Most MOHO assessments have protocols for administration as well as research on validity and reliability and thus could be categorized as structured assessments. However, MOHO assessments are ipsative referenced and thus are categorized as nonstandardized.

Evidence-Based, Client-Centered Practice and Nonstandardized Testing

Evidence is at the center of evidence-based practice, a movement driving many health care disciplines. Tomlin and Borgetto (2011) developed a new model of evidence-based practice for use in occupational therapy called the *Research Pyramid* (see Chapter 15, "Occupational Therapy Evaluation and

Table 8.2. Examples of Occupational Therapy Conceptual Models and Perspectives on Nonstandardized Assessments

Conceptual Models	Perspectives on Assessments
Model of Human Occupation (Kielhofner, 2008)	"Nonstandardized assessments take advantage of natural circumstances that arise for learning about a client. They can be adapted to unfolding situations in therapy, and the occupational therapist gains conceptual answers to questions unanswered during course of intervention" (Kielhofner, 2008, p. 157).
Ecological Models (Person–Environment–Occupation Model, Law et al., 1998; Person–Environment–Occupation–Performance Model, Christiansen, Baum, & Bass-Haugen, 2005; Ecology of Human Performance Model, Dunn, Youngstrom, & Brown, 2003)	"Evaluation process determines what features of the person, environment, and occupation support or interfere [with] occupational performance. Person is not viewed in isolation but is considered in terms of environment where occupational performance takes place. Practice should not be confined to protocols but requires a thoughtful, reasoned and collaborative process of evaluation and intervention" (Brown, 2014, p. 499).
Occupational Adaptation (Schultz, 2014)	Practice should be theory-driven and include assessments that not only measure static outcomes but also assess the impact of intervention on the client's engagement in personally meaningful life roles. Occupational adaptation–based interventions target the client's increased adaptiveness, regardless of condition, as a primary outcome. Assessment and intervention are process-oriented with an emphasis on the dynamic exchange that occurs between the therapist and the client (Schultz, 2014).

Evidence-Based Practice") that challenges the traditional, single-hierarchy, medical evidence model. The **Research Pyramid** puts descriptive research at its base and experimental, outcome, and qualitative research as its three sides. The added emphasis on the value of descriptive and qualitative studies in producing evidence addresses an essential component of occupational therapy practice: clients' day-to-day experiences (Tomlin & Borgetto, 2011).

Cook (2001) highlighted the methods of inquiry in practice needed to capture the complex, multidimensional, and moving picture of clients during their daily engagement in occupations. Nonstandardized assessments can provide a dynamic picture of clients as they perform and engage in occupations in clinical and natural settings.

In a study on the use of standardized assessments by occupational therapists in the United States, pediatric occupational therapists reported that standardized assessments were valued more highly in their practice setting than in adult practice settings (Piernik-Yoder & Beck, 2012). The study reported that occupational therapists practicing in adult settings tend to use nonstandardized assessments more. Occupational therapists in both adult and pediatric settings cited various reasons why they find standardized tests challenging to use. These reasons include the fast pace of the setting, high caseloads, amount of time available for assessments, and finding tests that accurately ascertain and portray their clients' abilities and levels.

Client-centered practice requires that practitioners understand the specific needs of each individual. Consequently, assessments need to focus not only on measurable components that relate to occupational performance but also on subjective experience and observable qualities of people's participation in occupations (Law & Baum, 2005), which likely require at least one assessment that is ipsative referenced.

Controlling Bias and Nonstandardized Testing

The goal of any type of testing—standardized or nonstandardized—is to understand one or more aspects of the person being evaluated. To achieve this goal, the evaluator is obligated to control for as much testing variance or bias as possible. The acronym *PIE* can help occupational therapists remember three aspects of **testing bias**:

> Nonstandardized tests provide a dynamic picture of clients as they engage in various occupations in clinical and natural settings. Nonstandardized tests provide means to capture the day-to-day experiences of clients.

1. **P**erson-related bias
2. **I**tem bias
3. **E**nvironment bias.

There are two types of person-related bias (the *P* in PIE): (1) evaluator or rater bias and (2) test-taker bias. To determine actual occupational performance, an evaluator must control for his or her expectations and rating tendencies that could result in error, that is, severity or leniency, central tendency, and halo effect. For the evaluator to gather critical information, the person being assessed must demonstrate genuineness in any performance and be a good historian (i.e., a person who provides the truth about a situation) when responding to questions. Remember that a good historian must have an adequate level of cognitive functioning.

Item bias (the *I* in PIE) involves the degree to which the specific element being tested fits the actual occupation the test taker performs in real life. Environment bias (the *E* in PIE) concerns the degree to which the testing context matches the appropriate natural environment. In addition to the three aspects of bias, there is a certain unnaturalness in the observation event itself, which can lead to testing variance and possible error.

To apply PIE to a testing situation, consider the example of Mr. O'Neill, an 83-year-old widower who usually brushes his teeth alone in the bathroom of his home. Janet, an occupational therapist testing the occupational performance of this task in a hospital setting, needed to control for all three aspects of PIE testing bias.

To reduce testing error, both types of person bias would need extra attention: Janet would need to control for her expectations and rating tendencies and determine Mr. O'Neill's genuineness and historian abilities in his response to her questions about toothpaste container (manual squeeze or pump) and toothbrush (manual, battery-operated, or electric). Janet's presence in observing Mr. O'Neill may result in him performing this seemingly mundane task differently than usual. Just by changing context (by observing Mr. O'Neill in his home), she could eliminate environment bias and most of the bias related to item and to person, especially to the person being tested. The variance corresponding to observer presence, however, would remain.

The outcomes (e.g., behaviors) of nonstandardized assessment must be double checked to make certain the findings are usual, typical, average, and representative (Brentnall & Bundy, 2009). Making nonstandardized testing as systematic as possible and controlling for bias can result in objective information that has great relevance to the client receiving occupational therapy services.

Organizing Structures and Nonstandardized Testing

Various naming systems *(taxonomies)* and theoretical approaches provide an organizing structure for evaluation, including the use of nonstandardized testing. The American Occupational Therapy Association (AOTA; 2014) provides a system of naming the various aspects of the occupational therapy profession's domain of concern in the *Occupational Therapy Practice Framework: Domain and Process* (3rd ed.; *Framework*). A therapist can use nonstandardized testing to assess the *Framework* aspects that include occupations, client factors, performance skills, performance patterns, and contexts and environments.

Nonstandardized assessment can be applied on a global scale by using the World Health Organization's (WHO's; 2001) *International Classification of Functioning, Disability and Health (ICF)*. In the *ICF*, areas for nonstandardized testing include assessment of a person's participation or involvement in a life situation, activity limitations or challenges a person may have in executing activities, participation restrictions or challenges a person may experience when engaged in life situations, and external and internal influences related to a person's functioning.

A therapist can also use nonstandardized testing with theoretical approaches that have an organizing structure. For example, the Canadian Model of Occupational Performance and Engagement (CMOP–E; Canadian Association of Occupational Therapists [CAOT], 1997; Polatajko, Townsend, & Craik, 2007) provides structure to allow assessment of person, environment, and occupation. For the CMOP–E, *Framework* (AOTA, 2014), and *ICF* (WHO, 2001), Figure 8.1 compares three aspects: (1) life areas (i.e., occupations), (2) foundational (i.e., body level) components, and (3) contextual factors. The content in these references portray the value and importance of theory in the development and implementation of appropriate assessments.

Nonstandardized Testing Components

When thinking about using a nonstandardized assessment, the occupational therapist should consider three important components: (1) elements of nonstandardized assessments, (2) operations of nonstandardized assessments, and (3) outcomes of nonstandardized assessments. Each component is discussed below.

Elements of nonstandardized assessments

Elements of nonstandardized assessments refers to the characteristics of assessments, including client centeredness, equipment and supplies, training, invasiveness, responsivity, needs, and expenses. Nonstandardized assessment should incorporate consideration of and clinical reasoning about the following concerns:

- *Client-centered approach:* The client is "a person, group, program, organization, or community for whom the occupational therapy practitioner is providing services" (AOTA, 1995, p. 1029).
- *Equipment:* The items needed are often highly portable and usually do not involve the purchase of additional supplies and equipment. Some standardized assessments require that buyers purchase additional equipment (e.g., a tricycle) not included in test kits.
- *Training:* Typically extensive training or certification for use is not required. For some standardized assessments, costs are incurred not only with the instrument but also for training in the use of the instrument.
- *Invasiveness:* Nonstandardized assessment is typically noninvasive and involves little risk.
- *Responsivity:* In cases when standardized assessment results might indicate that a client has reached a plateau, nonstandardized

Model	Life Areas (Occupations)	Foundational (Body-Level) Components	Contextual Factors
ICF (WHO, 2001) — *Activities and Participation (Daily Life Area Domains):* Activity is the execution of a task or action by a person; participation is involvement in life situations.	Community, social, and civic life; Major life areas; Interpersonal interactions and relationships; Domestic life; Self-care; Mobility; Communication; General tasks and demands; Learning and applying knowledge	*Body Functions and Structures:* Skin and related structures; Neuromusculoskeletal and movement related; Genitourinary and reproductive; Digestive, metabolic, and endocrine; Cardiovascular, hematological, immunological, and respiratory; Voice and speech; Sensory; Mental	**Personal factors** / *Contextual Factors* / *Environmental Factors:* Services, systems, and policies; Attitudes; Support and relationships; Natural environment and human-made changes to the environment; Products and technology
Occupational Therapy Practice Framework (AOTA, 2014) — *Occupation:* Occupations are central to a client's identity and sense of competence and have particular meaning and value to the client.	Social participation; Leisure; Play; Work; Education; Rest and sleep; Instrumental activities of daily living; Activities of daily living	Performance patterns—groups and populations; Performance patterns—person; Performance skills; Client factors	*Context and Environment:* Virtual; Temporal; Social; Physical; Personal; Cultural
CMOP–E (CAOT, 1997; Polatajko, Townsend, & Craik 2007) — **Occupational Performance and Engagement:** Occupations are composed of activities, which are composed of tasks, which are in turn composed of actions composed of voluntary movement or mental processes.	Leisure; Productivity; Self-care	*Person:* Spirituality; Affective; Cognitive; Physical	*Environment:* Social; Cultural; Institutional; Physical
	Life Areas (Occupations)	**Foundational (Body-Level) Components**	**Contextual Factors**

Figure 8.1. Comparison of the CMOP–E, Framework, and ICF.
Note. CMOP–E = Canadian Model of Occupational Performance and Engagement; ICF = International Classification of Functioning, Disability and Health.

assessment may be responsive enough to ascertain small outcome changes in the client's performance. In many cases, standardized instruments do not have enough sensitivity to detect small changes observed by the occupational therapist.

- *Fulfills unmet need:* Nonstandardized assessment expands upon the information obtained from standardized assessments and may be specific to a particular aspect of occupational performance for which a standardized assessment does not exist.
- *Expense:* Many standardized assessment instruments are costly. After the initial assessment is bought, individual test or scoring forms must be purchased on an ongoing basis. Nonstandardized assessment costs are typically much lower.

Operations of nonstandardized assessments

Operations of nonstandardized assessments refers to the manner of administering the assessment, including ease of administration, time, environment, ease of analysis, and reasoning:

- *Relatively easy to administer:* The procedural steps in administering nonstandardized assessments are usually straightforward compared with the complex procedures of some standardized tests.
- *Time:* Nonstandardized assessments take less time to administer compared with many standardized assessment instruments, although they may take more time to document because of the need to select unique language to describe testing and test results.
- *Environment:* Nonstandardized assessments are typically conducted in the client's natural environments to help control for the environmental aspect of PIE testing bias. For example, observing a child in the classroom provides assessment information about a student in an environment that is natural to the child.
- *Ease of analysis:* Nonstandardized assessments do not have the complex scoring procedures typical of standardized assessments. However, depending on the circumstances, topics, or

data obtained, the analysis may take considerable time and may be multidimensional.

- *Reasoning:* Interpreting nonstandardized assessments may require considerable clinical expertise and analytic reasoning to provide an understanding of multiple data points.

Outcomes of nonstandardized assessments

Outcomes of nonstandardized assessments refers to the manner of administering assessments, including validity of findings for an individual, control of PIE bias, validity of findings from natural environments, and the link between the outcomes of the nonstandardized assessment to theory. The specifics of these outcomes include

- *Validity of findings for the client:* Nonstandardized assessments capture the uniqueness of an individual, offering assessment results with strong internal validity for an individual client.
- *Control of PIE bias:* Nonstandardized testing offers opportunities to control for the person aspect of PIE testing bias, particularly evaluator or rater variance, by establishing rater reliability. A single occupational therapist can start with intrarater reliability by making sure to perform nonstandardized assessment methods the same way each time. Interrater reliability can be established across all therapists within a practice setting for commonly used nonstandardized testing methods. In fact, formalizing a system to ensure and document interrater reliability among therapists in a practice setting could serve to fulfill some requirements mandated by national agencies that accredit hospitals and clinics.
- *Validity of findings related to the natural environment:* Instead of testing performance in sterile conditions or contexts (sometimes associated with standardized assessment instruments), assessing behaviors that occur naturally in context can help control for the item aspect of PIE testing bias.
- *Link between outcomes of the nonstandardized assessment to theory:* The nonstandardized assessment should be administered and

interpreted consistent with the conceptual framework, model, or frame of reference so the therapist can decide whether the theoretical approach is a fit for the particular client.

WHEN TO USE
NONSTANDARDIZED TESTING

Nonstandardized testing is used throughout the occupational therapy process, both at the information-gathering stages of screening and evaluation and after the initial information-gathering stages during intervention planning, intervention, and reevaluation. During the screening and evaluating process, a therapist can use nonstandardized assessments to collect information for both parts of the *Framework's* evaluation process: the occupational profile and the analysis of occupational performance (AOTA, 2014). Even when a therapist merely observes a client within his or her natural setting, it is considered a nonstandardized assessment.

Screening

Using nonstandardized testing is common during screening, a time when occupational therapists collect information related to a potential client to determine the need for further evaluation and the possibility of intervention. Not intended as a comprehensive evaluation, **screening** provides preliminary information to determine whether further occupational therapy services are needed.

Screening often involves observation and interview, two nonstandardized assessment categories. Nonstandardized screening in a school setting may consist of observing a student on the playground or interviewing the teacher to gather information related to the basis for occupational therapy referral and the background of the child. In an adult day care setting, an occupational therapist might perform a screening during a group craft activity to identify participants who are interested and have the functional capacity to participate in a gardening group.

During evaluation, the other initial information-gathering stage, occupational therapists use nonstandardized testing alone or in an integrated approach by using nonstandardized assessment methods to supplement standardized assessments. Although the recommendations and examples of nonstandardized assessments provided later in this chapter can be used for either screening or evaluation, the level of detail of certain methods is more relevant for evaluation.

Use During Intervention Planning, Intervention, and Reevaluation

A therapist can use nonstandardized testing after the initial information-gathering stages: during intervention planning, intervention, and reevaluation. Occupational therapists interpret nonstandardized testing results to plan intervention and use nonstandardized methods—primarily observation, interview, and performance testing—to monitor progress during intervention. At the time of reevaluation, occupational therapists compare the client's performance with initial results to gauge improvement. Nonstandardized testing can play an important role in the area of reevaluation to determine the effectiveness of occupational therapy.

OCCUPATIONAL PROFILE
AS A GUIDE TO CHOOSING
ADDITIONAL ASSESSMENTS

The *occupational profile* is a summary of information that describes the client's occupational history and experiences, patterns of daily living, interests, values, and needs (AOTA, 2014). The purpose of developing an occupational profile is to understand the client's specific priorities and desired outcomes for therapy. Information gathered from the occupational profile can assist the therapist in deciding the most appropriate standardized and nonstandardized tests during assessment. The *Framework* contains a list of questions that a therapist can ask to efficiently develop an occupational profile for a client (Exhibit 8.1). Remember that this approach is not norm referenced in any way but uses an ipsative reference to identify the unique configuration of priorities for a given client and his or her family.

A few nonstandardized assessments can be used to provide a detailed occupational profile of a

EXHIBIT 8.1. IMPORTANT AREAS TO COVER IN AN OCCUPATIONAL PROFILE OF THE CLIENT

- Reasons for seeking services and concerns about performance of occupations and daily life tasks;
- Areas of perceived success and areas where improvement is desired;
- The influence of environment or context in supporting or inhibiting performance;
- Occupational history;
- Values and interests;
- Daily life roles;
- Patterns of occupational engagement and perceived changes over time;
- Priorities and desired targeted outcomes, relative to occupational performance, participation, roles, and quality of life.

Note. Adapted from "Occupational Therapy Practice Framework: Domain and Process," 3rd Edition, *American Journal of Occupational Therapy, 68*(Suppl. 1), p. S13. Copyright © 2014 by the American Occupational Therapy Association. Adapted with permission.

client. For example, for pediatric clients, the Short Child Occupational Profile (SCOPE; Bowyer et al., 2005) can be used, and for clients older than 12 years, the Occupational Performance History Interview II (OPHI–II; Kielhofner et al., 2004) can be used. More detailed descriptions of the SCOPE and OPHI–II are given in the later sections of this chapter.

USING NONSTANDARDIZED ASSESSMENTS

The appropriate and effective use of nonstandardized testing requires the occupational therapist to have a solid theoretical knowledge base and sound clinical reasoning, two of the three evidence-based practice approaches. Using nonstandardized assessment instruments appropriately and effectively is dependent upon selection and use of assessments in four major categories: (1) observation, (2) interview, (3) questionnaire, and (4) occupational performance assessment. For effective use of nonstandardized assessments, Table 8.3 provides questions and directions.

The two most common forms of nonstandardized assessments are (1) observation and (2) interview. The two remaining categories—(1) occupational performance assessments and (2) questionnaire—have less coverage in this chapter because observation is often used as a method of collecting occupational performance assessment information and interviews often include a questionnaire component.

Occupational therapists may use the following process before, during, and after evaluation to improve validity. Before the assessment, ask

- Am I biasing this assessment in any way?

During the assessment, monitor the client's autonomic nervous system functioning by asking

- Is the person unduly stressed (sweating, repetitive behavior, self-stimulating, fast breathing, blanching)?
- Are the responses consistent? Does the message from body language match messages from verbal statements?
- Are there signs of fatigue?

After the assessment, ask

- Was this assessment a novel experience for the person?
- Did an event occur that could change the findings of the nonstandardized assessment?
- Were the responses average and typical of how the person usually functions?
- How can the outcomes of this assessment be corroborated?

Observation

Observation, which comes from the Latin *observo* (meaning to watch, pay attention to, and take careful note of) has come to signify a systematic examination of some type of phenomenon. In occupational therapy, observation is probably the most common procedure for collecting knowledge for evaluation purposes. In fact, occupational therapists at all competence levels—novice to expert—include observation as an integral

Table 8.3. Effective Use of Nonstandardized Assessments

Question	Directions
What is the theory base?	Base all information gathering on theory. Because theory and practice must be linked consistently, theory needs to provide the foundation for evaluation and intervention. Theoretical knowledge is one of three approaches to providing evidence-based practice.
How does nonstandardized assessment relate to evidence-based practice?	Use an ipsative, client-centered approach to underpin nonstandardized information gathering. According to Ilott (2004), "The perspective of the patient, and their caregivers, is a critical component of experiential evidence, especially their views about what constitute[s] desirable or successful outcomes" (p. 348). Experiential evidence (the product of occupational therapy clinical reasoning) is one of the three approaches to providing evidence-based practice.
What organizing structure (e.g., taxonomy) is being used, and how is the nonstandardized assessment relevant?	Select the nonstandardized assessment method based on relevance to what is being measured and the organizing structure being used. For example, an occupational therapist using the *ICF* (WHO, 2001) would choose a method to assess either the two components of functioning and disability (activities and participation, body functions and structures) or the two components of contextual factors (environmental and personal factors). Another example is a therapist who uses the *Framework* (AOTA, 2014) to assess areas of occupation, client factors, performance skills, performance patterns, context and environment, and activity demands.
What are the sources of nonstandardized assessments, and how are assessment data triangulated?	Use multiple assessments in evaluating a client. Although a therapist-designed checklist can offer some information about a person, documenting observations adds to the richness of data collection. Using more than one assessment allows occupational therapists to triangulate the data collection process, fulfilling the nonstandardized assessment goal: determining the actual occupational performance of the person evaluated.
How will the client be monitored during nonstandardized assessment?	Use assessments as means to an end, never as ends in themselves. Occupational therapists should be sensitive to client cues and careful not to stress, fatigue, or invade the personal and cultural space of a client. Therapists can reschedule the session, stop and take a break, or switch to a different information-gathering approach if client cues indicate need for change.
How does nonstandardized assessment accommodate diversity?	Respect the diverse nature of humans who vary in gender, class, cultural background, and many other ways. Sensitivity to diversity can be addressed by selecting nonstandardized assessments that allow for variation in client response. Nonstandardized assessments provide individuated evidence, not class evidence. Therefore, when working with persons of diverse backgrounds, nonstandardized assessments may be the preferred method of evaluation to accommodate cultural differences and offer cultural sensitivity.
What is the secret of getting true nonstandardized assessment results?	Establish rapport with the client. When gathering information about people, especially through nonstandardized assessments, rapport is crucial. For a variety of reasons, an occupational therapist who is highly skilled in the interpersonal aspect of clinical reasoning may not be able to establish rapport that is optimal to the assessment session. Regardless of the level of rapport established, the documentation of nonstandardized assessments must include information about the status of rapport to help readers interpret adequacy and accuracy of evaluation information.

Note. AOTA = American Occupational Therapy Association; *ICF = International Classification of Functioning, Disability and Health;* WHO = World Health Organization.

part of their assessment information-gathering repertoire.

The following are examples of ways to observe phenomena (e.g., behaviors, activities, functions, participation, environments):

- Looking at the posture, symmetry, and fluidity of motion while someone engages in mobility activities;
- Looking at the posture, symmetry, and fluidity of motion while someone engages in any other type of activity;
- Examining a classroom for flow patterns, noise levels, and visual demands;
- Watching a person with a disability getting dressed in the morning at home or another appropriate site;
- Diagramming the way a person with a disability moves from one end of the occupational therapy clinic to the other while navigating around tables, people, and chairs; and
- Observing a person interacting with others.

Although the process of observation involves visually sampling phenomena, other senses (e.g., hearing, smelling, touching) often provide additional information. For example, using vision alone to sample a kitchen environment might involve a description of the physical layout, lighting level, and workstation efficiency. Other sensory information about a kitchen—a lingering natural gas smell, sticky counters that hinder horizontal movement of pots to the stove, or a sandy floor—may raise safety issues. For the purposes of this chapter, *observation* is synonymous with *visual sampling* and includes obtaining information through all senses.

Because of the nature of observation, occupational therapists must control for all three aspects of PIE assessment bias. Both types of the person aspect of PIE assessment bias must be controlled, particularly bias related to the evaluator. To control for the item aspect of PIE assessment bias, an occupational therapist must ensure that the specific element corresponds to the actual real-life occupation of the client being evaluated. Assessment of occupational performance conducted in a natural environment (e.g., client's home, church, public library, social

club) has built-in controls for the environmental aspect of PIE assessment bias.

Although not optimal, assessment of occupational performance also occurs in simulated contexts (e.g., clinic) when natural environments are not readily available. The validity of occupational performance assessment and its generalization to the natural environment are based on the match or fit of the simulated context to the natural environment. Test validity improves when a simulated context closely resembles the natural environment, increasing the probability that the client will be able to generalize skills practiced in the clinic to a natural setting such as home. In addition, therapists must account for the unnaturalness of the observation itself, which may lead to some testing variance and potential error in information gathering.

Therapists use varying degrees of formality and structure to systematize the procedure of collecting evaluation information through observation. Information collected through observation can include nonnumerical descriptions of characteristics that are qualitative, measurable information resulting in numerical data that are quantitative, or a combination of qualitative and quantitative aspects. The systematic, procedural component of observation affects the degree of formality, level of structure, and balance of the qualitative and quantitative information.

Observations related to standardized assessments are frequently formal and structured because therapists must follow specific protocols that were refined during instrument development. Results of information obtained through standardized assessments often start as qualitative but are then transformed into quantitative information. Observations are usually classified or ranked into categories, then assigned numerical values. The numerical values, based on observation of performance levels, factor into the scoring of the standardized assessment. For example, a therapist watches Mark, an 8-year-old second-grader, string 8 blocks within a 15-second time period and assigns a raw score of 8 blocks, which correlates with a point score of 7 on the Manual Dexterity subtest of the Bruininks–Oseretsky Test of Motor Proficiency (BOT–2; Bruininks & Bruininks, 2005).

Without a routine systematic procedure, an observation is likely to be classified as informal and unstructured. For instance, an occupational therapist used an informal, unstructured approach to observation when he entered the home of Mrs. Jameson, an 83-year-old widow who lived alone before hospitalization. The therapist watched her move from the foyer through the rooms and took notes for a home accessibility visit before her discharge. (Sometimes a home visit will be made prior to discharge to review safety, appropriateness, and functionality.) His observations probably included both qualitative and quantitative information (e.g., Mrs. Jameson's motor and praxis skill performance as she reached for drinking glasses on a top shelf, the size and number of throw rugs on the floor, the time she requires to move from the couch to the bathroom).

As procedures become more systematic and routine, observations become semiformal and semistructured. An occupational therapist who systematically works sequentially through a self-designed checklist as a guide to collecting observations is using a semiformal, semistructured approach. Although less official-looking because there are no written guidelines, the expert therapist who has an established routine for evaluating persons demonstrating similar occupational patterns is also using a semiformal, semistructured approach.

Observations that are semiformal or informal and semistructured or unstructured are not necessarily inferior to formal, structured observations. Formal, structured observation (which is part of standardized assessments) is frequently a sterile procedure with resulting outcomes that can be different from what happens under customary conditions in a natural environment. In other words, standardized conditions in a prescribed setting may yield reliable information but may not be valid for the person. For example, a person may be able to transfer in a simulated clinic bathroom but may have difficulty transferring in the home bathtub if the shower nozzle is in the opposite direction from that of the clinic shower. The clinic evaluation would provide documentation that the patient was successful in tub transferring.

Observation (i.e., visual sampling) that is less systematized often results in an increased richness of information. Interestingly, formal, structured observation that is part of the information-gathering process for a standardized instrument

is frequently augmented with less formal and structured observation. In the earlier example of Mark, the occupational therapist made additional observations as follows.

Mark, a right-handed boy, used his left thumb and finger pads to hold the string (1 inch from the end) in a vertical direction 6 inches in front of his chest. With his right hand, he picked up 3 blocks at once, placing 1 block at a time on the tip of the string while retaining the other blocks fisted in his middle, ring, and little fingers. As Mark dropped 1 block on the string, he grasped the string tip (above the block) in his right thumb and index finger pads, allowing gravity to move the block down the string held vertically. He then transferred the string back to his left thumb and finger pads to begin sliding another block onto the string.

The procedures developed during the standardization of the Manual Dexterity subtest of the BOT–2 resulted in observations about Mark that were formal, structured, and quantitative: Mark's raw score of 8 (blocks) equated to a point score of 7 for that subtest item. However, the supplemental nonstandardized assessment information provided valuable unstructured and informal information that was qualitative in nature. On the basis of the additional observations, the occupational therapist improved the richness of information related to Mark's ability to organize a task, sequence steps, and use strategies (in this case, a gravity-assist method).

Collection methods for observation information

To collect observation information, particularly in quantitative format, occupational therapists use four common methods: (1) event recording, (2) duration recording, (3) rate recording, and (4) time sampling. In occupational therapy, the two most common methods of collecting information are event recording and duration recording.

Event recording, the simplest of the four methods, provides a count of each occurrence of a specific type of phenomenon within an evaluation period. For event recording, an occupational therapist keeps a tally of occurrences, resulting in an understanding of the frequency of a phenomenon. In Mrs. Jameson's home accessibility evaluation, for example, an occupational therapist assisting in the decision of whether Mrs. Jameson can return home to live alone could keep a tally of unsafe acts, a form of event recording, by counting the number of times Mrs. Jameson slipped on throw rugs, used the towel bars in the kitchen and bathroom for stability in transitions, or steadied herself with both hands on the counter in preparation for reaching for a glass.

When therapists use timing devices such as stopwatches or kitchen timers, they are performing *duration recording.* For a particular phenomenon (e.g., behavior, activity engagement), duration recording determines the length of time of an occurrence, the amount of time needed for completion, the length of time spent, or latency (the length of time a phenomenon is not observed).

Using duration recording in Mrs. Jameson's case, the occupational therapist could measure how much time she required to move from the driveway into the house, how long she spent moving from her foyer to the kitchen, and the length of time she needed to complete the task of getting a glass of tap water. The occupational therapist could also use latency duration recording by measuring the time interval between unsafe acts.

To use duration recording, the therapist must determine which "end" of time is considered optimal by determining whether the focus is speed (a shorter time) or endurance (a longer time). For example, if the focus is speed, then the optimal end of the time scale is a low number of time units. In terms of speed, a person who assembled a five-piece work task in 10 seconds is 3 times faster than someone who took 30 seconds to assemble the same five-piece work task. If the focus of duration recording is endurance, then the optimal end of the time scale is a high number of time units. For instance, when working on increasing attention to task (a type of endurance), a student who attended to task for 12 minutes without becoming distracted performed 3 times better than another student who was able to pay attention without distractions for only 4 minutes.

Rate recording, a combination of event and duration recording, is calculated by dividing frequency (event recording) by length of time (duration recording). Mrs. Jameson's occupational therapist, who is interested primarily in determining whether she can return to living alone in her home, used event recording to keep a simple tally of the number of times she performed unsafe acts. A tally of one unsafe act provides little meaning unless duration of the home accessibility evaluation is known. For the case of an evaluation lasting 15 minutes, the rate recording is calculated by dividing the event recording of unsafe acts (1 act) by the duration recording of the evaluation (15 minutes).

In this instance, Mrs. Jameson performed 1 unsafe act every 15 minutes. Extrapolating that information to a 24-hour day, allowing 8 hours of sleep, Mrs. Jameson had the potential for 64 unsafe acts per day and 448 unsafe acts per week. On this basis, the occupational therapist may recommend that it is not safe for Mrs. Jameson to return home to live alone. One unsafe act during a 4-hour evaluation (1 per 240 minutes), however, results in an extrapolation of 4 possible unsafe acts per day and 28 potential unsafe acts per week.

Although 4 unsafe acts per day is better than 64, Mrs. Jameson's occupational therapist still would need to determine whether it is safe for her to return home alone. In this case, the quantitative information generated by rate recording may not be enough to make a final recommendation. If her occupational therapist supplemented the rate recording with qualitative information that indicates all 4 unsafe acts during the visit occurred when Mrs. Jameson tripped on throw rugs, a simple recommendation to remove the throw rugs would eliminate all 64 potentially unsafe acts per day predicted in the shorter evaluation, as well as the 4 possible daily unsafe acts observed during the longer evaluation.

According to Ottenbacher (1986), *time sampling* (also called *scan sampling, instantaneous time sampling, discontinuous probe time sampling,* and *interval sampling*) "involves recording the state of a behavior at specific moments or intervals in time" (p. 71). This most sophisticated method of collecting observation data requires signaling specified intervals by a timer, recorded cues, or other means. The observation times are interspersed with intervals of no observation, which are usually used for recording results of preceding observation intervals. Time sampling can be used in combination with event recording, duration recording, or rate recording.

To apply time sampling to Mrs. Jameson's case, her occupational therapist could use an audio recording indicating 5-minute observation times followed by 10-minute intervals of no observation to record the frequency (event recording) of unsafe acts within that observation interval. If the one unsafe act seen in the rate recording example earlier did not occur during the observation interval, then the occupational therapist would record observing no unsafe acts. As this example shows, time sampling (although a potent research strategy) can be time-consuming and burdensome, and has the potential to produce inaccurate information in practice settings.

An example of an occupation-based observational assessment is the SCOPE. The SCOPE, based on MOHO, can be used to observe individual or groups of children and provide a broad overview of children's occupational participation. The SCOPE identifies a child's strengths and weaknesses as well as factors based on MOHO concepts that facilitate or restrict occupational participation and engagement.

Although not formally classified as an assessment, the Dynamic Performance Analysis (DPA; Polatajko, Mandich, & Martni, 2000) is an observation-based framework developed for the Cognitive Orientation to Daily Occupational Performance (CO–OP; Polatajko & Mandich, 2004). The DPA and CO–OP were developed based on the treatment approach CMOP–E. During observations of clients, DPA analyzes performer and performance requisites and identifies sources of performance breakdown during participation and engagement in occupations.

Two other observational assessments, the Test of Playfulness and Test of Environmental Supportiveness (TOP and TOES; Skard & Bundy, 2008), are currently being used in pediatric occupational therapy practice. Both considered ecological assessments, the TOP and TOES are used to observe children from 6 to 18 years of age during free play and identify person-related and environmental influences on children's playfulness.

Format for observation

We have developed the following format to provide fundamental steps of observation-based nonstandardized assessment:

- *Step 1:* Describe the setting. Note whether the assessment is occurring indoors or outdoors; note whether the environment appears cluttered or noncluttered; note the number of people, animals, and objects in the setting; note the lighting, temperature, sounds or noise, and smells.
- *Step 2:* Assess the emotional and social tone of the setting, and provide a label that connotes the feeling evoked. For example, is the setting safe? Peaceful? Chaotic?
- *Step 3:* Conduct an activity analysis by making note of activities and actions.
- *Step 4:* Reflect on how the community would view the ongoing activities (i.e., is the behavior acceptable within that community?).
- *Step 5:* Make note of how long the observation occurred and during what time of day.
- *Step 6:* Summarize findings.
- *Step 7:* Make an interpretation, including actions recommended if necessary.

Interview

Interview refers to the process of inquiry during which one person asks another person one or more questions. Virtually all occupational therapists use interviewing—and more often than not, nonstandardized interview methods—to collect information about almost every client from the very first moment of meeting. Interviews often begin with prompts (e.g., "Describe how you are doing," "Tell me how it has been going") that lead to follow-up probes or additional questions (e.g., "Tell more about that," "And what did you do then?").

Using these types of prompts, probes, and questions reveals a great deal to the occupational therapist about the client's activities and participation in life and his or her challenges while engaging in life situations, including areas of occupation, client factors, performance skills, performance patterns, and contexts and environment (AOTA, 2014). The example questions are open-ended questions, which are designed to elicit information and allow the person being interviewed to express his or her own ideas and concerns without direction from the interviewer.

An alternative to open-ended questions is closed-ended questions, which have forced-choice options. An example of a forced-choice response format is selection of one item from an exclusive number of possible responses. Closed-ended questions are often found when specific information is required, such as asking a client his or her age, or on questionnaires, a nonstandardized assessment category that is discussed later in this chapter.

Like observations, nonstandardized interviews vary in degrees of formality (formal, semiformal, or informal), structure (structured, semistructured, or unstructured), and information type (qualitative vs. quantitative). Generally, as a format becomes increasingly systematic, the interview assessment is correspondingly considered more formal and structured. Some interview assessments are not done in a systematic manner and are therefore considered semiformal and semistructured, offering an integrated approach to the collection of qualitative and quantitative information.

Interviews factor heavily into an occupational therapist's clinical reasoning process. For most occupational therapists, interviewing provides the foundation for three forms of clinical reasoning: (1) interactive reasoning, (2) narrative reasoning, and (3) conditional processing. Occupational therapists use **interactive reasoning** (i.e., client-centered interchange) to piece together the fragments of a client's life story and the unique perspective of the client (i.e., **narrative reasoning**) into a holistic pattern that guides interpretation and intervention planning. The therapist's **conditional reasoning** integrates the therapist's understanding of the client's perspective and his or her understanding of the client's actual abilities to allow for selection of the instruments and questions needed for the interview (Schell, 2014).

Obtaining useful information during the data collection stage of an interview is contingent upon controlling for item and person aspects of PIE assessment bias. Because interviews involve the interaction of two people, the evaluator and the person being assessed, both types of person-related assessment bias require close attention.

Guidelines for interview
We view the following general guidelines as the fundamental steps of interview-based nonstandardized assessments.

- *Step 1:* Tell me about yourself. Who are you?
- *Step 2:* What is the issue or problem?
- *Step 3:* Why is it an issue or problem?
- *Step 4:* When is it an issue or problem?
- *Step 5:* What areas do you see as your strengths?

- *Step 6:* How have you addressed the issue or problem in the past? How can I, as a therapist, assist you with the problem?
- *Step 7:* Do you see a way that we can use your strengths in this process?

The series of questions provided in these steps may be easily adapted to switch the emphasis of the interview from a problem-based nonstandardized assessment to a different focus as needed.

Individualized interview assessments
Occupational therapy has several individualized interview assessments, including the OPHI–II and the Canadian Occupational Performance Measure (COPM; Law et al., 1998). Both interview assessments are occupation centered, and each is based on a different conceptual model.

The OPHI–II is an ipsative-referenced assessment based on the MOHO. The OPHI–II is an individualized, client-centered, semistructured interview that systemizes the collection of occupational history information that can be used in developing a person's occupational profile. Using the structure of the occupation-based OPHI–II to obtain client narratives, therapists help clients "integrate their past, present, and future into a coherent whole" (Kielhofner et al., 2004, p. 9).

The OPHI–II, which is designed to allow flexibility while exploring a client's occupational life history, includes three scales: (1) Occupational Identity, (2) Occupational Competence, and (3) Occupational Settings (Environment). Version 2.1 of the OPHI–II includes scale key forms (Kramer, Kielhofner, & Forsyth, 2008), designed using Rasch measurement, that convert Likert responses into interval measures. The OPHI–II manual (Kielhofner et al., 2004) has other reproducible forms, including the OPHI–II Clinical Summary Report Form and Life History Narrative Form.

The COPM is an ipsative-referenced assessment that is based on the CMOP–E. The COPM was designed to examine interactions among the person, environment, and occupation. A client-centered, occupation-based interview assessment, the COPM identifies problem areas in occupational performance, provides a rating of the client's priorities in occupational performance, evaluates performance and satisfaction relative to those problem areas, and measures changes in a client's perception of his or her occupational performance over the course of occupational therapy intervention (Law et al., 1998).

The COPM allows flexibility in interviewing clients. According to the COPM manual, "it is essential that therapists use their skills in interviewing, probing for full responses, validating assumptions and motivating respondents to obtain the most thorough and comprehensive assessment" (Law et al., 1998, p. 34). The test form provides additional directions as follows:

To identify occupational performance problems, concerns, and issues, interview the client, asking about daily activities in self-care, productivity, and leisure. Ask clients to identify daily activities which they want to do, need to do or are expected to do by encouraging them to think about a typical day. Then ask the client to identify which of these activities are difficult for them to do now to their satisfaction. (Law et al., 1998, p. 2)

Deceptively simple in appearance, the COPM is a powerful, time-saving assessment that gathers salient client-centered information. See Exhibit 8.2, which provides a SOAP note (**s**ubjective, **o**bjective, **a**ssessment, and **p**lan) for Sandy, a typical college student considered a member of the well population.

EXHIBIT 8.2. OCCUPATIONAL THERAPY INITIAL EVALUATION: THE SOAP NOTE FOR SANDY

S: Sandy indicated that she was relieved to be working on her occupational performance (OP), saying her "life was such a mess." She said that she can't seem to get anything done, is failing her business law course, and forgets simple things.

O: On the Canadian Occupational Performance Measure (COPM), a client-centered, interview-based assessment instrument that detects self-perceived change in OP over time, Sandy identified 9 OP problems. Of these, 2 (22%) were in self-care (taking too long in morning routine and forgetting to brush teeth); 5 (56%) were in productivity (decreased time management skills because of high levels of electronic social networking, misplacing homework, getting unorganized easily, running out of gas, and falling asleep in business law class); and 2 (22%) were in leisure (paying high communication bills and having no fun at all). Using the importance scale (COPM–I), Sandy prioritized her 5 most critical OP problems and then rated her performance (COPM–P) and satisfaction (COPM–S) for each. The table below lists Sandy's COPM scores, which indicate overall decreased performance and satisfaction levels associated with two underlying person components related to cognition: time management and organizational skill difficulties.

OP Problem	COPM–I Score	COPM–P Score	COPM–Score
1. Time management	10	2	1
2. Homework	10	3	2
3. Brushing teeth	9	4	3
4. Organizational skills	9	3	3
5. Paying bills	8	2	2
COPM Total Score (average)	9.2	2.8	2.2

Note. COPM–I = Client's perceived importance; COPM–P = Client's perceived performance score; COPM–S = Client's satisfaction with performance score. COPM–I, COPM–P, and COPM–S scales consist of a 1–10 rating, with 10 indicating the optimal level of each.

A: Rapport was established, and testing indicated that Sandy is a good historian, so the results of this evaluation reflect a reliable and valid estimate of Sandy's OP at the current time. Use of the COPM showed functional deficits in Sandy's OP related to self-care, productivity, and leisure performance and satisfaction, secondary to inadequate time management and organizational skills. Sandy's problem list consists of the 5 OP problems listed in the previous table. Sandy, who has excellent potential for improvement, would benefit from skilled occupational therapy to improve her OP through compensatory strategies.

P: Sandy is to be seen for 45-minute sessions semiweekly for 2 weeks for skilled occupational therapy instruction in compensatory time management and organizational strategies. By discharge, Sandy will exhibit independent use of these strategies, demonstrating improved self-care, productivity, and leisure performance and satisfaction as evidenced by improvements in COPM–P and COPM–S reevaluation scores compared with initial COPM–P and COPM–S scores. The table on the next page lists Sandy's long- and short-term goals.

(Continued)

EXHIBIT 8.2. OCCUPATIONAL THERAPY INITIAL EVALUATION:
THE SOAP NOTE FOR SANDY (Cont.)

OP Problem	Short-Term Goal (1 week)	Long-Term Goal (by discharge)
1. Time management	Decrease electronic social networking to a scheduled 5 times per day.	Decrease electronic social networking to a scheduled 3 times per day.
2. Homework	Place finished homework for one course in an expandable folder.	Place finished homework for all courses into color-coordinated expandable folders.
3. Brushing teeth	Brush teeth 1 time per day.	Brush teeth 2 times per day.
4. Organizational skills	Organize work related to school.	Organize work related to school and personal life.
5. Paying bills	Decrease monthly communication bill by $20.	Decrease monthly communication bill by $50.

Ashley Dodson, MS, OTR
DATE

Sandy is a right-handed, 21-year-old woman who is a junior at a Midwestern university and lives in a campus apartment with three roommates. A business major, Sandy became engaged to an engineer in Alaska on Valentine's Day and plans to be married the week after graduation. The SOAP note for Sandy shows application of the COPM and uses the person, environment, and occupation language of the CMOP–E.

Questionnaires

Questionnaires are used to collect information during the evaluation process and include client self-report measures that a client or caregiver completes by paper and pencil or instruments administered with electronic devices such as computers. Because this type of assessment can be completed with or without an occupational therapist present, selection of completion method may help control for person-related PIE assessment bias that involves the evaluator.

Questionnaires have the potential to control for the person-related assessment bias involving whether the client or caregiver is a good historian, can read and comprehend the information requested, has the requisite motor skills (using a writing instrument or a computer), and makes appropriate decisions among choices. Medical histories that patients complete in a medical setting are an example of questionnaires that document a person's past.

In occupational therapy, the Occupational Self Assessment (OSA; Baron, Kielhofner, Iyenger, Goldhammer, & Wolenski, 2006), which is based on the MOHO, is one example of an ipsative-referenced questionnaire. The OSA was "developed to assess the MOHO concepts of occupational competence and value for occupation through self report" (Kramer et al., 2008, p. 173). The individualized, client-centered questionnaire consists of two primary self-assessment forms: OSA Myself and OSA My Environment. The OSA helps clients establish priorities for change, which translate into intervention goals. Included in the assessment are reproducible forms for planning and implementing goals and showing progress and outcomes.

Occupational Performance Assessments

Occupational performance assessments are different from questionnaires. Rather than rely on self-report, an occupational therapist uses his or her strong activity analysis skills to use performance assessments as a means of collecting information about how a client carries out a task in context. From a nonstandardized perspective, observation is a primary assessment in the collection of data related to occupational performance. Therefore, an occupational therapist who uses this method of collecting information must control for the three aspects of PIE assessment bias. Additionally, the occupational therapist must take into account the unnaturalness of the observation itself, which can lead to testing variance.

Examples of nonstandardized occupational performance assessments include activities such as cooking lunch in a kitchen, buttering a piece of toast while seated at a dining table, changing the sheets on a bed, or creating a pinch pot out of clay. Occupational performance assessment can be based on the client's real-time performance of predetermined criteria such as making a sandwich, operating the stove efficiently and safely, moving from one room to another and within rooms, or preparing a space for completion of a specified craft project. In this situation, the client demonstrates an aspect of occupational performance that is rated qualitatively and quantitatively by the occupational therapist.

SUMMARY

In occupational therapy, both nonstandardized and standardized assessments are important. Standardized assessments must be used within the restricted and prescribed conditions, which often impose sterile or artificial conditions on the client. Furthermore, standardized assessment instruments sometimes provide little usable information related to the complexity of the occupational therapy domain of concern. Nonstandardized assessment, however, produces ipsative-referenced results that may offer stronger internal validity and more sensitivity for a client than information produced by standardized instruments.

Occupational therapists should consider nonstandardized assessment as a sound method of gathering rich information about clients, and are challenged to improve the reliability and validity of nonstandardized assessment use. Any assessment—standardized or nonstandardized—should be used in systematic ways to provide consistency and control for all three aspects of PIE assessment bias. Making the nonstandardized assessment process as systematic as possible should provide equally valid results every time it is used, regardless of the person conducting the evaluation. Nonstandardized assessment can be used alone effectively to gather information during evaluation.

For various reasons, nonstandardized assessment may be the only way an occupational therapist can perform a particular evaluation.

An optimal method of data collection uses nonstandardized and standardized assessments in an integrated approach. Integration of nonstandardized assessment offers ipsative-referenced information about individual clients to supplement standardized assessment information that compares clients' performance with criterion-referenced standards or with norm-referenced peer groups.

Occupational therapists must have a solid theoretical knowledge base, sound clinical reasoning, and an understanding of evidence-based practice approaches to appropriately and effectively use nonstandardized assessments. Therapists who wish to implement evidence-based practice should consider Ilott's (2004) reminder that all sources of evidence—empirical research, experiential evidence, and theoretical knowledge—are equally valid.

QUESTIONS

1. Discuss the role of theory in nonstandardized assessment.
2. Discuss the role of clinical reasoning in nonstandardized assessment.
3. Describe 3 actions the occupational therapist can take during nonstandardized assessment that incorporates PIE to ensure validity of the evaluation.
4. Describe and discuss 3 clinical situations in which nonstandardized assessment would be appropriate.
5. When does a standardized assessment become nonstandardized?
6. What are the benefits and drawbacks of evaluating a client in his or her natural environment (e.g., home, work, school)? What are the benefits and drawbacks of evaluating a client in a specialized intervention environment (e.g., hospital, clinic, outpatient rehabilitation center)?

References

American Occupational Therapy Association. (1995). Service delivery in occupational therapy. *American*

Journal of Occupational Therapy, 49, 1029–1031. http://dx.doi.org/10.5014/ajot.49.10.1029

American Occupational Therapy Association. (2014). Occupational therapy practice framework: Domain and process (3rd ed.). *American Journal of Occupational Therapy, 68*(Suppl. 1), S1–S48. http://dx.doi.org/10.5014/ajot.2014.682006

Anastasi, A., & Urbina, S. (1997). *Psychological testing* (7th ed.). Upper Saddle River, NJ: Prentice Hall.

Baron, K., Kielhofner, G., Iyenger, A., Goldhammer, V., & Wolenski, V. (2006). *A user's manual for the Occupational Self Assessment (OSA; version 2.2).* Chicago: Model of Human Occupation Clearinghouse.

Bowyer, P., Kramer, J., Ploszaj, A., Ross, M., Schwartz, O., Kielhofner, G., & Kramer, K. (2005). *A user's manual for the Short Child Occupational Profile (SCOPE).* Chicago: Model of Human Occupation Clearinghouse.

Brentnall, J., & Bundy, A. C. (2009). The concept of reliability in the context of observational assessments. *OTJR: Occupation, Participation, and Health, 29*(2), 63–71.

Brown, C. (2014). Ecological models in occupational therapy. In B. A. B. Schell, G. Gillen, & M. E. Scaffa (Eds.), *Willard and Spackman's occupational theraphy* (12th ed., pp. 494–504). Philadelphia: Lippincott Williams & Wilkins.

Bruininks, R. H., & Bruininks, B. D. (2005). *BOT–2: Bruininks–Oseretsky Test of Motor Proficiency (second edition) examiner's manual.* Circle Pines, MN: AGS.

Canadian Association of Occupational Therapists. (1997). *Enabling occupation: An occupational therapy perspective.* Ottawa: CAOT Publications ACE.

Christiansen, C. H., Baum, C. M., & Bass-Haugen, J. (2005). *Occupational therapy performance, participation, and well-being.* Thorofare, NJ: Slack.

Cook, J. (2001). Qualitative research in occupational therapy. In J. V. Cook (Ed.), *Qualitative research in occupational therapy: Strategies and experiences* (pp. 3–9). Albany, NY: Delmar.

Coster, W. (2008). Embracing ambiguity: Facing the challenge of measurement [Eleanor Clarke Slagle Lecture]. *American Journal of Occupational Therapy, 62*, 743–752. http://dx.doi.org/10.5014/ajot.62.6.743

Donnelly, C., & Carswell, A. (2002). Individualized outcome measures: A review of the literature. *Canadian Journal of Occupational Therapy, 69*, 84–94. http://dx.doi.org/10.1177/000841740206900204

Dunn, W., Youngstrom, M. J., & Brown, C. (2003). Ecological Model of Occupation. In P. Kramer, J. Hinojosa, & C. B. Royeen (Eds.), *Perspectives on human occupation* (pp. 222–263). Philadelphia: Lippincott Williams & Wilkins.

Ilott, I. (2004). Challenges and strategic solutions for a research emergent profession. *American Journal*

of Occupational Therapy, 58, 347–352. http://dx.doi.org/10.5014/ajot.58.3.347

Gillen, G. (2013). A fork in the road: An occupational hazard [Eleanor Clarke Slagle Lecture]. *American Journal of Occupational Therapy, 67*, 641–652. http://dx.doi.org/10.5014/ajot.2013.676002

Hinojosa, J. (2007). Becoming innovators in an era of hyperchange. *American Journal of Occupational Therapy, 61*, 629–637. http://dx.doi.org/10.5014/ajot.61.6.629

Kielhofner, G. (2008). *A Model of Human Occupation: Theory and application* (4th ed.). Baltimore: Lippincott Williams & Wilkins.

Kielhofner, G., Mallinson, T., Crawford, C., Nowak, M., Rigby, M., Henry, A., & Walens, D. (2004). *A user's manual for the Occupational Performance History Interview (OPHI–II; version 2.1).* Chicago: Model of Human Occupation Clearinghouse.

Kramer, J., Kielhofner, G., & Forsyth, K. (2008). Assessments used with the Model of Human Occupation. In B. J. Hemphill-Pearson (Ed.), *Assessments in occupational therapy mental health: An integrative approach* (2nd ed., pp. 159–184). Thorofare, NJ: Slack.

Law, M., Baptiste, S., Carswell, A., McColl, M. A., Polatajko, H., & Pollack, N. (1998). *Canadian Occupational Performance Measure* (3rd ed.). Ottawa: CAOT Publications ACE.

Law, M., & Baum, C. (2005). Measurement in occupational therapy. In M. Law, C. Baum, & W. Dunn (Eds.), *Measuring occupational performance: Supporting best practice in occupational therapy* (2nd ed., pp. 3–20). Thorofare, NJ: Slack.

Ottenbacher, K. J. (1986). *Evaluating clinical change: Strategies for occupational and physical therapists.* Baltimore: Williams & Wilkins.

Piernik-Yoder, B., & Beck, A. (2012). The use of standardized assessments in occupational therapy in the United States. *Occupational Therapy in Health Care, 26*, 97–108. http://dx.doi.org/10.3109/07380577.2012.695103

Polatajko, H. J., Mandich, A., & Martini, R. (2000). Dynamic performance analysis: A framework for understanding occupational performance. *American Journal of Occupational Therapy, 54*, 65–72. http://dx.doi.org/10.5014/ajot.54.1.65

Polatajko, H. J., & Mandich, A. (2004). *Enabling occupation in children: The Cognitive Orientation to Daily Occupational Performance (CO–OP) approach.* Ottawa: CAOT Publications ACE.

Polatajko, H., Townsend, E., & Craik, J. (2007). Canadian Model of Occupational Performance and Engagement (CMOP–E). In E. A. Townsend & H. J. Polatajko (Eds.), *Enabling occupation II: Advancing an occupational therapy vision of health, well-being, and justice through occupation* (pp. 22–36). Ottawa: CAOT Publications ACE.

Schell, B. A. B. (2014). Professional reasoning in practice. In B. A. B. Schell, G. Gillen, & M. E. Scaffa (Eds.), *Willard and Spackman's occupational therapy* (12th ed., pp. 384–397). Philadelphia: Lippincott Williams & Wilkins.

Schultz, S. (2014). Theory of occupational adaptation. In B. A. B. Schell, G. Gillen, & M. E. Scaffa (Eds.), *Willard and Spackman's occupational therapy* (12th ed., pp. 527–540). Philadelphia: Lippincott Williams & Wilkins.

Skard, G., & Bundy, A. (2008). Test of playfulness. In L. D. Parham & L. S. Fazio (Eds.), *Play in occupational therapy for children* (2nd ed., pp. 71–93). St. Louis: Mosby/Elsevier.

Tomlin, G., & Borgetto, B. (2011). Research Pyramid: A new evidence-based practice model for occupational therapy. *American Journal of Occupational Therapy, 65,* 189–196. http://dx.doi.org/10.5014/ajot.2011.000828

World Health Organization. (2001). *International classification of functioning, disability and health.* Geneva: Author.

CHAPTER 9

Reliability and Validity: The Psychometrics of Standardized Assessments

Patricia Crist, PhD, OTR, PC, FAOTA

Highlights

- Selecting valid and reliable assessments
- Standardized assessments
- Overview of basic assessment and measurement concepts
- Reliability of assessments
- Internal consistency
- Scorer reliability
- Validity of assessments
- Assessment responsiveness
- Final thoughts about reliability and validity.

Key Terms

Alternate-form reliability
Ceiling effect
Communication
Concurrent validity
Construct validity
Content validity
Convergent validity
Correlation
Correlation coefficient
Criterion-related validity
Cronbach's α
Discriminant validity
Ecological validity
Face validity
Factorial validity
Floor effect
Goodness

Inter-item internal consistency
Internal consistency
Interrater reliability
Intrarater reliability
Kuder–Richardson method
Measurement
Negative correlation
Objectivity
Odd–even reliability
Pearson product–moment correlation coefficient
Positive correlation
Precision in measurement
Predictive validity
Psychometrics
Quantification
Reliability
Scientific generalizations

Score band of uncertainty	Test reliability
Scorer reliability	Test results
Sensitivity	Test–retest reliability
Specificity	Test stability
Split-half reliability	Uniformity
Standard error of measurement	Validity
Standardized assessment	Validity coefficient
Standardized procedures	Verdicality
Test blueprint	Verisimilitude

No one wants a car mechanic to work on his or her car without a good diagnostic procedure. No one wants a physician to perform surgery without first carrying out definitive diagnostic tests. No parent wants his or her child screened for developmental problems without use of an accurate test. Likewise, no one would want to receive occupational therapy without first undergoing an evaluation process. In each scenario, confidence in the outcomes of the evaluation is dependent on both the skill set of the evaluator and the quality of evaluation assessments chosen.

Evaluation should result in the accurate definition of the occupational performance deficit to support professional decision making in these areas:

- *Diagnostic:* Determine the presence and severity of a problem
- *Descriptive:* Give details regarding the current state of the problem
- *Comparative:* Monitor progress or current status compared with previous status
- *Predictive:* Provide a prognosis based on current conditions or performance problems
- *Conclusive:* Determine the effectiveness of or outcomes from intervention for individuals or programs.

SELECTING VALID AND RELIABLE ASSESSMENTS

Occupational therapists are responsible for choosing the best assessments available for their practice and accurately scoring and interpreting the results. Confidence in test results is critical in identifying problems in people needing attention, planning intervention, monitoring changes as a result of occupational therapy intervention, and determining accumulated outcomes at the termination of services. Assessments that are reliable and valid provide better and more accurate information related to the purpose and intended use of the assessment.

> Confidence in test results is critical when identifying problems in people needing attention, planning intervention, monitoring changes as a result of occupational therapy intervention, and determining accumulated outcomes at the termination of services.

The purpose of this chapter is to provide an overview of the psychometric characteristics of standardized assessments, referred to primarily as *reliability and validity*. As stated in Chapter 1, "Evaluation: Where Do We Begin?" psychometrics of an assessment directly relates to the degree of accountability or confidence in one's test results. **Validity** is whether the assessment measures what it is intended to measure, whereas **reliability** is whether there is consistency between two scores. Validity is more critical than reliability for any assessment used in clinical practice. However, both reliability and validity support the quality, accuracy, and generalizability of assessment outcomes for intervention planning, program evaluation, outcomes measurement, and research to support evidence-based practice.

Assessment manuals report reliability, validity, and related statistics about the development and use of the assessment. Often, additional information is reported in journal articles, research summaries, and reviews. This chapter provides a foundation for clinical reasoning and professional confidence in assessment selection, application, and interpretation of the evaluation results across the intervention process. Occupational therapists must be familiar with measurement, or psychometric, concepts to evaluate and defend the "goodness"

Validity is more critical than reliability for any assessment used in clinical practice. However, both reliability and validity support the quality, accuracy, and generalizability of assessment outcomes for intervention planning, program evaluation, outcomes measurement, and research to support evidence-based practice.

of the assessments they use daily.

A well-done evaluation process is based on the "art" of administration as well as the science, called *psychometrics,* underlying assessment use. **Psychometrics** is the science of testing (Cohel & Swerdlik, 2010; Thorndike & Thorndike-Christ, 2009). Additionally, there is a science of assessment selection, and use is based on the theory of test and measurements, which determines the **goodness** of a standardized test, that is, a reflection of an assessment's reliability, validity, and accuracy. These issues form the guiding questions each therapist needs to ask about the assessment he or she is using or planning to use:

- *Validity:* Does the test measure what it is supposed to measure?
- *Reliability:* Does the test consistently yield the same or similar score rankings (with all other factors being equal)?
- *Accuracy:* Does the test score fairly closely approximate a person's true level of ability, skill, or aptitude. (Kubiszyn & Borich, 2013, p. 326)

Occupational therapists should use only assessments that yield sufficient evidence supporting these three dimensions. Occupational therapists are responsible for knowing the technical adequacy of the assessment (the psychometric qualities), the purpose of the assessment, and the population for which the assessment was intended, and using that assessment competently.

STANDARDIZED ASSESSMENTS

From a clinical perspective, the goodness of an assessment is a combination of its quality ("science") and the skills ("art") of the evaluator. The psychometrics supporting the intended use of the assessment determines the assessment's quality. A standardized assessment has reported norms from a specific population; relevant reliability and validity studies to support the assessment's intended

clinical use; and, most important, interpretation guidelines for test scores to report individual assessment outcomes, called **test results.**

Uniformity, consistency, and competency in administering assessments are essential during the evaluation process. **Uniformity** in assessment procedures means that the evaluator consistently administers the assessment the same way each time and gets the same or similar outcomes, called **intrarater reliability,** which is discussed later. To maintain uniformity, an assessment must have (at the very least) comprehensive published instructions for administration and scoring. The evaluator must be well versed, trained, and consistent in administering the assessment according to these specified instructions. Some assessments require that an occupational therapist be certified in the administration to ensure that the assessment is administered and used accurately.

An occupational therapist must realize that a screening or assessment with published administration and scoring procedures may have

Standardized assessments must have published procedures for administering and scoring, along with reliability and validity studies to support the intended use of the assessment during service delivery.

standardized procedures but may not necessarily be a standardized test (i.e., ipsative assessments; see Chapter 8, "Nonstandardized Assessments"). A **standardized assessment** has published procedures for administering and scoring, along with reliability and validity studies to support the intended use of the assessment during service delivery. A standardized assessment provides

- **Objectivity** (i.e., a measure that is not dependent on the personal opinion of the examiners);
- **Quantification** (i.e., numerical precision enabling finer discrimination in performance or characteristics and interpretation);
- **Communication** (i.e., enhancement of interprofessional use); and
- **Scientific generalizations,** including program evaluation, outcomes studies, and reimbursement documentation (Nunnally & Bernstein, 1994).

A standardized assessment is an instrument that has undergone rigorous psychometric procedures to support its intended purpose and use.

All standardized assessments publish their standardized administration and scoring procedures, sometimes including normative data and suggested interpretations of results in the form of a test manual. A standardized assessment also will have information about its reliability and validity studies as evidence that, when using this assessment, therapists are measuring the same way every time (i.e., reliability) and measuring what they intended to measure (i.e., validity). Studying the reliability and validity of an assessment contributes to evidence-based practice. An instrument is fully standardized when two different evaluators observe the same assessment of a person and independently arrive at the same score. Thus, the foundation for having confidence in a standardized assessment is reliability and validity as a result of methodological research.

OVERVIEW OF BASIC ASSESSMENT AND MEASUREMENT CONCEPTS

Some important concepts in basic tests and measurements are psychometric properties of an assessment resulting from methodological research, including reliability, validity, and test score interpretation frequently reported in some type of correlation coefficient. Understanding these concepts is critical to being a competent evaluator.

Psychometric Properties of an Assessment

Understanding the psychometric qualities of a standardized assessment requires a foundational knowledge of statistics, especially correlation, and the basic approaches used to demonstrate the goodness or various qualities of an assessment. Table 9.1 lists key statistical terms used in reporting the reliability and validity of assessments.

Measurement

The basis of all assessment is the meticulous and precise **measurement** of what the assessment is evaluating. Measurement contributes to the reliability of scoring processes through methodically defining and thoroughly labeling what is being measured. Objective measures give predictable meaning and accuracy to these measurements. Explicit rules for assigning numbers to assessment observations are an inherent component of the standardization process. Occupational therapists must follow these standardized rules during the scoring. Using standardized measures enhances therapists' ability to communicate their findings accurately, and the assignment of numbers allows for more specific reporting of outcomes. Thus, measurement is a systematic way to report assessment findings and reflects therapists' adherence to professional traditions regarding measurement.

Test Scores

Ideally, test scores reflect what is being measured by the assessment, frequently a person's ability. In reality, however, a person's score on a test is not always accurate; it is a combination of the person's "true score" plus the negative influence of testing error that influences test outcomes:

Obtained score = True score + Testing error

Errors in measurement are the disagreement between a person's true score and the obtained score. Measurement errors are random, unpredictable influences on test scores. However, using standardized procedures for administering assessments increases the chance that a person's real abilities have been identified because consistent assessment delivery decreases outside distractions or influences on performance. The goal for occupational therapists during assessment is to decrease the influence of error on testing results.

For example, a student may experience the concepts of true score and error when taking a test. Does the score on an exam accurately reflect the student's degree of knowledge or ability? This question can only be answered affirmatively when outside influences are not present to introduce inaccuracies (testing error) that might negatively influence or mask the student's actual capabilities (true score). Testing errors might include insufficient sleep before a test, having the flu on the day of a test, test items based on

Table 9.1. Basic Statistical Terms Used in Tests and Measurement

Term	Description
Correlation	The degree of relationship between two sets of scores. It implies the degree of relationship or association but does not imply causality.
Correlation coefficient	A statistical indicator that quantifies the degree of relationship between two sets of scores. The coefficient varies from –1.0 to +1.0. The strength of the relationship is represented by how close the correlation is to a perfect +1 or –1. The direction of the relationship indicates if the variables are related to each other positively (+) or negatively (–). • *Positive correlation (+1):* A high score on one assessment is related to a high score on another, or two low scores are related. • *Negative correlation (–1):* A high score on one assessment is related to a low score on another.
Measurement research	The rules for assigning numbers to behavior, characteristics, or performance to quantify the results of an assessment.
Methodological research	Approach used to study and report norms, reliability, and validity to establish evidence of the quality of an assessment's outcomes for practice-related planning and decisions.
Psychometrics	Test and measurement statistics provided to support the technical or scientific quality of an assessment.
Reliability	The degree of precision consistency between two scores; reliability indicates that a tester comes up with the same results each time he or she conducts an assessment, given that there are no intervening variables.
Test score	A person's current obtained score (Os) on a test is a combination of his or her true score (Ts) plus the negative influence of testing error (Te) from sources that prevent the current score from fully reflecting the person's true abilities: $Os = Ts + Te$.
Test statistic	The reported statistical/numerical result from a study to describe a type of reliability or validity.
Validity	The degree to which a test accurately measures the specific construct, trait, behavior, or performance it was designed to measure.

Note. From "Reliability and Validity: The Psychometrics of Standardized Assessments," by P. Crist, p. 182. In J. Hinojosa, P. Kramer, and P. Crist (Eds.), *Evaluation: Obtaining and Interpreting Data* (3rd ed.), Bethesda, MD: AOTA Press. Copyright © 2010 by the American Occupational Therapy Association. Used with permission.

content not covered in class, the test room being too noisy or too cold, a major stressful life event occurring before or during the test, and so on. Thus, the obtained score is only an estimate of the student's real (or true) capability. A true score (by definition) contains no error; this evaluation goal is never obtained because error can be reduced but not eliminated.

The occupational therapist's goal is **precision in measurement.** Precision in measurement is reduced and replaced by error when there is variability caused by inconsistencies in the therapist's ratings or scores, including delivery; measurement tool calibration and accuracy; environmental conditions; and a test taker's physiological, emotional (mood and motivation), and current health condition. A therapist can have precision in measurement and reduce errors by

- Using standardizing measurement methods;
- Having appropriate and sufficient training in assessment procedures (including certifying and rechecking periodically);

> The obtained score (Os) is only an estimate of the student's real (or true) capability. A true score (by definition) contains no error; this evaluation goal is never obtained because error can be reduced but not eliminated. Where Ts is the true score and Te uncontrolled error influencing the score, $Os = Ts + Te$.

- Having experience in administering and scoring the instrument (learning standardized procedures, reliability, validity); and
- Repeating the measurement to verify evaluator, test taker, and instrument consistency (Hulley, Cummings, Browner, Grady, & Newman, 2013).

If the score obtained is closer to a true score, the better the assessment's overall reliability and validity. Because true scores are constant or never change between one test administration and another, reliability reflects the degree of true score differences contributing to the observed score and the portion of performance or function that will remain constant over time if conditions remain the same. Likewise, the more sources of error influencing test results, the less the true score will make up a person's obtained score. As a result of the degree of error influencing testing outcomes, intervention decisions might be based on incorrect or misleading information.

Reliability and Validity

The two most important concepts arising from psychometric or measurement theory are reliability and validity. *Reliability* refers to consistency between two scores. Typically, an assessment's reliability is established by correlating the scores from a person on the same test given at two different times using equivalent sets of items or testing conditions (Anastasi & Urbina, 1997). Reliability contributes to predictability and reproducibility of results if the evaluator administers the assessment without changes in the person or conditions for testing.

Validity is ensuring that what is measured is what is intended to be measured, or the degree to which the test measures what it purports to be measuring. An assessment's validity is established by comparing scores on a given assessment of a specific construct, trait, behavior, or performance with another measure of the same construct. Specific types of reliability and validity are discussed later in this chapter.

The author or publisher of an assessment, or an interested professional, performs the studies of reliability and validity that occupational therapists use in selecting quality tests or interpreting results.

Often, an author of an assessment establishes the types of reliability and validity that support the purpose and application of his or her assessment. Occupational therapists in practice do not establish test reliability or validity but depend on studies conducted by third parties and published manuals and articles to learn about the reliability and validity of a particular assessment. A therapist gains confidence in the use of a particular assessment for evaluating a client by referring to the published reliability and validity. Moreover, a therapist can determine whether the assessment is appropriate for identifying deficits or dysfunction, intervention progress, or outcomes.

Correlations and the Correlation Coefficient

Correlation statistics establish many types of reliability and validity. *Correlation* (*Merriam–Webster's Online Dictionary*, n.d.) is defined as "the degree of association of two random variables." A brief introduction to the concept of correlation is provided to assist with understanding the remaining content of this chapter. Readers should refer to statistical texts for more extensive explanations (e.g., Howell, 2014; Portney & Watkins, 2009; Weinberg & Abramowitz, 2008).

Correlation does not imply causality, only that a relationship exists between two measures or variables; a third external factor may be the cause. For example, the number of sexual overtures increases markedly when college women sunbathe in bikinis. Although these two positively correlate, a third factor—seasonal weather changes (hot vs. cold temperatures)—might be the causal factor in these two occurrences increasing or decreasing in frequency at the same time.

The *correlation coefficient* (indicating the degree of agreement between two measures) is another important statistic in tests and measurements. Most assessments use a specific statistical test to arrive at a correlation coefficient called the *Pearson product–moment correlation coefficient*, reported as *r*. However, there are many other correlation coefficients, and each uses a different symbol other than *r*. Test manual correlation reports do not have to be overwhelming. Just remember, a statistician selects a particular correlation approach based on how the assessment converts an observation to a number and scores responses, and the correlation approach adopted is not as important as the final coefficient value, which is what actually appraises test quality.

Correlation coefficients can range from –1.00 to +1.00. A correlation of 0.00—the midpoint of the continuum between the two extremes—indicates that the two sets of test scores are unrelated. As the scores move to the ends of the continuum, the magnitude or strength of correlation increases. In other words, the relationship between the two variables of measures —how much they have in common or share with each other—increases.

> Correlation approaches vary widely, and many correlation coefficients are used to evaluate assessments, but correlation approach and coefficient symbol are not as important as the final coefficient value, which ranges from –1.00 to +1.00

A second important correlation concept is the direction of the relationship, indicated by a positive or negative coefficient. A *positive correlation* is an association between two variables going in the same direction. As one variable becomes large, the other also becomes large, and vice versa. Positive correlation is represented by correlation coefficients greater than 0 (0 to +1.0). A *negative correlation* is an inverse association between two variables. As one variable becomes larger, the other becomes smaller. Negative correlation is represented by correlation coefficients less than 0 (–1.0 to 0).

The labels + and – have nothing to do with the quality of the correlation. For example, a therapist would expect a positive correlation coefficient between the degree of deformity and the reported pain for arthritis. The hypothesis is that as hand deformity increases, reported pain increases, and as hand deformity lessens, less pain will be reported. A therapist would expect a negative correlation between the amount of pain and increases in pain medication in arthritis. In this case, a therapist hypothesizes that as pain medication is increased, reported pain decreases. Likewise, a therapist would want a negative correlation between calorie consumption and weight loss and a positive correlation between food calorie intake and weight. Always analyze whether the coefficient is in the direction desired by thinking through the expected direction of the relationship when the two variables are compared. A therapist will not see a perfect prediction from correlation (+1.00 or –1.00), because this means the scores are error free, which can never happen when evaluating human performance. For example, the correlation between eating pickles and dying is +1.0, because 100% of persons who eat pickles die. The same relationship can be found with drinking bottled water and dying!

The strength of the correlation found between two measures is also central to determining the quality of the reliability or validity of an assessment. The higher the correlation coefficient (ignoring the + or – sign), the greater its strength. As a general guideline, industry standards use the following coefficient ranges to judge reliability and validity studies reported by test developers and publishers:

> The terms *positive* and *negative* do not evaluate the quality of the correlation but the direction of the correlation. Positively correlated values will increase or decrease together (0 to +1.0) depending how much characteristics or information is in common or agreement between two measures, whereas negatively correlated values will have an inverse relationship (–1.0 to 0) depending on the amount of dissimilarity or uniqueness. Correlations given the value of 0 are not correlated.

- *.90–.99*: High and preferred, but not frequently observed
- *.80–.89*: Satisfactory or adequate
- *.70–.79*: Weak or minimally acceptable
- *Less than .70*: Caution—inadequate or unacceptable.

The correlation statistic measures the amount of agreement between two assessment methods. Therefore, if the reported correlation coefficient between two versions of the same test is .90, and one squares the coefficient to determine the percentage of agreement, or explanation in common, between the two tests, the result is 81% [(correlation coefficient)^2 = $(r)^2$ = $(.90)^2$ = 81%]. In other words, performance on the second test will be 81% in common with the first, but 19% of the performance variance remains unexplained by the two measures.

Some people do not consider r^2, but it is another way to understand results. For example, an occupational therapist and a physical therapist each administers different but widely used, self-reporting pain scales. The supervisor asks the two therapists to use a single measure to increase efficiency. The literature comparing the two scales states that the correlation between them is .25. Using r^2, this means that approximately only 6% of the information gained from both assessments is in common, leaving 94% that is explained differently by each assessment. In this case, a loss of information may occur if only one assessment is selected. On the other hand, if the coefficient is .90, r^2 is equal to 81%, and there is great overlap in information across the two assessments. In this case, the therapists could afford to drop one, choosing whichever has other features most relevant to their practice needs.

RELIABILITY OF ASSESSMENTS

Reliability is the extent to which an assessment captures a person's true score despite limiting error possibilities. Reliability has two important properties:

1. The part of a person's performance that remains constant over time (i.e., score reliability).
2. The part of the obtained score variance among test takers that is the result of true score differences (i.e., test reliability; Thorndike & Thorndike-Christ, 2008).

Score Reliability: Standard Error of Measurement

The **standard error of measurement (SEM)** is a measure of the reliability of the obtained score. The *SEM* is the standard deviation of the distribution of error in measurement (Bolton, Parker, & Brookings, 2008). *SEM* reflects the degree of true score versus error in an obtained score from a person. It supports the notion of accuracy in assessment and answers the question, How closely does the assessment score approximate the true score of a test taker? (Kubiszyn & Borich, 2013).

The *SEM* estimates the possible deviation of a test taker's observed score from his or her true score. If a test is repeatedly given to the same person under similar conditions, his or her observed score will vary within a certain range of total scores. The statistical average of all these observed scores is a good indicator of one's true score. As a result of the variance between true and observed scores, the occupational therapist needs to treat the final test score as an estimate, not as a definitive true score. A therapist can use the published *SEM* for the assessment to increase the accuracy and interpretation of an individual score obtained during an assessment.

The *SEM* is an estimate of the reliability of the obtained score; in other words, a measure of the inconsistencies (attributed to various sources of error or pure chance) calculated from the standardization sample. The *SEM* is the measurement error for a particular assessment and is likely to be the gap between the observed score and one's true score. A smaller *SEM* indicates that the observed score better reflects the true score. In practice, if an assessment has a small *SEM*, the occupational therapist can be confident that the client's observed score is close to the true score provided the therapist followed standardized procedures for administration and scoring. If the score does not reflect a person's true score, the *SEM* will likely be larger than published and will not be an accurate estimate, because more error may be contributing to the observed score than what was found in the standardization sample.

The *SEM* is established during the standardization of the assessment by accumulating repeated scores from the standardization sample to see how much scores in performance or function stay constant over time, when nothing has occurred that could cause change. The *SEM* is reported in test manuals or other measurement publications. In practice, one uses the reported *SEM* to describe the degree of consistency or preciseness related to obtaining a true score. Other resources to calculate the *SEM* statistically are beyond the scope of this chapter.

The importance of the *SEM* score is that it indicates the degree of confidence that a therapist can have that a client's obtained score is a reflection of his or her real performance ability rather than some random influence or error. The *SEM* is usually reported in the test manual accompanying the assessment. Adding the *SEM* to the obtained score, then subtracting the *SEM* from the obtained score, gives the boundary of confidence (the **score band of uncertainty**) within which the client's true score is likely to lie. For example, if the obtained score is 50 and the reported *SEM* for the test is 3, the estimate of a client's true score is somewhere between 47 and 53. A therapist would have less confidence in this estimate of true score if the *SEM* were large, meaning that more error contributes to the obtained score. In the previous example, imagine the implications if the *SEM* was 12, giving a much larger range of uncertainty regarding the client's true score.

Although the *SEM* is important for interpreting an individual score, it has additional utility to the occupational therapist. An assessment often is used to determine a person's eligibility for criteria-based services or programs; the obtained score can determine whether a person qualifies for occupational therapy or other related services. For example, many developmental programs require that a person have an intelligence quotient (IQ) score less than 70 to participate. A child may not qualify for this program if a recent IQ test reported the child has an IQ of 72. However, if the IQ test manual reports an *SEM* of 6, then the child's score could range from 66 (72 – 6) to 78 (72 + 6). This lower score would mean that the child would be eligible for services. If a therapist felt that the child might benefit from the program, the therapist could use the assessment's *SEM* as evidence to support program admission.

A therapist sometimes administers a retest to see whether the person receives the same or different result. Of course, if the same therapist administered the retest, he or she could be biased, so it would be best if the same therapist did not conduct the repeat test. In such a case, having another therapist administer the retest would mean that the new score is more defensible.

Test Reliability

There are several types of **test reliability.** Authors or psychometricians emphasize only certain reliability types that support the purpose and use of a given assessment. Because the purpose of this chapter is to provide an overview of common approaches, only the most common types of reliability are discussed here. The reader is reminded that

- *Reliability* is the consistency with which an assessment performs.

- All reliability is established by test developers or others to improve the quality of the assessment. Therapists use this information to select tests and help interpret individual scores; typically, they never do their own local reliability studies to support intervention decision making.
- Therapists should report the assessment's reliability in the evaluation report or summary. They should provide the information that supports the intended purpose and use of the assessment. For example, if the purpose of a test is to measure intervention changes, then test–retest reliability must be reported.
- All reliability is reported using some type of correlation coefficient.

Table 9.2 summarizes the forms of reliability typically reported for assessments used in occupational therapy. Each type of test reliability is listed according to the various names typically used in the literature. A brief description and the preferred reliability coefficient required for satisfactory reliability also are included. The next two sections discuss two different aspects of reliability: (1) test–retest reliability and (2) alternate-form reliability.

Test–retest reliability or stability

Test stability is established by giving the same test to the same person in the same context at two different times. This procedure is repeated until data from a large group of similar people have been collected. A sufficient amount of time must pass between the administrations of the test and retest in order for the test taker to forget his or her responses to test items, as well as to prevent other intervening factors from influencing the second set of scores. Typically, the average time between tests is 1 to 2 weeks. The first set of scores is compared with the second set of scores to derive a correlation.

Occupational therapists often look for **test–retest reliability** on tests they will use to measure change over time as a result of intervention. Therapists want the test to be a stable measure of what is expected to change and not be easily influenced by other outside events. With good test–retest reliability, therapists have increased confidence that any changes in the score reflect true changes in the area measured, not unreliability entering from external sources.

Table 9.2. Types of Reliability

Type	Description	Coefficient Standard
Standard error of measurement	The inconsistency or unreliability of the obtained score for an individual. (Also noted as *SEM.*)	.90 or greater
Test–retest reliability or stability	A measure of test score stability on the same version of the assessment over 2 occasions.	.90 or greater
Alternate, parallel forms of reliability or equivalence	The correlation in scores using 2 different forms of the same assessment.	.85 or greater
Internal consistency	*Split-half reliability:* The extent to which the score from one half of an assessment correlates with the other half. *Kuder–Richardson (KR):* The extent to which any 1 item on an assessment correlates with other items on the same assessment. *Coefficient alpha:* Similar to KR, but used when an assessment has items with multiple response options.	.70–.95
Scorer reliability	*Interrater reliability:* The degree of agreement between 2 raters after observation of the same person during an assessment. *Intrarater reliability:* Administering and scoring an assessment consistently the same way each time it is administered.	.90 or greater

Note. From "Reliability and Validity: The Psychometrics of Standardized Assessments," by P. Crist, p. 189. In J. Hinojosa, P. Kramer, and P. Crist (Eds.), *Evaluation: Obtaining and Interpreting Data* (3rd ed.). Bethesda, MD: AOTA Press. Copyright © 2010 by the American Occupational Therapy Association. Used with permission.

Alternate-form or parallel forms of reliability or equivalence

The assessment developer can obtain an estimate of the reliability of an assessment by using two equivalent forms of the assessment. The developer gives two groups of people both assessments at the same time and correlates their scores to establish equivalence between two forms of the assessment. This approach eliminates the influence of practice and memory present in the test–retest situation. However, developing two equivalent assessments with different items testing the same information or skill is not easy. When test security is an issue, alternate forms of assessments are used, such as with large-scale tests like the SAT or the GRE.

Occupational therapists should look for assessments with **alternate-form reliability** when responses to items are easily remembered, stimulate learning, or possibly even practice specific skills. For example, during an assessment of motor abilities with a child, a therapist might ask the child to model skipping as a test item. Afterward, the therapist observes the child practicing this skill regularly during recess. Asking the child to skip during the reassessment would result in measuring the effects of practice in addition to the effectiveness of the intervention provided.

In this case, having two forms of a test of motor ability would be beneficial. If the therapist administers the assessment to determine whether a change has occurred because of intervention, the therapist needs to know whether the assessment will teach or whether the person will remember the items. If the assessment uses scenarios that trigger specific memories, then having two equivalent forms of a test to determine intervention effectiveness is beneficial.

INTERNAL CONSISTENCY

Internal consistency determines the degree of agreement or commonality between items in an assessment that measures a single concept or skill. It is logical that if a person gets one item correct on an assessment, he or she should get other items correct also, if the assessment truly measures a single concept. Test items are then internally consistent with each other. The goal in designing a reliable instrument is not only for scores on similar items to be related (internally consistent) but also for each score to contribute some unique information. A commonly accepted rule is that an alpha (α) coefficient of .6–.7 indicates acceptable reliability and .8 or greater indicates good reliability. High reliabilities (.95 or greater) are not necessarily desirable, because they indicate that the items may be redundant.

Split-Half Reliability for Assessment

Split-half reliability involves splitting a single form of an assessment into two equivalent, shorter forms. One method for doing so is creating one form of the assessment using the first half of items and a second form using the second half of items of the assessment. Another approach is to put all even-numbered items into one test and all odd-numbered items into another. An assessment developer uses this approach when varying item difficulty is not evenly spread throughout the assessment, for example, in assessments in which items get increasingly difficult. Reliability of this form of an assessment is called *odd–even reliability*. An assessment developer should examine the internal consistency to find alternate form reliability or shorten an assessment by 50%.

Split-half reliability information is important to occupational therapists in three situations. First, a therapist may find that this method was used to create a new shorter form of the assessment and, as a result, may want to know how it was done and to what degree the new shorter test correlates with the longer version that is no longer available. Second, both the short form and the long form of the test may be available and an occupational therapist might want to have options in choosing the short versus long form when clients fatigue easily or when a lesser amount of time can be allocated to a specific assessment than at other times. Third, this method may result in two equivalent forms of the same assessment, giving the therapist a choice of which to use, like forms developed through alternate reliability.

Inter-Item Internal Consistency

An occupational therapist is interested in **inter-item internal consistency** reliability to ensure that the same skill, ability, or knowledge is measured with each item on the assessment. Items that do not contribute to the overall score because they measure something else lower a test's reliability and, as a result, the ability to identify problems warranting intervention or measuring change. The following are measures of internal consistency:

- *Kuder–Richardson (KR) method* refers to the item–total correlation, called the KR20 and KR21. The KR only handles responses that can be scored as correct or incorrect (i.e., objective answers).
- *Cronbach's α* statistic, or coefficient, is used when multiple responses to the same item can be made. This method is used on assessments when responses are acquired using response scales such as *never, some of the time, most of the time,* and *all of the time.*

SCORER RELIABILITY

Scorer reliability is important because occupational therapists do not want to be responsible for introducing error into an assessment process. Therapists' scorer reliability improves through training in the assessment's standardized procedures and rechecking skill maintenance over time.

As an assessment is used repeatedly, unintentional deviations in delivery and skill occur, which may modify the standardized approach. As a result, it is important that therapists periodically recalibrate their skills on a specific assessment as well as compare outcomes from other raters.

Intrarater Reliability

Intrarater reliability is supported through a therapist's professional values and ethical commitment to providing quality occupational therapy evaluation. It is not a formal type of reliability used in tests and measurements. This type of reliability is reflected in behaviors that ensure continuous competence in the use of the assessments. When therapists are trained in an assessment according to published standardized procedures, intrarater reliability is ensured.

Therapists also need regular recalibration for all assessments—used frequently and infrequently—because consistency in their skills varies over time. Recalibration includes, but is not be limited to, restudying standardized procedures and fine-tuning skills, having another trained evaluator review and critique current administration skills, and attending a workshop on the administration of the assessment. Only regular recalibration gives therapists the competence to use assessments consistently as they were designed and intended to be used. Scorer reliability is the fundamental requirement underlying intrarater reliability.

Interrater Reliability

Test manuals report **interrater reliability** to demonstrate that, with adequate training (as described in the test manual), practice, and recalibration, two different raters will consistently arrive at essentially the same score. The key is that training and adherence to published standardized procedures will produce similar scores for both raters.

Occupational therapists should look for interrater reliability information when more than one therapist in a setting or across settings might assess or reassess the same client over time. Interrater reliability also may be important when multiple therapists evaluate different clients but come together to assign these clients for intervention purposes into like groups based on similar test scores. Preferably, a therapist also should determine his or her own interrater reliability periodically by conducting assessments simultaneously with another trained colleague to compare their independent scoring results.

In assessment training and recalibration, the two raters compare scores and discuss those that are different to arrive at the one expected by the test publisher. Later, a therapist might want to score an evaluation of the same client without discussion. Next, the therapist computes the percentage of agreement between the two raters' scores. When this informal approach to establishing interrater reliability approaches the published numerical value, the therapist can be confident that he or she is trained or recalibrated sufficiently in the standardized procedures for administration and scoring. Once interrater reliability has been established, the therapist can feel confident that regardless of who sees a client for evaluation, he or she would arrive at the same scores.

Sometimes in a setting, it is necessary, and even valuable, to establish interrater reliability between two therapists who work in two different areas where clients are transferred to and from. With interrater reliability established between two therapists, the necessity to reevaluate assessment scores when a client is transferred may be eliminated, or the current therapist's scores may be directly compared with previous scores to determine changes in ability or to modify the intervention plan.

> Interrater reliability information is important when more than one therapist in a setting or across settings might assess or reassess the same client over time, or when multiple therapists evaluate different clients but come together to assign these clients for intervention purposes into like groups based on similar test scores.

Score Reliability: Standard Error of Estimate

Just as the *SEM* indicates the margin of error as a measure of unreliability across the standardization sample, the standard error of estimate (*SEE*) is the result of the margin of error that gives imperfect reliability in determining a person's score as correct. The *SEE* is not a major measure used in score reporting and is seldom mentioned for the assessments that occupational therapists might use.

VALIDITY OF ASSESSMENTS

Assessment validity provides support that the assessment measures the correct target construct, trait, behavior, or ability. Table 9.3 outlines the major types of validity found in assessments used by occupational therapists. The validity of an assessment is supported when the assessment demonstrates that it actually measures what it claims to measure. Typically, the correlation between two assessments of the same trait, behavior, or ability provides evidence that supports the validity of an assessment. A validity coefficient of an assessment enables therapists to assess how well the individual assessment results compare with an external

Table 9.3. Types of Validity

Type	Description
Standard error of estimate	The inaccuracy or invalidity in determining a person's true score. (Also noted as *SEE*.)
Face validity	Established through the appearance of the items as related to the purpose of the assessment. It is not based on statistical proof.
Content validity	The extent to which the items on the assessment represent a sufficient, representative sample of the domain or construct being examined.
Criterion-related validity	*Concurrent or congruent validity:* The extent of agreement between 2 simultaneous measures of the same behavior or trait. *Predictive validity:* The extent to which scores on an assessment forecast future behavior, abilities, or performance.
Construct validity	*Convergent validity:* The degree to which 2 tests being conducted measure the same ability or behavior; the amount of agreement between the 2. *Discriminant validity:* The degree to which each of 2 assessments being conducted measure a different ability or behavior; the amount of disagreement between the 2.
Ecological validity	Degree to which the assessment relates to or predicts the real world. *Veridicality:* Degree to which test results will predict performance in natural context. *Versimilitude:* Similarity between the natural context and the assessment context.
Factorial validity	The identification of interrelated behaviors, abilities, or functions that contribute to collective abilities or functions. Sometimes referred to as *multitrait–multimethod validity*.

Note. From "Reliability and Validity: The Psychometrics of Standardized Assessments," by P. Crist, p. 194. In J. Hinojosa, P. Kramer, and P. Crist (Eds.), *Evaluation: Obtaining and Interpreting Data* (3rd ed.). Bethesda, MD: AOTA Press. Copyright © 2010 by the American Occupational Therapy Association. Used with permission.

criterion measure. Occupational therapists want to know that they are measuring validly what they want to measure, not some undesirable aspect contributing to performance. Usually, therapists are concerned with assessment reliability once they know the assessment validity.

Face Validity

In assessment manuals, **face validity** usually presents the subjective and logical judgment used by the author or experts to declare that a test is going to measure what one wants to measure. Face validity of an assessment also is important for the client. As long as the assessment appears to address the client's health concerns meaningfully, the client will be motivated to do it well. Face validity is not testable because it rests in the eyes of the beholder, and it can be considered a primitive form of content validity.

Content Validity

Content validity examines how well an assessment represents all aspects of the phenomenon being evaluated or studied (Hulley et al., 2013). The assessment developer establishes an assessment's content validity by examining the degree to which items on the assessment are an accurate representation of content; the test developer examines test items to see how well they cover the content. Content validity is simple to establish as long as what is being assessed is not complex.

To analyze content validity, the test developer must use specific objectives for the test or a test blueprint. A ***test blueprint*** is an outline of the major content areas covered in an assessment. The test blueprint often includes the percentage of items from each subcategory to be included in the final draft of the assessment. This percentage can be supported by the literature, analysis of experiences, or some desired goal. For example, the national certification examination in occupational therapy is derived from a test blueprint that allocates the number of items to be included based on the percentage of time in activities, such as evaluation and intervention, that were reported by the participants in a national study of entry-level practice. Thus, the content validity of the national certification examination is established by confirming whether the number of items on the exam reflects current practice percentages.

Content validity is based on logical judgment using assessment objectives, a blueprint, literature-supported criteria, or some other systematic resource on which to evaluate the presence and degree of content validity. In fact, interjudge agreement increasingly is becoming a popular method of supporting content validity claims. The published assessment manual or other scientific publications should provide sufficient descriptive information about the process used to arrive at content validity assertions.

Criterion-Related Validity

Criterion-related validity is the extent to which one measure is related to a specified set of criteria or systematically related to a similar measure. To establish criterion-related validity, the scores from one assessment are correlated with an external criterion, typically an already used, usually well-established or widely accepted measure or assessment of the same criterion. This practice often is referred to as "comparing to the gold standard." Assessment developers also use a correlation statistic, called a *validity coefficient,* to verify criterion-related validity. Two types of criterion-related validity are concurrent validity and predictive validity.

Concurrent or congruent validity
Concurrent validity compares a new assessment with one that is considered a measurement standard, sometimes referred to as *the gold standard* in measurement tools. Determining the concurrent validity across tests is useful in occupational therapy to validate occupational therapy's specific professional assessments with others outside the field. The assessment developer compares the scores of a new test to an established test of the criterion by conducting both assessments at the same time. When an assessment has good concurrent

validity with another, one assessment can be eliminated. Reasons to select an assessment are because

- It is more cost-effective,
- It takes a shorter amount of time to administer,
- It has better face validity to encourage participation, or
- Its results reflect greater congruence with program goals or purpose.

Predictive validity
A test's **predictive validity,** or the ability of an assessment to predict future abilities or outcomes, is important to occupational therapists. Typically, this kind of validity relates a current characteristic to anticipated future abilities or settings. Predictive validity is established by taking a measurement at one point in time and correlating it with later findings. A therapist can develop these findings by assessing the status of a client with respect to an important skill or ability and then conducting another test of that skill or ability at a future point to see what portion of the earlier test predicted the current abilities of the client.

If the purpose of an assessment is to forecast future abilities, problems, or outcomes based on the assessment results, then the predictive validity of an assessment is important. In early intervention, occupational therapists want to know the relationship between a client's current developmental abilities and future academic or social competence issues that may arise without intervention. An occupational therapist might use a coma scale in acute care to predict future rehabilitation potential and aptitude tests to predict future work options. The therapist would want to know the predictive ability of a coma assessment or aptitude test because the results might give or limit access to services or limit the client to certain types of care systems.

Sometimes, predictive validity can guide the selection of a frame of reference as therapists study intervening variables or activities. Test manuals may compare interventions through their discussion of

> Predictive validity is important when the purpose of an assessment is to forecast future abilities, problems, or outcomes based on the assessment results, but it is difficult to establish. Construct validity is a valuable alternative when predictive validity is not possible.

the outcomes from their predictive validity sample. However, predictive validity is a challenge to establish. When predictive validity is not possible, a therapist would find construct validity valuable.

Construct Validity

Construct validity is how well a measurement conforms to theoretical constructs. This validity is established by providing evidence supporting the relationship of a given assessment and a given theory. Construct validity is established through a review of the items in the assessment and determining how well it aligns with the set of predictions of a particular theory. For example, if a theory states that certain improvements in handwriting will occur after certain interventions, then a construct validity assessment using a pre- and postintervention study can determine whether the theoretically expected changes actually occurred. If the theory predicts that handwriting is related to a child's grasp and the test administered supports the importance of the grasp, then the assessment will have good construct validity. In other words, scores on the first assessment correlate with the second. Convergent validity and discriminant validity are two specific forms of construct validity.

Convergent validity

Convergent validity occurs when there are high positive correlations between two assessments. When a new assessment becomes available, occupational therapists may compare it with an established assessment to determine the amount of agreement between the two assessments. If a high validity coefficient is achieved, then both tests measure the same construct and, consequently, a therapist can choose the assessment that best meets his or her needs. However, if the two assessments for the same construct have poor convergent validity, each measures something different, a therapist should try to uncover the reason for the difference. This information will support a therapist's decision to conduct both assessments because each assessment provides different kinds of information.

Discriminant validity

Discriminant validity is the opposite of convergent validity. With discriminant validity, high negative correlations between the two assessments are desirable when measuring the same general content or construct in very different areas. An assessment that has good discriminant validity will detect only persons with similar conditions or abilities and rule out all others. The more consistently the assessment rules out others, the better the discriminant validity.

Meaningful comparisons are essential. For example, occupational therapists would expect a test of cognition to better identify cognitive deficits in people with Alzheimer's disease rather than those without it. Or, if the assessment is designed to isolate cognitive dysfunction in the presence of Alzheimer's disease, a meaningful discriminant validity test should be able to detect a worsening of cognitive abilities at each stage of the illness. Another approach could be to compare the performance of individuals experiencing various illnesses, such as multiple sclerosis or Parkinson's disease, with different cognitive issues to see whether assessment results accurately separate these people according to their cognitive performance.

Ecological Validity

Ecological validity relates to the generalizability of study findings to other similar events or activities in everyday life; in tests and measurements, it has to do with an assessment's ability to measure, collect, and record behaviors or observations that would be observed in a typical, daily living context. Ecological validity has only recently been getting increased attention in measurement sciences. This form of validity aligns very well with occupational therapy values because it involves attention to function and quality of life, which are the concerns of clients and their families, other professions, and third-party funding or employment sources. Additionally, attention is shifting to the importance of context, not just in practice but also in evaluation.

For practice, ecological validity is important when considering current or predicted level of independence, discharge criteria, and even community functioning. Widely accepted within occupational therapy, the potential utility of an observation or behavior gathered during an evaluation or by an assessment (ecological validity) is framed within the cues associated with natural contexts or habitats.

Ecological validity has two components: verdicality and verisimilitude. **Verdicality,** the first characteristic stated to be important to ecological validity, is how well test results predict real-world performance. More recently, **verisimilitude,** the degree to which the assessment process is similar to the real-world conditions, has gained prominence.

In an occupational therapy assessment, ecological validity is important because therapists want to know how much scores and observations from a test reflect the client's current or predicted performance abilities in natural contexts. For example, if a therapist measures cognition in the clinic, knowing the ecological validity of the test to predict cognitive capacities or deficits at home or work would be useful (i.e., verdicality). Verdicality is observed during the majority of assessments that measure body functions, body structures, and performance skills.

Ecological validity is important to our evaluation processes and outcomes for intervention planning and documentation. Verisimilitude comes into play when, for example, the therapist conducts instrumental activity of daily living assessments in a clinic apartment simulation unit instead of in a client's home environment. In research using a subtest of the Assessment of Motor and Processing Skills (Fisher & Jones, 2012) to measure occupational performance first in the clinic and then immediately in the home, and vice versa, a different composite of problematic skill patterns was evidenced (Park, Fisher, & Velozo, 1994), leading one to question this assessment's verisimilitude.

Ecological validity of an assessment can be established two ways: (1) performing the assessment of function in a controlled clinical setting and then repeating it as soon as possible in the client's home to see whether scores vary because of the natural cues in the home versus the controlled, distraction-free environment during clinical assessment; or (2) correlating the assessment with accepted

> Ecological validity helps to determine an assessment's ability to measure, collect, and record behaviors or observations that would be observed in a typical, daily living context and is important when considering current or predicted level of independence, discharge criteria, and even community functioning.

assessments of functional performance in natural contexts. Occupational therapists can use the reported ecological validity of an assessment to provide reference between clinical observations and potential for community or independent living. In other words, ecological validity is the relevance of the assessment to daily living.

Factorial Validity

Factorial validity is a preferred approach to establish the validity of measures for complex behaviors. This type of validity is not necessary when an assessment looks at isolated, single-performance abilities or problems. However, an occupational therapist is interested in occupations and daily living activities, which are complex and require multiple occupational performance abilities. For an assessment to have factorial validity, it should be correlated with various other assessments that measure common traits, typically one factor or variable at a time. Sometimes, only the portion of the complex assessment that is similar to a single factor or construct is correlated with another, not the entire assessment. Factorial validity is also referred to as *multitrait–multimethod validity*.

ASSESSMENT RESPONSIVENESS

The bottom line on reliability and validity is the quality of the assessment to consistently and accurately measure a behavior or ability. The next most critical issue is responsiveness to measure change as a result of intervention, called *sensitivity* and *specificity*. **Sensitivity** is the ability to accurately detect people with a condition; **specificity** is the ability of assessment to not identify or detect people who do not have a condition. Responsiveness is related to both the reliability and validity of an assessment. It relates to the extent to which the assessment can practically or theoretically measure the current state of a person to determine current status. Most important, responsiveness determines whether and how much change has occurred.

The degree of fit between the construct and what is actually measured is important. For example, applying assessment scores with a similar construct, but one that is not reflective of the person's demographics as compared with those in the standardization sample (a question of specificity), may alter the sensitivity of an assessment.

In addition, responsiveness to change may be related to avoiding ceiling and floor effects and having scales in assessments that are unable to detect changes in performance. *Ceiling effect* is when the assessment is not able to detect additional changes at the top (ceiling) of the scale, whereas *floor effect* is when the assessment is not able to detect additional changes at the bottom (floor) of the scale. Assessments with good reliability and validity, used as intended in terms of standardization sample and procedures, have a wide enough scale to detect changes without a ceiling or floor effect and will enhance the chance of detecting change that is due to intervention (Domholdt, 2005).

FINAL THOUGHTS ABOUT RELIABILITY AND VALIDITY

This chapter has primarily focused on reliability and validity from conceptual (definition and description), methodological (research), and applied (practice) perspectives. Some additional considerations related to determining the quality of different measurement approaches need to be raised. Two timeless questions must be asked and the therapeutic value of the answers understood clearly:

1. Can an assessment have good reliability but poor validity?
2. Can an assessment have poor reliability but good validity?

The answers demonstrate one's understanding of these critical assessments and measurement concepts. Establishing the validity of assessments is more important than establishing reliability. Validity is a check against some established external criterion, demonstrating that the assessment measures what it is designed to measure (Anastasi & Urbina, 1997).

SUMMARY

Quality assessments are critical to occupational therapists' decision-making process. Therapists must seek all possible avenues to explore the quality of the assessments they use. Ensuring the quality of an assessment is no easy task. Much of the time and financial responsibility rest on the test developer until a test publisher becomes invested in marketing the assessment. Both test developers and publishers are bound by ethics, but occupational therapists must always be slightly skeptical when an assessment is being marketed, because an unethical publisher may choose to withhold certain reliability and validity studies that do not support its particular assessment. Occupational therapists should not rely solely on a test manual or even the knowledge that the assessment is frequently used by occupational therapists, and they should always conduct their own investigations. Before selecting a new assessment or reusing an existing test, occupational therapists should look at external reviews of these instruments reported in the profession's literature as well as critical reviews from outside the profession.

QUESTIONS

1. How can error in testing results be controlled or dampened to ensure accurate measurement of a person's condition or change as a result of intervention? Compare reliability and validity. Can an assessment be reliable but not valid? Can an assessment be valid but not reliable? What is the clinical relevance of using a reliable assessment? Of using a valid assessment?
2. What strategies or approaches can an occupational therapist use to make sure the final score of an assessment is more true score than error?
3. What guides an occupational therapist in looking for the right or best type(s) of established reliability or validity during the selection of an assessment?
4. What is ecological validity, and how is it important in occupational therapy evaluation? Applying the American Occupational Therapy Association's (2014) *Occupational Therapy Framework: Domain and Process,* what is the ecological validity of the assessments commonly used in practice, such as the Timed Up-and-Go test (Shumway-Cook, Brauer, & Woollacott, 2000)?

5. How can test specificity and sensitivity be enhanced or supported during assessment in practice?

6. Describe the differences in measurement among standard deviation, standard error of measurement, and standard error of estimate. What do they mean, and how are they applied in interpreting a person's performance after assessment?

7. For each type of reliability and validity, summarize the following: How and why an assessment developer would want to establish this type of validity, why knowing that the assessment had this characteristic would be important to an occupational therapist, and why this type of reliability or validity is important to know when interpreting the scores obtained from a person for diagnostic or intervention planning purposes.

References

American Occupational Therapy Association. (2014). Occupational therapy practice framework: Domain and process (3rd ed.). *American Journal of Occupational Therapy, 68*(Suppl. 1), S1–S48. http://dx.doi.org/10.5014.ajot.2014.682006

Anastasi, A., & Urbina, S. (1997). *Psychological testing* (7th ed.). Upper Saddle River, NJ: Prentice Hall.

Bolton, B. F., Parker, R. M., & Brookings, J. B. (2008). Scores and norms. In B. F. Bolton (Ed.), *Handbook of measurement and evaluation in rehabilitation* (4th ed., pp. 3–28). Austin, TX: Pro–Ed.

Cohel, R. J., & Swerdlik, M. E. (2010). *Psychological testing and assessment: An introduction to tests and measurement* (7th ed.). Boston: McGraw Hill.

Crist, P. (2010). Reliability and validity: The psychometrics of standardized assessments. In J. Hinojosa, P. Kramer, & P. Crist (Eds.), *Evaluation: Obtaining and interpreting data* (3rd ed., pp. 179–200). Bethesda, MD: AOTA Press.

Domholdt, E. (2005). *Rehabilitation research: Principles and applications.* St. Louis: Elsevier/Saunders.

Fisher, A. G., & Jones, K. B. (2012). *Assessment of motor and process skills* (7th ed., rev.). Fort Collins, CO: Three Star Press.

Howell, D. C. (2014). *Fundamental statistics for the behavioral sciences* (8th ed.). Belmont, CA: Wadsworth/Cengage Learning.

Hulley, S. B., Cummings, S. R., Browner, W. S., Grady, D. G., & Newman, T. B. (2013). *Designing clinical research* (4th ed.). Philadelphia: Lippincott Williams & Wilkins.

Kubiszyn, T., & Borich, G. (2013). *Educational testing and measurement: Classroom applications and practice* (10th ed.). New York: Wiley.

Merriam-Webster's online dictionary. (n.d.). Correlation. Retrieved from http://www.merriam-webster.com/dictionary/correlation

Nunnally, J. C., & Bernstein, I. H. (1994). *Psychometric theory* (3rd ed.). New York: McGraw-Hill.

Park, S., Fisher, A. G., & Velozo, C. A. (1994). Using the assessment of motor and process skills to compare occupational performance between clinic and home settings. *American Journal of Occupational Therapy, 48,* 697–709. http://dx.doi/10.5014/ajot.48.8.697

Portney, L. G., & Watkins, M. P. (2009). *Foundations of clinical research: Applications to practice* (3rd ed.). Upper Saddle River, NJ: Pearson/Prentice Hall.

Shumway-Cook, A., Brauer, S., & Woollacott, M. (2000). Predicting the probability for falls in community-dwelling older adults using the Timed Up and Go Test. *Physical Therapy, 80*(9), 896–903.

Thorndike, R. M., & Thorndike-Christ, T. (2008). Reliability. In B. F. Bolton (Ed.), *Handbook of measurement and evaluation in rehabilitation* (4th ed., pp. 33–56). Austin, TX: Pro–Ed.

Thorndike, R. M., & Thorndike-Christ, T. (2009). *Measurement and evaluation in psychology and education* (8th ed.). Upper Saddle River, NJ: Prentice Hall.

Weinberg, S. L., & Abramowitz, S. K. (2008). *Statistics using SPSS: An integrative approach* (2nd ed.). New York: Cambridge University Press.

CHAPTER 10

Scoring and Interpretation of Results

Patricia Crist, PhD, OTR, PC, FAOTA

Highlights

- Scoring
- Response methods for test items
- Norm-referenced and criterion-referenced tests
- Essential statistical concepts for scoring and interpretation
- Item analysis
- Norms
- Reporting scores
- Controlling error in test scores for better interpretation
- Steps in scoring and interpreting performance on a standardized assessment.

Key Terms

Ambiguity error	Halo effect
Assessment validity	Inclusive range
Ceiling	Interpretation of assessment scores
Central tendency	Interval scale
Central tendency errors	Intraindividual error
Checklist scales	Item difficulty
Contrast error	Item discrimination
Criterion-referenced testing	Likert scales
Cross-validation	Local norm groups
Derived score	Logical error
Developmental age-equivalent scores	Marking system
Extreme groups validation	Mean
False acceptances	Measurement science
False rejections	Median
Fixed reference group norms	Metric data
Forced-choice scales	Metric scale
Generosity or leniency error	Mode
Grade equivalents	Multiple norm group comparisons

National norms
Nominal scale
Norm-referenced testing
Normal curve
Normal distribution
Norms
Observation of performance
Obtained score
Ordinal scale
Percentile equivalent or rank measures
Percentile scores
Proximity error
Psychometrics
Q-sort
Range
Rasch analysis
Rating scales
Ratio scale

Raw score
Response methods
Response scale
Semantic differential scales
Semi-interquartile deviation or range
Sensitivity
Severity error
Significance
Special group norms
Standard deviation
Standard score
Standardization sample
Stanine scores
t scores
Test validity
Variability
Variance
z score

The primary goal of evaluation is to determine intervention needs or changes in an established assessment-based intervention. Abilities, attitudes, cognitions, perceptions, motivations, and other constructs, including environmental influences related to occupational performance, require not only reliable and valid measures but also accuracy in translating the measures for understanding and use in occupational therapy. A critical aspect of the evaluation process for an occupational therapist is the ability to interpret assessment results accurately.

Applying evaluation conventions to scoring processes and interpretation of results leads to effective evaluation documentation and facilitates best practices in intervention planning. Additionally, scoring and interpretation approaches are the basis of describing program outcomes. Therefore, skilled scoring and interpretation provide a valid measurement of client performance. Further, individual results grouped together can provide compelling measures of program outcomes.

At the foundation of this understanding is the occupational therapist's knowledge of the psychometrics underpinning scores and the degree of measurement accuracy in relation to the influence of error. Knowing reliability, validity, accuracy, and error related to scoring and interpreting measures contributes to the degree of confidence one can assume in reporting assessment results. This chapter provides the knowledge required to give meaning

to scores, called the ***interpretation of assessment scores.*** Using measurement principles leads to assessment accuracy that underpins professional confidence in reporting scores.

SCORING

The goal of scoring an assessment is to transform an observed or acquired performance on a test item to an accurate, defensible, and meaningful interpretation that can contribute to clinical reasoning and provide understandable assessment results for problem solving, intervention planning, and communication purposes. Converting an observed performance during an assessment to a usable result follows a systemic process:

$$\text{raw score} \rightarrow \text{derived or obtained score} \rightarrow$$
$$[\text{standard score}] \rightarrow \text{test interpretation}$$

The evaluator's first step in scoring a test behavior is marking a **raw score** for the observed performance or response. Then in typical practice, the assessment manual provides a **response scale** or **marking system** to

> The goal of scoring an assessment is to transform an observed or acquired performance on a test item to an accurate, defensible, and meaningful interpretation that can contribute to clinical reasoning and provide understandable assessment results for problem solving, intervention planning, and communication purposes.

transform the raw score into meaningful information for intervention purposes. This score is called a *derived* or *obtained score.* One of the few times raw scores are used, other than the initial step of scoring an assessment, is during research data collection, because a raw score is a pure score without other transformations.

In some instances, assessment manuals (or the therapist as an evaluator) convert the derived score to a **standard score,** which sometimes makes scores even more meaningful to stakeholders. Standard scores allow comparisons between assessments that use different scoring scales. The brackets around this step in the diagram reflect the optional nature of the conversion to standard scores because a therapist can accurately interpret from either obtained or standard scores. Certainly, the ability to complete all these steps in scoring is dependent on the development and standardization of procedures published for the assessment.

A score or test result is only a snapshot of current abilities or conditions. In intervention planning and clinical decision-making processes, a therapist should consider other important evaluation-related information, such as observations, records, reports from other disciplines, client and program resources, predictions regarding recovery or skill development, and, most importantly, the client's goals and needs.

The compelling goal of any assessment is to identify definitively and accurately what needs to be measured. This is called *test validity.* The validity of an assessment is an indication of how well it measures what it says it does. Validity is a primary determinant in a therapist's decisions. According to Anastasi and Urbina (1997) and Urbina (2004), there are essentially four decisions from assessment that are the outcome of a test's validity; two are correct decisions and two are wrong decisions:

- Two correct decisions:
  1. Assessment correctly detects a condition that truly exists.
  2. Assessment correctly does not find a condition that does not exist.

- Two wrong decisions:
  1. Assessment wrongly finds a condition that truly does not exist (i.e., **false acceptances**).

2. Assessment wrongly does not find a condition that truly exists (i.e., **false rejections**).

With the first wrong decision (false acceptance), an assessment result would support providing unneeded interventions that could be harmful, such as taking a drug for an illness a client does not have, risking uncomfortable side effects for no benefit. With false rejections, the client does not receive treatment from which he or she could have benefited. False acceptances are a waste of valuable resources and add unnecessary health care costs. False rejections are a more serious testing failure.

Thus, along with the reliability and validity of the obtained scores, scoring interpretation (i.e., **assessment validity**) becomes very important so the frequency of correct findings is maximized and wrong decisions minimized. Assessment validity indicates that the results are correct and true to ensure accuracy in what is being measured, to identify the best intervention approach, and to provide cost-efficient health care. These factors are the essence of assessment validity.

RESPONSE METHODS FOR TEST ITEMS

When selecting an assessment with the best quality for a given program need, the occupational therapist has several choices. Ultimately, the quality of test scores begins with the type of response method or rating scales included in the assessment. **Response methods** or **rating scales** provide a mechanism for gathering information on the strength of a response, feeling, or performance. In addition, the quality of the method or scale influences the value of the information obtained for future intervention or program evaluation purposes. Although covering all rating scales or response methods is impossible, the following are typical ones seen in occupational therapy:

- *Observation of performance* uses a standardized protocol that directs attention to preidentified issues, some not relevant to the evaluation needed.
- *Likert scales* are a highly used response type in which specific rank-ordered responses

are presented in the scale. Likert scales are response rating scales with 3 to 7 linearly related test response options differentiating the degree of response. The response anchors vary, and include *strongly disagree* to *strongly agree, very much like me* to *not at all like me,* and *0% of the time* to *100% of the time.* Likert scales with midpoints, especially those that read *don't know* or similar, are test-taker friendly but give no real response for the basis of diagnosing or interrupting problems. A midpoint, for *no response, not sure,* or *no opinion,* increases test-taker comfort, but repeated use as a selected response greatly limits a therapist's understanding of the client's problems or needs. When the assessment does not provide a midpoint item (especially one that allows fence sitting), the test taker is forced to choose a side. This set-up ultimately will give the therapist better information about the client's true needs or interests. However, this approach to testing may lower test-taker motivation to complete the test.

- *Checklist scales* include all the possible adjectives or characteristics relating to the purpose of the assessment, using a *present* or *absent* response format. Checklists can give wide coverage of characteristics but cannot give information regarding the strength of contribution of the ones that are marked present.
- *Forced-choice scales* attempt to reduce bias in responses by forcing the test taker to choose one of the assessment items. There is no midpoint for no decision or a *no response, not observed,* or *not present* category. Forced-choice scales provide an evaluation of strength of response, for example, "Indicate the degree to which the following statement describes your interest."
- *Semantic differential scales* allow subjective evaluation of concepts along a continuum with end anchor words such as goodness descriptors (good–bad, fair–unfair), potency or strength responses (heavy–light, hard–soft), or activity dimensions (active–passive, fast–slow). These scales are most effective when a multipoint scale is provided for marking answers, if the midpoint is not *don't know* or *not sure.*

- *Q-sort* asks the responder to sort a series of items such as pictures or words into specific stacks according to stated criterion categories such as *which activities you currently engage in* or *do now, used to do, would like to do in the future,* and *not interested in doing.*

These response or rating scales are the major types seen in occupational therapy; there are many more. The best scales most clearly approximate what the therapist wants to assess and use a method that thoroughly elicits potential responses. Nevertheless, the most important rule to increase response rate, ensure a true score, and provide validity is to ask only about what one wants to know.

NORM-REFERENCED AND CRITERION-REFERENCED TESTS

It is important to understand the two major types of assessments, norm-referenced and criterion-referenced, before discussing scoring. **Norm-referenced testing** compares the results of the person being tested against the population or representative sample. Norm-referenced testing allows a therapist to place or rank the individual's performance in relation to others who have taken the test. Norm-referenced testing

- Compares individual results to the population or a representative sample,
- Allows ranking of individual performance against other test takers,
- Broadly tests behaviors or abilities, and
- Is more useful when requesting additional intervention from third-party payers.

Criterion-referenced testing uses a criterion or a standard of performance or skill attainment to measure mastery. Criterion-referenced testing provides an occupational therapist with knowledge regarding the test taker's level of proficiency or mastery of the skill or ability that the assessment measures. Two other common labels for criterion-referenced testing are (1) *competency* or (2) *competency-based testing.* Criterion-referenced testing

- Compares individual results to a criterion or standard of performance,

- Measures client mastery of skill or ability,
- Narrowly tests a specific area of mastery, and
- Is important for discharge decisions and determining learning group or therapeutic group placement.

All of us are familiar with both types of testing. The college entrance boards compare each test taker to the standardization group to score performance. Most classes use norm-referenced testing, assuming that getting an earned score of 95% means that student knows about 20% more information than a student with an earned score of 75%. Criterion-referenced approaches are used in high school physical education classes (when a student has to demonstrate a certain level of physical condition before passing) and in schools that require a student to achieve a certain minimum test score to graduate.

In occupational therapy, the national evaluation for Level II fieldwork is based on mastery learning or acquiring competency to be an entry-level therapist. The occupational therapy national certification examination is criterion-referenced, because the test taker must accumulate enough correct answers out of the total number of valid test items to demonstrate that he or she is at least minimally competent to be an entry-level occupational therapist. Similarly, the American Occupational Therapy Association (AOTA)–developed occupational therapist and occupational therapy assistant's Level II fieldwork student assessments are competency based. To ensure score validity, only a pass–fail grade (i.e., competent or not competent) is accurate, not a letter grade (i.e., levels of competency).

Norm-referenced assessments provide comparative information from a **standardization sample** of people with defined demographic characteristics. On campus, all the scores earned by one class on one midterm are interpreted as "the normative group" for that one exam. For an assessment used in practice, the outcomes from the standardization sample are called **norms.** Norms are the comparative basis for interpreting the results of the person the therapist assesses.

To make a valid comparison, the test taker's characteristics must be similar to the demographic characteristics of the norm sample. In creating a norm-referenced assessment, the developer selects test items that promote variance and spread performance results along a continuum of complexity.

Norms provide a comparison of the possible range of scores rather than simply showing the presence or absence of a characteristic, ability, or skill as criterion-referenced approaches do. Norm-referenced assessments permit a broader testing of behaviors or abilities, whereas criterion-referenced testing measures a narrow, frequently very specific, area of mastery.

When creating a criterion-referenced assessment, the developer chooses items that reflect different levels of mastery. Thus, content validity is very important. Criterion-referenced or mastery tests are important in occupational therapy when deciding whether to discharge a client or place him or her in certain learning or therapeutic groups based on similar capabilities or deficits. Criterion-referenced assessments are useful in measuring skill or performance attainment of activities of daily living because an occupational therapist simply wants to know what a person can and cannot do. Although a therapist can use the findings from this type of assessment to request more intervention time from third-party payers, norm-referenced information usually is more effective in supporting the need for intervention.

Both types of tests can be standardized in terms of test items, administration, and scoring. To ensure the quality of the assessment processes and have confidence in scores, an occupational therapist must always

- Read the test manual before administering the assessment,
- Practice delivering the assessment before using it to assess a client,
- Adhere exactly to the published administration and scoring instructions in the assessment manual without deviating or adapting the assessment to a specific situation, and
- Convey the importance of the assessment to clients so they will be encouraged to do their best.

If a therapist deviates from the published procedures for any reason, he or she must use caution when reporting the results. When a therapist does not follow the standardized procedures, he or she has no way to determine the effect of this choice on the obtained scores. The results received are not necessarily accurate because of the deviation from the standardized procedure. When writing a report after deviating from the standardized procedures, the therapist must describe the deviation and what occurred, indicating that it might affect the results, and caution against using these data.

ESSENTIAL STATISTICAL CONCEPTS FOR SCORING AND INTERPRETATION

A test score is typically the sum of responses to test items or tasks. The goal in scoring is to convert an observation to a numerical quantity so that a therapist can record, analyze, and meaningfully interpret the results. Interpreting scores requires that the therapist understands this process and applying related statistics, called **psychometrics** or **measurement science.** With increased accountability expected in practice, an occupational therapist must understand the statistics used in tests and measurements.

This textbook provides only a conceptual understanding of certain test statistics applied to the evaluation process. The next section is a review of the psychometrics that are essential to a competent evaluator. Readers are advised to use other resources for a more thorough discussion on statistics and a deeper understanding of what is discussed here. The concepts discussed in the following section are defined or described in Table 10.1.

Measurement Scales

Tests and measurements use four different measurement scales. These levels or scales are important to know in testing because the required response or answer method dictates the boundaries for quantifying and reporting test results. The scales (and

Table 10.1. Basic Statistical Concepts for Scoring and Interpretation

Concept	Description
Score	*Raw score:* A test taker's response to a specific test item before it is converted to some other number following test manual instructions; what is marked by the test taker or evaluator during the process of the evaluation. *Obtained or derived score:* Conversion of the raw score to some other form using a method published for the test. *Standard score:* Conversion of the derived score to a form that permits comparison of the test results with others.
Levels of measurement	*Nominal:* Score that identifies a test taker as having or not having the characteristic. *Ordinal:* Score that rank orders a given characteristic across all test takers. *Interval:** Score that reflects the magnitude of difference between responses; contains a standard unit of measurement, making it possible to quantifiably measure differences between test takers. *Ratio:** Score that is like an interval scale but is ratio based using a scale with a zero point (i.e., complete absence of characteristic).
Normal distribution	Mathematically determined curve representing the theoretical distribution of scores or some other characteristic across the population that clusters around a central point called a mean or average.

Note. *Can be combined to create a "metric scale."
From "Scoring and Interpretation of Results," by P. Crist. In J. Hinojosa, P. Kramer, and P. Crist (Eds.), *Evaluation: Obtaining and Interpreting Data* (3rd ed.), Bethesda, MD: AOTA Press, p. 206. Copyright © 2010 by the American Occupational Therapy Association. Used with permission.

examples) are presented from the simplest to the most sophisticated (Exhibit 10.1).

Nominal scale

Nominal scale scores identify a person as having or not having a particular characteristic. Test items with responses resulting in mutually exclusive categories, such as yes or no, male or female, marital status (single, married, widowed, divorced), pain or no pain, having a symptom or not, being able to run or not, and being able to fix breakfast or not are nominal. The condition, characteristic, ability, or whatever the test item is measuring is marked as either present or not present.

Checklists and Q-sort response scales result in nominal data. One example is the assigned number for a Special Olympian because the number identifies a competitor and has no relevance other than tracking competitors. Other examples include indicating whether loss of sensation is present or not present with carpal tunnel syndrome and sorting different activities into "Preferred," "Not Preferred," and "Do Not Know" categories.

Ordinal scale

An **ordinal scale** ranks the characteristic measured along a continuum. Ordinal scales provide information only about position, not magnitude or degree of a condition or ability. Some examples of ordinal ranking are tallest to smallest, most to least pain, total number of medications, and high to low stress. The condition, characteristic, ability, or attribute the test item is measuring must vary in a linear progression and along a continuum with anchors at each end being polar opposites.

The use of Likert or semantic differential response scales results in ordinal data. Examples are winning a gold, silver, or bronze medal or reporting sensation loss in one, two, or three fingers with carpal tunnel syndrome.

Interval scale

An **interval scale** has a standard unit of measure in response sets that allow a person to estimate the magnitude of difference between responses. It is an ordinal scale with equal units along its length. For instance, when measuring the number of minutes it takes a worker to sort hardware into three different canisters, the person who finishes the test item in 5 minutes is twice as fast as a person who does the same tasks in 10 minutes. Other examples are temperature and time to run a 50-meter race.

Ratio scale

A **ratio scale** is like the interval scale with an underlying measurement, but a major difference is that a ratio scale has a true zero point (ratio based). Some examples are miles per hour and feet per second. For an occupational therapist, ratio scales are often physical measures, such as top running speed in the 50-meter race or rate of nerve conductance with carpal tunnel syndrome.

EXHIBIT 10.1. TYPES OF SCALES

Nominal scale	Either having or not having a particular characteristic questions • Male or female • Marital status • Pain or no pain
Ordinal scale	Ranked along a continuum; position information, not magnitude or degree • Tallest to smallest • Most to least pain • Total number of medications • High to low stress • Winning a bronze, silver, or gold medal
Interval scale	Magnitude estimations (ordinal scale with equal units along its length) • Temperature • Time to run the 50-meter race
Ratio scale	Interval scale with a true zero point; usually used for physical measures • Miles per hour • Feet per second

Measurement scale summary

Most measurement scales use either ordinal or interval scales to gather responses to test items. Some experts argue that there is no real difference in response data tabulated using an interval or ratio scale, and so they combine the two and call it a ***metric scale.***

Understanding the item response method and the related scale of measurement used to gather scores is important because it influences how an occupational therapist interprets scores. For instance, a checklist collects nominal data on characteristics. All a therapist knows when scoring this test is which characteristics the client reports or identifies to describe himself or herself or some activity. A therapist does not know the strength of the response, which likely varies from one checklist item to another.

Central Tendency

With a normal curve, all three measures of **central tendency**—the mean, median, and mode—are equivalent (i.e., at the peak of the normal curve; Exhibit 10.2). Figure 10.1 contains a normal curve, which will be discussed extensively later. Each of the three measures of central tendency is a different approach to describing the most common or average characteristic in a group or set of scores. Exhibit 10.2 describes the different types of central tendency.

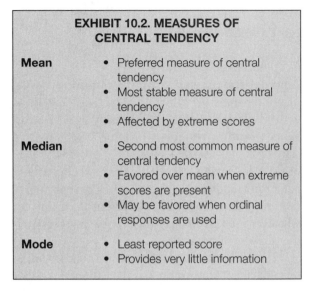

EXHIBIT 10.2. MEASURES OF CENTRAL TENDENCY

Mean
- Preferred measure of central tendency
- Most stable measure of central tendency
- Affected by extreme scores

Median
- Second most common measure of central tendency
- Favored over mean when extreme scores are present
- May be favored when ordinal responses are used

Mode
- Least reported score
- Provides very little information

Mean

The ***mean*** ($\bar{X}$) is the average of the group of scores. Some texts use M rather than $\bar{X}$ (referred to as "bar X") as the symbol for the mean or mathematical average. The formula is

$$\bar{X} = \frac{\Sigma X}{N} \quad \text{or} \quad \text{average} = \frac{\text{sum of all scores}}{\text{total number of scores}}$$

where

- Σ (the sigma symbol) indicates sum of the scores obtained
- X indicates the scores obtained, and

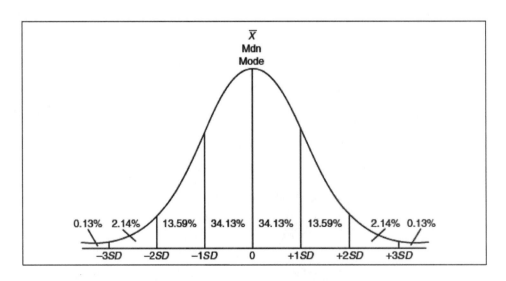

Figure 10.1. Normal distribution.
Note. Mdn = median; *SD* = standard deviation; $\bar{X}$ = mean.

- *N* indicates the total number of scores gathered.

The mean has several features that make it the preferred measure of central tendency. It is the most stable because each score contributes to the calculation, but it is greatly affected by extreme scores. The implications of this characteristic of the mean are discussed later in this chapter.

Median

The **median** is the second most frequently encountered measure of central tendency. It evenly divides the population in half, with 50% above the median and 50% below. The median is favored over the mean when extreme scores are present, as discussed later in this chapter. Also, it may be favored with ordinal response items on a test. The measurement abbreviation for the median is *mdn*.

To calculate a median, a therapist orders scores from low to high and then selects the score that divides the group equally in half. If there is an even number of items, then the median is the average of the two center-most numbers. Following are examples of the calculation:

$$\frac{(56 + 62)}{2} = 59$$

		45
45	45	52
52	56	56
56	56	62
62	56	75
109	62	109
mdn = 56	mdn = 56	mdn = 59

Mode

The **mode** is the least reported score, used only when it permits the author to make an important point regarding the interpretation of the results. The mode is not often used because it provides very little information beyond which scores occur most frequently. If two scores occur most frequently, it is a bimodal distribution. If each score appears an equal number of times, then there is no mode.

Following are examples of the calculation:

Scores

- 1 6 9 8 2: No mode
- 5 1 2 5 6 5: Mode = 5
- 1 5 1 5 5 1: Mode = 5
- 1 5 1 5 6 1: Modes = 1 and 5

Variability

Variability is the spread of scores around a measure of central tendency. Variation provides information regarding how condensed or widely spread the scores are in the distribution. Variation is important because a smaller variation around the measure of central tendency indicates that the score is accurate (i.e., a true score) and not due to random variation (i.e., error).

To calculate variability (i.e., range) in a group of scores, subtract the smallest score in the group from the largest, as shown below:

Highest score	Lowest score	Variability
95	65	30
95	15	80
95	85	10

Standard deviation

The **standard deviation** is the estimate of variance that accompanies the mean. The notation for the standard deviation is *SD*. Standard deviation is powerful because it considers every score obtained. Standard deviation as a measure of test variability is discussed under the normal distribution section below. The standard deviation provides the basis to compare results from different tests taken by a person. Essentially, the variance is similar to the standard deviation. If item responses are collected using ordinal scales of measurement, extreme caution must be taken in reporting the mean and related standard deviation, because the initial data are not sophisticated enough to warrant this application.

The calculation for a standard deviation is more difficult to do than calculating the other types of variances. Most assessment manuals report the standard deviation, and calculators make it easy to determine. Here are the two approaches to calculating standard deviation:

$$SD = \frac{\sqrt{\Sigma(x - \overline{X})^2}}{N}$$

Or, because $x - \overline{X} = \overline{x}$

$$SD = \frac{\sqrt{\Sigma \overline{x}^2}}{N}$$

Semi-interquartile deviation or range

The **semi-interquartile (SIRQ) deviation or range** is based on the range of the middle 50% of the scores around the median instead of the entire range of scores. It is noted as the SIQR. Like the median, this variance measure compensates for extreme scores and is preferred when test items are gathered using ordinal response scales.

Calculation of the SIQR is even more complex than calculating variance and standard deviations and is a bit more challenging. Because test developers provide a table in most test manuals with which to match your obtained score, only the formula is presented here:

$$SIQR = \frac{Q_3 - Q_1}{2}$$ where 75% of the scores are below Q_3 & 25% of the scores are below Q_1

One disadvantage of the SIQR is that it uses only half of the acquired scores, so it is more stable than the range but not as good as the standard deviation, which considers all scores.

Range

Range is the easiest estimate of variance but also the least sophisticated. The notation for range is R. The range is calculated by subtracting the lowest score from the highest score. Sometimes, the range is called an *inclusive range.* The inclusive range is calculated by subtracting the lowest score from the highest score and adding 1.

The following are ways to calculate and inclusive for the range set of scores 33 45 47 51 62 79 88 93:

- Range = 93 – 33 = 60
- Inclusive range = (93 – 33) + 1 = 61

Range is must often written in reports in the following ways:

- "The scores range from 33 to 93."
- Range: (33 < x < 93)
- Range: = 33 to 93

An occupational therapist seldom sees the calculated range reported to describe variance in scores because it provides little valuable information. What a therapist usually sees is the lowest and highest score reported, so he or she knows the general spread and, if the therapist has an individual score, would know where it would generally fit in the norm sample results.

The reported range also may be interesting for seeing whether anyone passed all items on an assessment; if a person does so, then there is a **ceiling.** The presence of a ceiling in norm-referenced testing is problematic because the therapist will not see any differences between individuals in the ceiling score area. Likewise, in norm-referenced testing, a therapist wants a range as wide as possible with no extreme score outliers, giving the best possible variation to detect differences between scores.

Normal Distribution

The **normal distribution** is a standard developed in 1733 by Abraham de Moivre from theory and mathematical calculations (Pearson, 1924; see Table 10.1 for the definition). For test and measurement purposes, the underlying premise is that if a person gathered responses to any variable from a very large number of people, the numbers of people achieving each score most likely would distribute themselves in a **normal curve,** the model used to make comparisons among scores or statistical decisions. Normal distribution is shown in Figure 10.1.

EXHIBIT 10.3. CENTRAL TENDENCY AND VARIABILITY IN SCORING

Central tendency
- *Mean:* Average of a group of scores; noted as $\bar{X}$ or M.
- *Median:* Score that splits the distribution in half; 50% of the scores are above and 50% are below the median; called the *midpoint score*; noted as *mdn*.
- *Mode:* Score that occurs most frequently in the distribution of scores.

Variability
- *Standard deviation:* Estimate of variability that normally accompanies the mean because of accumulated error; noted as *SD, S,* or σ.
- *Variance:* Also called the *mean square deviation*, is a variation on the *SD*; noted as *MSD*.
- *Semi-interquartile deviation or range:* Based on the range of the middle 50% of the scores around the median instead of the entire range of scores; noted as SIQR.
- *Range:* Usually the high and low score are given as the range; another method is to subtract low score from high score, giving one number for the range; noted as R.

In the normal distribution, the mean $(\bar{X})$, median *(mdn)*, and mode are all equal because the distribution is symmetrical on both sides. The previous section included a description of the measures of central tendency (Exhibit 10.3). In addition, the percentages of scores represented under each area that equate to each standard deviation is a standard derived from the normal curve. Each standard deviation is set at a place where the direction of the curve changes mathematically.

Remember that standard deviation refers to an error in measurement. If there is no error (which does not occur in testing), an occupational therapist could dismiss the concept of standard deviation altogether, but because error is present in any assessment administered, a therapist always will introduce some measurement of variance into the interpretation of results.

This simple curve should be committed to memory because recalling this information with ease will help immensely in listening to and giving reports in team meetings or reading client records regarding assessment outcomes. Some helpful information from the normal curve includes

- The percentage of scores between 0 and +1 *SD* or 0 and –1 *SD* is 34.13% (commonly referred to as 34%),
- The percentage of scores between +1 *SD* and +2 *SD* or –1 *SD* and –2 *SD* is 13.59% (commonly referred to as 14%),

- The percentage of scores between +2 *SD* and +3 *SD* or –2 *SD* and –3 *SD* is 2.14% (commonly referred to as 2%), and
- 99% of the scores fall between –3 *SD* and +3 *SD*.

Typically, all scores on an assessment will be between –3 *SD* and +3 *SD*. Further, a therapist can add the areas under the curve to gain reference information:

> 68% of the scores are between –1 *SD* and + 1 *SD* (34% + 34% = 68%).

Alternatively, a therapist can calculate the percentage of scores above or below a standard deviation: What percentage of people scored less than +2 *SD*? Add the areas to the left of this mark: 2% + 14% + 34% + 34% = 84%. These numbers always correlate with **percentile scores** (cumulative percentages). Therapists who understand the standard deviation in relation to the normal distribution can easily convert scores to percentile scores because they are equivalent to the areas under the curve. So in the last example, the individual score was in the 84th percentile.

The therapist should never automatically interpret a score left of the center of the normal distribution as being bad or negative. Sometimes a therapist would prefer scores to be on that side of the mean, with a negative

> Never automatically interpret a standard deviation score left of the center of the normal distribution as being bad or negative. Always interpret assessment data or norms with reference to the direction of the measure used.

EXHIBIT 10.4. TYPES OF SCORE REPORTING

Measurement scale
- Metric (ratio or interval)
- Ordinal
- Nominal

Central tendency
- Mean
- Median
- Mode

Variance
- Standard deviation
- Semi-interquartile deviation or range
- Not applicable

Note. From "Scoring and Interpretation of Results," by P. Crist. In J. Hinojosa, P. Kramer, and P. Crist (Eds.), *Evaluation: Obtaining and Interpreting Data* (3rd ed.), Bethesda, MD: AOTA Press, p. 213. Copyright © 2010 by the American Occupational Therapy Association. Used with permission.

SD reported, for example, if the normal distribution reflects the degree of disability present, the current cholesterol level, or bone density score. Always interpret assessment data or norms with reference to the direction of the measure used.

Relationships Between Central Tendency and Variation in Testing

The mean and standard deviation are the most sophisticated and sensitive measures for evaluating data because they are based on the assumption that the obtained scores are based on interval or ratio levels of measurement and all scores in the distribution are used. The simplest measure is the mode because it gives little information; thus, modes are seldom reported. More often, the upper and lower limits of the range are reported to indicate the variation of the scores. The level of difficulty is related to the way in which responses are gathered (i.e., the level of measurement; Exhibit 10.4).

When a response to a test item results in interval or ratio data, sometimes combined and called **metric data,** it is legitimate to calculate a mean and standard deviation. However, with ordinal data, a therapist can use only the median or mode, and the mode only with nominal data. An interval or ratio measure can be converted to the less sophisticated

forms related to ordinal and nominal items; an ordinal response can be converted to a nominal response. However, one category cannot be converted to a more sophisticated one because there is not sufficient information to make a valid conversion.

Skewing in Score Curves

In the real world of testing, many tests result in skewed curves, which affect the use of the normal distribution and related measures of central tendency. Figure 10.2 shows examples of positively and negatively skewed assessments. As illustrated and discussed previously, the mean is the most sensitive to clustering at one end of the curve and to extreme scores. The median is not as unstable. Thus, using the mean is problematic when extreme scores skew a curve.

One area where skewed distributions get much attention is in the classroom. Grade-conscious students realize two things:

1. Everyone prefers a negatively skewed test over a positively skewed one, especially if the instructor sticks to the published grading scale in the syllabus, because scores cluster toward the high end of the scale.
2. When a test is positively skewed, everyone in the class is shocked by their low grades and hopes that the instructor does not use the earned grade without somehow adjusting the scores (i.e., through bonus points or curving).

Instructors who are more sophisticated use test and measurement principles and statistics to aid in fair, accountable decision making regarding test scores and logical communication to others using standards accepted in testing practices. When the instructor uses test statistics with skewed test results, decision making should center on the median, not the mean. Sometimes an instructor is lenient and curves the test using the mode, instead of the median or mean, and applies the test's standard deviation to determine the cutoff score needed for each percentage or letter grade.

When an assessment has skewed results, the author of the assessment usually will address this issue in the manual and provide a guide for interpreting the assessment outcomes.

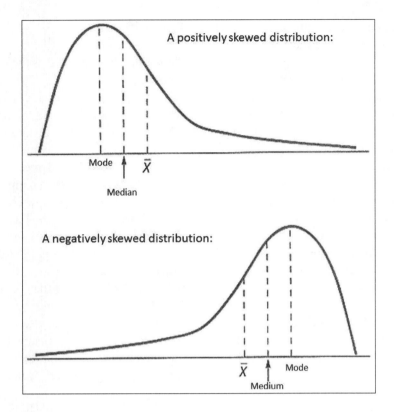

Figure 10.2. Impact on central tendency with skewed curves.
Note. Mdn = median; $\overline{X}$ = mean.
Source. J. Hinojosa. Used with permission.

Sensitivity

Sensitivity relates to the stability or the pull on a variable away from the mode of the curve. In skewed curves, the mean is pulled faster than the median, and the median is always between the mean and mode, so the mean is more sensitive.

What is the clinical importance of this concept? If an occupational therapist has a group of scores and there are a few very high or low outliers, reporting the mean will misrepresent the scores. Thus, the median is more suitable to use with outlying scores.

An administrative example applying the concept of skewed distributions shows the effect of outliers on the measure of central tendency. An administrator challenged an occupational therapy department to prove that average department salaries were below market value. He included the salary of the department head (an outlier; it was much higher than those of frontline staff) with all other occupational therapy salaries to arrive at a department average. According to the administrator's monthly expense printout, the average occupational therapist salary in the department was $50,100, which was $8,000 above the average reported by area hospitals. When the salary of the department head was removed from the average, however, the average occupational therapist salary was only $37,000. The staff explained their rationale using statistical information about outliers and was rewarded a permanent $5,000 salary increase!

ITEM ANALYSIS

The reliability and validity of an assessment are important, but another quantitative feature to consider is item analysis. The effectiveness of any item on a test can be studied by analyzing responses to it. Item analysis reflects two different features: (1) item difficulty and (2) item discrimination. Item analysis is used to perfect a test, or in other words, to improve its reliability and validity. Item analysis can shorten the test by eliminating test items that do not contribute significantly.

The **significance** of a test measures what the assessment purports to measure (i.e., validity) and whether it does it accurately (i.e., more true than error score). Some assessment developers try to use random selection for this process, which is better than serendipity, but it is not the best approach to adding or removing test items. For instance, a test item may be very difficult and the majority of test takers will not be able to answer, but if the high scorers on the test always get it correct, then it is a good item to retain because it discriminates this group from the rest.

According to Miller, Linn, and Gronlund (2012), item analysis is designed to answer questions such as

- Did the items function as intended?
- Were the test items of appropriate difficulty?
- Were the test items free of irrelevant clues and other defects?
- Was each of the distracters effective (in multiple-choice items)? (p. 362)

The assessment developers ask these questions when constructing their test, but these questions also are good for an occupational therapist to consider when choosing an assessment for practice. It is important for the therapist to look for this information in the assessment's standardization manual and reflect on subjective feelings or experiences with the assessment in the context in which it will be used.

In practice, it is useful to review items that the client did not answer correctly. This review may give the therapist clues as to what the client does not understand and what skills the client has not yet acquired. This reflective review of missed or wrong responses to items can include

- Discussing with the client to discover what he or she does not know,
- Looking for groupings of similar problems to focus intervention on skills that do not seem to have been acquired during a given time,
- Uncovering how a therapist might improve the intervention approach to prevent recurrence in future clients, or
- Looking for another assessment that better relates to the goals of the intervention program.

Item Difficulty

Item difficulty is defined as the percentage of people who pass it. An item that 75% of test takers pass is easier than one that only 15% pass. In the process of test construction, a spread on item difficulty is usually desirable. Easier items are frequently placed at the beginning of the assessment to build the test taker's confidence and motivate the person to continue with the assessment when items get more difficult.

A common rule is to choose a set of items with a spread in difficulty but with the average of the spread to be about 50%, or 0.50, if the goal is to maximize differentiation between people. On the other hand, screening tests might cluster around 0.20 to 0.30 to ensure that people are not missed initially (false rejections) by this quick method. In mastery testing, the item difficulty should be about 0.80 to 0.90 to ensure that the person has adequately mastered the desired skill consistently. Item difficulty can be calculated as

$$p = 100 \, (R/T)$$

where p is the statistical notation for item difficulty, R is the number of people who got the item right, and T is the total number who responded to the item.

Item Discrimination

Item discrimination is the degree to which an item differentiates correctly among test takers for the behavior or skill that the assessment is designed to measure (Anastasi & Urbina, 1997). On a criterion-referenced assessment, items may be selected only because of their ability to discriminate between having mastered or not mastered the desired level of competency. There are two ways to establish item discrimination: (1) The assessment can be given to people who have known varying levels of mastery in a criterion, or (2) each item can be studied in reference to the rank orders of how each person performed on the assessment overall.

For instance, professors who use computerized scoring on a test

> *Item difficulty* is a calculated percentage of people who pass a given item, whereas *item discrimination* is the degree to which an item differentiates among subgroups of test takers (e.g., high scorers vs. low scorers, mastery vs. nonmastery), making it a powerful tool to improve test fairness, reliability, and validity.

get item discrimination statistics that reflect each item's ability to predict who was most likely to get the answer right. If an equal number of low scorers and high scorers on the test answered the item correctly, then the item is a poor discriminator. On the other hand, if only the high scorers got the item right and low scores got it wrong, the item discrimination index would be very high.

If a professor is examining a test from a norm-referenced perspective, he or she would not necessarily throw out a question if a large number of students did not answer it correctly; he or she would first consider the item's discrimination statistics. Also, the professor can get response discrimination statistics that would tell him or her which responses were good distracters and which were not. The higher the distraction value of all wrong answers, the better the item will differentiate the scorers. Creating a good test is hard work, and it takes multiple efforts to refine good questions. Each improvement to a test improves test takers' chances of receiving a final score that reflects a true score rather than random error.

There are many specific statistical approaches to testing item difficulty and discrimination. One easy formula for calculating item discrimination is

$$D = (RU \times 2 \times RL) / (0.5T)$$

where D is item, RU is the number of students in the upper group who answered the item correctly, RL is the number of the students in the lower group who answered correctly, and 0.5T is half of the total group who took the test item. This approach is not a measure of true item validity because it compares the item not against an external criterion but against an internal criterion based on how the current test takers performed.

Items with low discrimination power should be studied for misleading clues, vagueness, or other technical problems. Typically, this information is presented in an assessment manual. Therapists need to understand conceptually how item difficulty is determined to use the assessments appropriately and when discussing this issue in practice.

Two other methods to provide support regarding the value of the scores obtained from a group of test takers are (1) extreme groups validation and (2) cross-validation. In **extreme groups validation,** the responses of the lower 27% to 33% of scores on a test are correlated with the responses of the top 27% to 33% of scores. In **cross-validation,** a different sample of individual responses is used to determine test validity than the sample used to study item difficulty. Conceptually, items with the highest negative correlation are retained. This difficult process is made easier and test precision is improving with new computer-assisted approaches.

Rasch Analysis

Rasch analysis is not really an item analysis procedure but is included because it is a method to arrive at standard results on assessments that are highly reliant on evaluator observation, in which all items have a variance in individual task difficulty (such as complex daily living tasks) or items require analysis of multiskilled activities (not single-focus test items). Rasch is a method to stabilize your reliability and validity as a scorer.

Rasch analysis or scoring is valuable in occupational therapy because therapists must subjectively observe complex task performance, which creates a greater chance for bias to enter errors into scores. (If judges of ice skating, gymnastics, or diving competitions used Rasch analysis, the raters would have fewer crises related to scoring discrepancies and final decisions.) Each task, especially daily living tasks, has its own level of difficulty. In occupational therapy, Rasch analysis of scores sees wiping a spill on a kitchen counter as less difficult than cleaning a spill on a carpet. The Rasch approach to item analysis reflects

- The performance ability of the person observed or tested,
- The item or task difficulty in comparison with other test items,
- The severity or leniency of the rater in scoring the task performance, and
- The degree of difficulty in declaring a rating for the task.

Each item on an inventory has a Rasch score calculated from repeated studies of the consistency of ratings for a test item. Each evaluator is standardized in becoming a reliable, valid scorer through training on standardized administration procedures that also includes interrater reliability checks with test experts. This process is followed by an independent rating of observed performance in which the average error of severity or leniency in scoring on the test is calculated for every time the scorer administers the test in the future.

Anyone who goes through training to use the Assessment of Motor and Processing Skills (AMPS; Fisher, 2012) understands this approach once he or she has been calibrated on the test. The AMPS is computer scored using the raw data the administrator provides, mixed in with the item difficulty pretested for each daily living task item and the administrator's calibration as an evaluator (accounting for scorer error) using this specific test. Thus, a client's score on the test reflects his or her true score because the score has been adjusted for typical common scorer errors attributed to task difficulty and evaluator misjudgments.

NORMS

In norm-referenced assessments, the comparison of scores to a well-defined group is expected. This group is referred to as the test's *norm group* or *norms*. To establish norms, the standardized test is given to a large group of people for whom the assessment was developed, or groups or individuals likely to use the test because of its stated purpose. These norms are published in the assessment manual, allowing future evaluators to compare the results of their individual scores to those of a larger norm group. Ideally, the more the norm group data parallel the assumptions of the normal curve, the better.

Norms frequently use one or more standard ways to report findings from an assessment, which are discussed in the next section regarding the reporting of scores. Norms are helpful in defining a person's strengths or weaknesses or describing the amount of skill or ability (progress) within a given intervention sequence or across time. To use norms accurately, the evaluator must ensure that a test taker has characteristics similar to those of the norm group; otherwise, a new source of error is introduced into data interpretations.

The evaluation report should specify the type of norm group, each of which has implications for interpreting the client's test score:

- *Multiple norm group comparisons* enable comparison of one person's score on a test to more than just a single norm group. For example, an evaluator might compare a test taker's results on a vocational readiness inventory to the norms of several different occupational groups.

- *Local norm groups* provide information for norms using only local test takers. These groups are used frequently in schools where curricula are unique, either within a school or within a school district or region. Sometimes, rehabilitation agencies find that a certain assessment is very useful but that no norms are specific enough to their group; they may establish local norms for comparisons of individual scores with those from their group. This process is not simple, but it can be done validly, especially if agencies consult a psychometrician. Over time, local norm groups can provide new evidence for practice.

- *National norms* represent people from across the country. Test developers may conduct a national norm standardization study. Because a thorough national norm study is impossible to conduct (it would be too complicated and expensive), the evaluator must consult the manual to identify the rationale and process used to establish the national norms and to judge the quality of the approach. Although it is difficult and costly to establish true national norms, most tests are perceived to be of higher quality if their norms are at the national, rather than local, level.

- *Special group norms* are norms for a test that may be used with more than one population of like individuals whose performance may vary because of their special problem or condition. Some call this *fixed reference group norms.* This type of norm often is used in occupational therapy evaluation. For instance, a test measuring social adjustment may be valid for people with social adjustment problems who also fit one or more disability groups or social conditions. Separate norms should be presented for each special group or use.

Other terms you might hear are *developmental norms, mental age norms,* and *national anchor group norms.* Reading the test manual closely should give the rationale for the norm group selection and process. For interpretation purposes using norms, a client's characteristics should be similar to those reported in the norm group.

REPORTING SCORES

An obtained score reflects a known distribution of test scores, including central tendency and variance estimates. Such scores can be found in most, if not all, assessments. Obtained scores only have meaning when considering the assessment itself, and when a therapist reports tests to clients, family, other therapists, and third-party payers, he or she needs to give scores that are easily communicated and possibly permit comparison with other assessment results. The scores offered by standardized tests and standard scores are two ways to report score results. Standard scores provide an easy way to report how a person performs in relation to others on the assessment as well as a simple way to compare the outcomes of different tests.

To review: The number assigned to a test taker's performance on a test item is the *raw score*. The assessment manual will instruct the therapist on which, if any, method should be used to convert the raw score to an *obtained* or *derived score,* which is usually incorporated into the evaluation report. Sometimes raw and obtained scores are the same; other times, they are not. Then a third, optional step is translating the derived score to a *standard score.* Sometimes the assessment manual publishes a table explaining how to convert the obtained score into a derived score. Other times, if needed, a therapist can convert the test score into a standard score as long as he or she knows the score's standard deviation. This may make it easier to communicate assessment results of similar problems.

Table 10.2. Types of Scores

Concept	Definition
Percentile	Scores are assigned that indicate what percentage of the sample scored above and below the test taker.
Stanine	Scores are assigned on the basis of an underlying scale broken into 9 standard sections. The basis for this scale is 5 ± 2.
Reporting Equivalencies in Some Standardized Tests	
Grade equivalent	Scores are assigned on the basis of data gathered from children in several different grades to identify what level of grade performance a student is currently exemplifying.
Developmental age	Scores are assigned on the basis of data gathered from children in several different grades to identify what level of developmental performance a student is currently exemplifying.
Percentile ranks	Scores are assigned on the basis of a comparison of expected performance from children in the test taker's same grade.
Standard Scores	
z scores	Scores relate to the standard deviation of the normal distribution; midpoint is 0, and 1 SD = *z scores* of 1.0; the basis is 0 ± 1.0.
t scores	Scores relate to the standard deviation of the normal distribution; midpoint is 50, and 1 SD = *t scores* of 10; the basis is 50 ± 10.

Note. SD = standard deviation.
From "Scoring and Interpretation of Results," by P. Crist. In J. Hinojosa, P. Kramer, and P. Crist (Eds.), *Evaluation: Obtaining and Interpreting Data* (3rd ed.), Bethesda, MD: AOTA Press, p. 221, Copyright © 2010 by the American Occupational Therapy Association. Used with permission.

Scores From Standardized Assessments

Standardized tests frequently convert their results into some type of externally accepted standard, such as percentages or grade or age equivalence. Table 10.2 provides brief definitions of the types of standardized scores, and Figure 10.3 presents typical standard score reporting methods in relation to the normal distribution, showing how the scoring methods relate to the distribution and to each other.

Percentile scores

A **percentile score,** sometimes called a *cumulative percentage score,* correlates exactly with the percentage areas under the normal distribution. A percentile score indicates the percentage of the norm group's test results below the test taker's score and the percentage above it. It explains one's relative standing within a larger group who also took the assessment. For instance, in a test of motor ability given to a child, the number of items passed and a score of the child's ability are compared with the number of tasks the norm group of children of the same age are able to pass. This percentile score for completed motor ability tests allows for interpretation of how the child performed in relation to peers in the norm group.

Percentile equivalent or rank measures

Percentile equivalent or rank measures are considered to be better than age or grade equivalents, because the comparisons are made only with children in the same grade and are not subject to error based on differential teaching across multiple grades. This type of score reporting avoids problems with unequal growth and differential learning experiences that are common to children. If an occupational therapist uses percentile equivalent or rank measures, he or she cannot simply explain that it is a percentage correct (percentile scores) approach. It is different and reflects the variance within the normal distribution.

Stanine scores

Stanine scores were developed by the military, the first group to promote testing for aptitude. The objective was to get the best match between the skills of applicants and the skills the military needed. Because of the positive outcomes in the military, education was the next group to actively pursue testing for describing performance and making decisions.

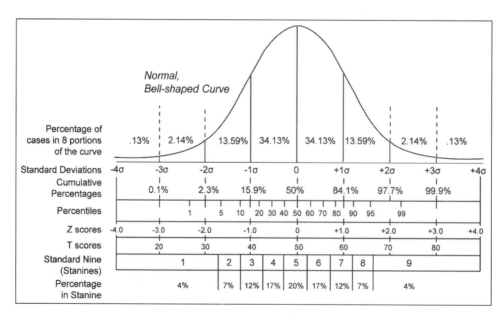

Figure 10.3. Types of score reporting.

The distribution of stanine scores is divided into 9 segments, with 5 as the midpoint and 5 ± 2 as nearly equivalent with −1 and +1 *SD*. Note in the normal curve illustrated in Figure 10.3 how the percentage within each of the stanines changes in relation to its location within the normal curve. Another similar linear scale is sten, in which the bottom line is divided into 10, not 9, segments.

Reporting Equivalencies in Standardized Tests

Norm-referenced standardized tests frequently compare their findings to external scales to give meaning to their scores.

Grade equivalents
Grade equivalents are established by issuing a test to students in a specific grade. These norms then can be used to compare a student's score with the expected patterns for the norm group. The performance of a student is compared with the norms for a grade equivalence test to describe the his or her current academic abilities common to a specific grade.

Much dissatisfaction is created by grade equivalencies, which are norms and not standards. Equal differences in scores do not necessarily mean equal differences in performance abilities, and grade equivalents are not comparable across schools. A detailed discussion is beyond the scope of this chapter, but the issue of grade equivalence is currently undergoing great debate in this country because of the high-stakes educational testing now widespread after following passage of the No Child Left Behind Act of 2001. Although the intentions of the policy sound positive, the reality is that a local or state group might not be able to design the correct tools to administer an assessment that fully meets the program criteria.

Developmental age-equivalent scores
Developmental age-equivalent scores are determined similarly to grade-equivalent scores. In this case, the goal is to determine how close the test taker's performance is to patterns of people from a certain developmental age. Frequently, these tests measure one developmental issue at a time, such as

physical, cognitive, or social growth and development. This scoring procedure has weaknesses similar to those of age equivalence.

As can be seen in Figure 10.3, all the major types of scores relate to the normal distribution including standard deviation. Studying this chart shows the relationship between the reported scores that can use this distribution.

Standard Scores

Standard scores provide an easy way to report how a person performed in relation to others on the assessment as well as a simple way to compare the outcomes of different administrations of a test. The therapist can convert the derived score into a standard score if he or she obtained the score's standard deviation from the test manual.

z scores
When a therapist has information about the standard deviation of a person's score, he or she can easily calculate a *z* score and *t* score (see Figure 10.3).

The basis for the *z* score is 0 ± the equivalent number associated with the identified standard deviation for the person from the test. The formula for transforming an obtained score into a *z* score to tell how far above or below the mean the *SD* units lie is:

$$z = \frac{x - \bar{X}}{SD}$$

where *z* is the *z* score, *x* is the obtained or raw score, $\bar{X}$ is the mean score, and *SD* is the standard deviation. For example, occupational therapists measure for improvements in activities of daily living and physical therapists measure for improvements in mobility after 1 week of intervention:

Occupational therapy	Physical therapy
$x = 85$	$x = 90$
$\bar{X} = 75$	$\bar{X} = 140$
$SD = 10$	$SD = 25$
$z = +1.0$	$z = -2.0$

The difference in *z* scores does not mean that one therapy is better than the other; what it means is that the client showed more positive improvement in activities of daily living than in mobility after 1 week of therapy.

t scores

At times, the *z* score can be confusing if it is a negative value; **t scores** avoid this problem because the midpoint of the *t* score is 50 ± 10 from each *standard deviation*. Using the above example,

Occupational therapy	Physical therapy
$t = 10(SD \text{ or } z) + 50$	$t = 10(SD \text{ or } z) + 50$
$= 10(1.0) + 50$	$= 10(-2.0) + 50$
$= 10 + 50$	$= -20 + 50$
$= 60$	$= 30$

One can report either a *z* score or *t* score, depending on preference. If one test reports a *z* score and the other a *t* score, the therapist can convert one so that the results can be compared, giving meaning to the obtained scores between two assessments.

CONTROLLING ERROR IN TEST SCORES FOR BETTER INTERPRETATION

So far in this chapter, we have reviewed issues in scoring, generic interpretation concerns, and effective reporting of results. This section provides a brief review of error and explains how to control its intrusion into testing administration and interpretation. The goal is to ensure that test scores consist of true scores, with limited error. (Chapter 9, "Reliability and Validity: The Psychometrics of Standardized Assessments," discusses the makeup of any given test score.) Sources of error include the test takers themselves, the testing instrument, the procedures used in administering the test, and the scoring of results. Just as one must fast before blood glucose tests to achieve a more accurate reading of one's blood glucose level, evaluators must consider how to reduce error before and during testing related to occupational therapy assessment.

Error Attributed to Test Takers

Error attributed to test takers is called **intraindividual error** and includes factors that a person brings to a test, or experiences as a result of completing the test, that negatively alter the obtained score. For instance, fatigue, illness, or a distracting stressful event, such as a personal or medical crisis or intense rehabilitation session just before the evaluation, are some of the test-taker factors that can introduce error. In occupational therapy, regional, ethnic, or language barriers and differences may contribute to errors.

Entry-level occupational therapists, and even some more experienced ones, sometimes fail to ensure that test takers can hear them, can clearly see test items, and are familiar with test objects and requests. Therapists must make sure that clients have their eyeglasses, hearing aids, mobility aids and splints, false teeth (if they are undergoing an eating evaluation), and so on, before beginning an assessment. It is surprising how many people will attempt to complete tests without these devices and announce afterward that they believe that this negatively influenced their test results. Readministering assessments wastes precious time and also may be problematic because test takers have already been exposed to the test items.

Error Introduced by the Test

Though error introduced by the assessment should be removed through good test standardization procedures, some always will exist because total perfection is not achievable, even though it is a worthy goal. An error may occur through poorly written items that may be too difficult. Furthermore, an error may happen because of unclear standardization procedures, such as using oral instructions with the test taker when his or her reading level is not adequate. Even though a test has been standardized rigorously for client populations similar to the one a therapist is going to use it with, the test still may not work for some reason. Always consider unexpected errors that arise from the test itself.

Error in Test Administration

Errors may be introduced during test administration by simply not following the published standardized instructions or the administrator not training himself or herself adequately in the assessment's standardized procedures. In addition, physical discomfort for either the test taker or examiner, the therapist's attitude toward the test, or problematic instructions or explanations also can negatively influence the score a client obtains on a test.

Error in Scoring

Errors in scoring can result from not recording the correct responses to test items but also by not closely following the published scoring instructions in the test manual. The errors—sometimes referred to as *personal bias errors* (Miller et al., 2012)—are classified as the following types:

- **Generosity or leniency error** occurs when there is a tendency to rate performance favorably or use only the high end of the scale.
- **Severity error** is the opposite of generosity error, when there is a tendency to unfavorably rate performance or use lower scores more frequently than warranted.
- **Central tendency errors** occur when a rater tends to give midpoint ratings, or ratings in the middle of the distribution of responses that effectively mean no rating, ultimately preventing a true score.
- **Halo effect** occurs when the evaluator's general impression of the test taker affects the accurate rating of performance.
- **Logical error** occurs when behaviors or performance is rated as more alike or dissimilar than they actually are because of evaluator information bias from other sources (e.g., insufficient opportunity to observe test behavior, prior knowledge that is inaccurate, test performance that does not relate to the current situation).
- **Proximity error** occurs when an unexpected event immediately preceding an assessment or something highly unusual triggers a reaction to the next test item and, as a result,

uniquely contributes error to test results. Remember, proximity error is already accounted for by using standardized administration procedures, so the expected influence of previous test items was calculated into the norms through the standardized administration to a sample.

- **Ambiguity error** occurs when, for some unknown reason, the rater's interpretation of a response to a test varies from the typical interpretation made by others.
- **Contrast error** occurs when the evaluator's subjective response to certain characteristics of the test taker influences scoring or results. It may start with the evaluator feeling negatively about the particular characteristic of the test taker.

These sources of error can be very perplexing. However, by following standardized procedures and reflecting on how and when you see these errors creeping into your scoring, you can at least limit, if not prevent, their negative influence, ensuring the maximum contribution of true score to the obtained score (Exhibit 10.5).

Controlling Error in Scores

Occupational therapists can control the influence of various errors by maximizing the percentage of true score in an obtained score. They begin with constant awareness of error sources and vigilance to prevent their intrusion. In addition, therapists should ensure that they

- Are properly trained and qualified to perform a specific assessment;
- Recalibrate their skills regularly on both frequently and infrequently used assessments;

EXHIBIT 10.5. SOURCES OF ERROR			
Test Takers	**Test**	**Test Administration**	**Scoring**
• Fatigue • Illness • Stress • Regional or language barriers • Lack of patient devices or aids	• Poorly written items • Inappropriate difficulty level	• Improper training • Physical discomfort • Attitude	• Incorrect response recording • Personal bias errors

- Follow standardized procedures, adapting tasks as infrequently as possible; and
- Avoid test-taker pretesting and testing conditions, including environmental concerns, that might negatively affect performance.

These conditions are refined by both artful skill and applied science during testing procedures.

STEPS IN SCORING AND INTERPRETING PERFORMANCE ON A STANDARDIZED ASSESSMENT

Interpreting individual outcomes from an assessment requires translating published standardization into meaningful interpretation of assessment results for treatment planning and outcomes. This process requires both the art and science of evaluation. In the evaluator role, the occupational therapist uses a standard set of 6 steps to translate scores.

1. Verify that the assessment is an appropriate choice to use by checking
   - That the purpose of the test matches the desired need to describe client performance;
   - The similarity between the person being tested and the demographic characteristics of the standardization sample in the test manual (e.g., age, diagnosis, condition, norms);
   - That the evaluator has the proper administration preparation, calibration, and training, and adequate resources, to deliver the assessment in a standardized manner; and
   - The best order, if doing more than one assessment.
2. Assess the client:
   - Control for fatigue and other factors that may affect the client.
   - Note any exceptions related to modifying standardized assessment delivery procedures or unexpected responses to assessment activities.
3. Debrief the client at the end of the assessment session and after the final report regarding assessment outcomes (oral and written).
4. Review the manual to
   - Follow scoring instructions, including transforming raw data into derived scores and standard scores.
   - Compare scored results to the appropriate standardization sample in the published manual. Sometimes more than one set of norms is available. Choose the one that most closely approximates the person being evaluated, noting any exceptions.
   - Use the interpretation guidelines that apply to obtained scores to describe the evaluation results and related interpretations.
5. Document outcomes in client records:
   - Include the results from the assessment.
   - Provide meaningful interpretation related to occupational therapy intervention planning and documentation of outcomes (state which norm sample was used; use clinical reasoning and critical thinking).
   - Note any deviation from standardized procedures, including using a norm-referenced group that does not approximate the person who has been evaluated (when deviation occurs, state cautionary use of results along with how this change may have affected outcomes or influenced intervention planning).
   - Recommend any further action, including additional testing, reevaluation, and referral.
6. If you are going to an intervention planning or goal-setting meeting, be prepared to comment on the scores obtained in reference to standard scores and standard deviation, and include assessment recommendations so that you can contribute to discussions and prioritization during team intervention planning.

SUMMARY

The purpose of assessment is to quantify the skills or abilities observed in a client. The information presented in this chapter provides the science for administering, scoring, and interpreting assessments in occupational therapy. Much of the art of being an evaluator is woven throughout this text. Both art and science are fundamental requirements to qualify as a competent evaluator in occupational therapy.

Ethical, professional, legal, and political concerns will always influence our use of assessments. Occupational therapists cannot acquiesce to these pressures without considerable negative impact on ourselves as professionals. Through a scientific or psychometric-based approach to assessment, therapists ensure professional-level competence and the valuable contribution that our evaluation process provides to our clients, as well as serving as accountable partners in the health care system.

QUESTIONS

1. Select 1 behavior, characteristic, or function that occupational therapists evaluate. Try writing an assessment item using the following response methods:
   - Observation scale
   - Likert scale
   - Forced-choice scale
   - Checklist scale
   - Semantic differential scale
   - Q-sort
   - Rasch scale.

   What challenges did you face in writing good items using each of these methods?

2. Apply the 4 different measurement concepts (nominal, ordinal, interval, and ratio) to something that you could measure in each of the following situations:
   - Running a marathon race
   - Determining upper-extremity edema
   - Coping with stress
   - Describing a child's ability to cut a shape out of paper with scissors
   - Reporting experience with pain
   - Making a peanut butter and jelly sandwich.

   What did you find in trying to apply these concepts to the variables to be measured?

3. Calculate the mean, median, and mode for the following set of test scores: 8, 1, 3, 14, 35, 5, 4, 8, 9, 10, 11, 2, 10, 9, 8, 7, and 6. Plot these scores on a graph and label the mean, median, and mode. Remove the score of 35 and redo the exercise. What happened to the measures of central tendency? What is the clinical relevance of this exercise?

4. Referring to the types of score reporting in Table 10.2, determine the following standard scores for a client's score that result in the following standard deviations reported on two different tests: $SD = +5$ and $SD = -2$.
   - z score
   - t score
   - Stanine
   - Cumulative percentage
   - Percentile.

   What percentage of people scored above and below each of these scores?

5. Why control for error in scoring tests? Choose a situation in which you score a test. Give an example of how the errors in scoring might influence the scores you assigned to a client's performance or that might influence the client's response on a questionnaire. What are 5 ways to control error in scoring?

References

Anastasi, A., & Urbina, S. (1997). *Psychological testing* (7th ed.). Upper Saddle River, NJ: Prentice Hall.

Fisher, A. G. (2012). *Assessment of motor and process skills* (7th ed., rev. ed.). Fort Collins, CO: Three Star Press.

Miller, M. D., Linn, R. L., & Gronlund, N. E. (2012). *Measurement and assessment in teaching* (12th ed.). Upper Saddle River, NJ: Merrill/Pearson.

No Child Left Behind Act of 2001, Pub. L. 107–110, 115 Stat. 1425 (2002), 20 U.S.C. 6301.

Pearson, K. (1924). Historical note on the origins of the normal curve of errors. *Biometrika, 16,* 402–404.

Urbina, S. (2004). *Essentials of psychological testing.* Hoboken, NJ: John Wiley & Sons.

CHAPTER 11

Interpretation and Documentation

Aimee J. Luebben, EdD, OTR, FAOTA
Rondalyn V. Whitney, PhD, OTR/L, FAOTA

Highlights

- Solving patient mysteries through documentation
- Interpretation
- Documentation.

Key Terms

DAP note	Interpretation
Deidentified	PIE
Design formats	Process stages
Documentation	Screening
Federal Educational Rights and Privacy Act of 1974	Settings
Formative evaluation	SOAP note
Guidelines for Documentation of Occupational Therapy	Summative evaluation
	Synthesize
Health Insurance Portability and Accountability Act of 1996	Testing bias
	Timing types

This chapter focuses on the interpretation and documentation aspects of the evaluation process. The section on interpretation includes information on factors that contribute to the transition from interpretation to intervention planning, including applying a theoretical foundation, accounting for testing bias, synthesizing multiple data points, and defending evaluation results. The section on documentation discusses purposes and classification, information confidentiality and privacy, and general recommendations.

The chapter features a documentation mystery that is woven throughout the sections to highlight key points. The lessons learned from solving the mystery of one client's evaluations are included throughout this chapter and focus on two aims: (1) interpreting assessment findings and (2) disseminating discoveries through documentation.

SOLVING PATIENT MYSTERIES THROUGH DOCUMENTATION

Occupational therapists often need to solve mysteries. For example, why might a person who appears eligible for services not be recommended for direct occupational therapy? **Documentation,** the only permanent record remaining after services are rendered, is often the key to solving patient mysteries. Much like a detective attempts to solve a cold case by poring over evidence, occupational therapists can resolve dilemmas by combing through documentation.

Take the mystery of 19-month-old Morgan and how documentation was used to refute not one but two direct service ineligibility decisions. Our mystery began when Al, a senior pediatric occupational therapist, received an impassioned plea from Morgan's parents, who asked for an evaluation for their daughter. Certain that she would benefit from direct early intervention services, the parents disclosed that evaluations performed within the previous 4 months by two facilities in different states had indicated Morgan was not eligible for direct occupational therapy services.

The mystery of Morgan's ineligibility for services deepened when Al learned that Morgan was a twin born at 36 weeks' gestation. Hesitant about evaluating the same child a third time within 4 months, Al opted to first review the previous evaluations. The documentation evidence included reports from interdisciplinary teams. Al's detective work revealed the testing had been adequate and the quantitative evidence from the standardized assessment tool used did not substantiate the eligibility decision of either facility.

The mystery was solved when Al determined that neither facility had provided satisfactory interpretation of the assessment findings. Morgan did not require a reevaluation; instead, the reports of both facilities needed reevaluation in the form of reinterpretation of results.

> Occupational therapists solve mysteries by profiling clients, examining clues within contexts, and synthesizing multiple data points to give order to the complexities of life. Occupational therapists are also masters of generalization who are adept at interpreting and applying information.

Occupational therapists are lifestyle detectives who search for clues, test hypotheses, interpret findings, determine conclusions, and disseminate discoveries, and so, "solving mysteries" is an appropriate metaphor for the practice of evaluation in occupational therapy.

INTERPRETATION

Interpretation is a primary part of the occupational therapist's job. Although many standardized assessment instruments have computer applications that score a client's performance and are advertised as capable of interpreting scores, interpretation is a principal realm of occupational therapists. Interpreting assessment information is an art that requires reflection, theoretical knowledge, clinical reasoning, and practice.

During the evaluation process, interpretation is key to making meaning of information collected through various assessment methods, including standardized assessment instruments, nonstandardized testing, and an integrated approach that uses nonstandardized assessment techniques to supplement standardized assessments. Making informed service delivery decisions requires accurate interpretation. Furthermore, precise assessment interpretation is fundamental to intervention planning.

Multiple factors contribute to interpretation, which is then translated into intervention planning. Applying a theoretical foundation, accounting for testing bias, synthesizing multiple data points, and defending evaluation results contribute to the transition from interpretation to intervention planning.

Al used a deductive approach to guide his decision-making process about intervention planning. Although both facilities determined that Morgan was ineligible for direct service intervention, Al applied a theoretical foundation, accounted for testing bias, synthesized multiple data points, and reevaluated standardized evaluation results as guided by his advanced clinical knowledge to ultimately solve a mystery for Morgan's family.

Applying a Theoretical Foundation

To consistently link theory and practice, intervention planning must rely on a theoretical foundation. Occupational therapists use theory to organize thinking and begin the clinical reasoning process.

In the case of Morgan, Al quickly determined the theoretical foundation was a developmental approach, which was appropriate and understandable considering that both facilities performing the evaluations were pediatric facilities. Because Morgan's evaluating therapists used a reasonable theoretical foundation, the mystery of her ineligibility for direct services was not solved.

Accounting for Testing Bias

The goal of testing is to determine the actual performance of the person being evaluated, but **testing bias** can influence an evaluation and must be accounted for in the interpretation. Optimal conditions are not always possible, but the occupational therapist should strive to achieve them. Optimizing testing conditions involves controlling for as much testing variance or bias as possible.

Designed to be used during the testing process, the **PIE** acronym also helps therapists identify in written documentation three sources of bias: **p**erson, **i**tem, and **e**nvironment.

Applying PIE to Morgan's reports, Al found little supporting evidence that indicated difficulties related to the two types of person-related testing bias (the *P* in PIE). Al presumed the prior evaluators controlled for their expectations and rating tendencies that could result in error. After meeting the family, Al believed that Morgan demonstrated genuineness in her performance and that her parents were good historians. As for item bias (the *I* in PIE), both facilities used a typical pediatric standardized criterion-referenced and norm-referenced assessment instrument that tests children as they play with toys, a natural occupation for Morgan.

The only extraordinary testing bias aspect was the environment (the *E* in PIE). For Morgan, arriving at each facility for testing was the first time she visited either place. Morgan was not only out of her natural environment, she was also observed by teams of people who were unfamiliar to her. The fact that Morgan was expected to perform typically in front of strangers in an unfamiliar environment was the first loose end Al found, but this aspect of testing bias was not enough to unravel the full mystery of her ineligibility.

Synthesizing Multiple Data Points

To interpret assessment findings, summarizing multiple data points is not enough. Occupational therapists must **synthesize** multiple data points, making certain that qualitative and quantitative information collected during evaluation provides a holistic and accurate picture of occupational performance.

The mystery of Morgan demonstrates how easily interpretation can go awry. Although therapists in both facilities used an integrated approach, using nonstandardized testing (observation, in particular) to supplement the standardized assessment information, therapists at each facility based the direct service decision on the standardized instrument's age equivalents that were available for each scale, but not for individual subtests. Using age-equivalent scores to determine service delivery presents a substantial potential for misinterpretation and should be handled with caution.

For individual subtests, each facility also reported percentile ranks that represent a normalized derived scale with unequal intervals, but neither facility provided any interpretation of these norms. Beyond style variations, the differences were many. One facility provided raw scores and adjusted for preterm birth, and the other facility supplied a normalized standard score with equal intervals, but neither did both.

For the facility reporting normalized standard scores but no corresponding interpretations or raw scores, Al was able to reconstruct subtests and scale scores. The narrative part of the report, what initially looked like detailed clinical observations of Morgan, was actually the language of individual test items from the assessment instrument. Further, the standardized protocol was not followed; the facility staff had not performed hand calculations required by the standardized instrument manual for raw scores lower than the upper limit of the smallest percentile rank in the table. Al was able to determine that the reconstructed raw scores showed that normalized standard scores for the total scale and one subtest were incorrect and as a result, an erroneous finding was reported.

Al gave Morgan's parents a document that included reconstructed raw scores, hand-calculated standard scores, and interpretations of all derived scale scores along with a narrative report documenting important clinical observations of Morgan. Al told the family that the reports should have included, at minimum, raw scores and normalized standard scores with equal intervals. To compare Morgan's performance with children in her age group, the interpretation of her performance and eligibility decision should have been based on the standard scores with equal intervals.

The mystery of Morgan was solved. She was eligible for direct services because she had serious developmental delays that were evident in the evaluation documents from two facilities but not identified because of interpretation errors. Solving the mystery showed that Morgan's other therapists summarized but did not *synthesize* their testing findings into an accurate interpretation. In the case of both facilities, Morgan did not qualify for direct service delivery because of therapist error in interpreting testing information collected through a standardized instrument.

Defending Evaluation Results

Once occupational therapists have finalized and disseminated evaluation reports, their jobs are not done. The reports, which live forever in records, must be defensible. Dissection of Morgan's reports led to a third report to the parents that defended the validity of the testing but not the accuracy of the interpreted findings. Morgan had been denied direct services on the basis of results from indefensible evaluations.

Solving the mystery of Morgan's previous evaluations revealed the power—both positive and negative—of interpretation. Al embarked on a crusade against the common use of norms based on age to determine developmental delay and eligibility for occupational therapy services. After analyzing Morgan's two evaluation reports, Al realized that using chronological age and age equivalents (or perceptual age, motor age, or whatever form or terminology age-based scores take) is not a good choice because older children who are delayed are penalized because both chronological age and age equivalents start at zero and keep increasing. An older child would have to be many more months behind age level compared with a younger child, although the percentage of delay could be the same. To examine this phenomenon in action, see Table 11.1, which summarizes the effects on delay percentages of being 5 months behind for 5 girls at various chronological ages.

The mystery of Morgan and the examples in Table 11.1 show that using chronological age and age-based norms can result in turning away people who really need occupational therapy. The ethical

Table 11.1. Effects of Being 5 Months Behind on Delay Percentage at Various Chronological Ages

Child	Chronological Age (Months)	Age Equivalent (Months)	Delay %
Lily	6	1	83
Mei	12	7	42
Hannah	18	13	28
Callie	26	21	19
Michaela	45	40	11

implications of using age equivalents to calculate developmental delay are therefore serious.

DOCUMENTATION

The purpose of documentation, according to the *Guidelines for Documentation of Occupational Therapy* (American Occupational Therapy Association [AOTA], 2013), is to

- Communicate information about the client from the occupational therapy perspective;
- Articulate the rationale for provision of occupational therapy services and the relationship of this service to the client's outcomes, reflecting the occupational therapy practitioner's clinical reasoning and professional judgment; and
- Create a chronological record of client status, occupational therapy services provided to the client, and client outcomes. (p. S32)

Without a doubt, the primary purpose of documentation—evaluation reports, in particular—is communication. Documentation is also important for public relations, education, reimbursement, and research. If care is taken in writing reports and descriptions, documentation can serve as an advertisement for the value of occupational therapy services and teach people outside the profession more about occupational therapy. For third-party payers, documentation is the sole source of determining whether to reimburse for occupational therapy services.

Documentation serves as the basis for research, including outcome studies, quality assurance, and other forms of program review. On a smaller scale, an outcome study at the case report level can be completed each time an occupational therapist delivers services. With many reimbursement sources mandating meaningful practical improvement in a person's function, occupational therapists are obligated to demonstrate improvement as an outcome if services are authorized (Smith, 2013). Although some occupational therapists believe a fine line divides research and evaluation, the line is more likely to represent an investigation continuum with research at one end and evaluation at the other. Documentation indicative of best practices is located in the middle of the research–evaluation continuum.

Documentation using single-case reporting with empirical data can provide evidence of meaningful clinical change resulting from occupational therapy services. Like single-subject research designs, single-case reports have inherently strong internal validity but correspondingly low external validity; generalizing to others may be difficult. To improve external validity, single-case reports need to be replicated and accumulated. The technology of electronic health records offers an integrated way of accumulating information. If occupational therapists collect similar information and report findings in a consistent format, the data-mining capabilities of electronic health records can provide opportunities to capture information on similar people, aggregate results, analyze outcomes, and demonstrate irrefutable evidence of the effectiveness of occupational therapy (Smith, 2013).

Classification

Documentation varies. Most documentation can be classified according to four aspects: (1) **process stages,** (2) **timing types,** (3) **setting and styles,** and (4) **design formats.**

Process stages
Because the occupational therapy information-gathering process consists of two process stages, documentation often is classified according to the stage: (1) screening or (2) evaluation. *Screening,* which provides preliminary information to determine whether further occupational therapy services are needed, is not intended as a comprehensive evaluation. A formal document related to a screening should be labeled as such—a *screening report.* In practice, many occupational therapists begin with gathering information by screening; quickly determining whether a formal evaluation is warranted; and when potential performance problems are discovered, start gathering more definitive information through various assessments. An evaluation report summarizes and synthesizes the findings of multiple assessments.

Timing types
Because evaluation reports provide snapshots of a client's occupational performance at a particular time, evaluation documentation often is classified according to the following timing types: initial, progress, or discharge (sometimes called *discontinuation*). If treatment is recommended in the initial report, then the other types of report correspond with intervention timing. Often, at least one other reevaluation report is completed during treatment before discharge, and a discharge (or discontinuation) evaluation is performed, usually as part of the final intervention session.

Initial and progress evaluation reports are considered formative evaluation; discharge documentation is considered summative evaluation. If the initial evaluation recommendation is "no services are needed," the first report also serves as a discharge or discontinuation document. An initial evaluation report that does not recommend occupational therapy services can be considered summative.

Setting and styles
Evaluation documentation can also be classified according to two general settings (medical model and community based) and three styles (acronym, narrative, and template based). Although originally designed to serve as progress notes, acronym-style documentation is often used in documenting evaluation findings. Several varieties of acronym-style documentation are used in medical-model settings. One example is the **SOAP note,** named for the letters that compose the section labels: *S*ubjective, *O*bjective, *A*ssessment, and *P*lan. Another example is the **DAP note:** *D*escription, *A*ssessment, and *P*lan. The DAP combines the *S* and *O* of the SOAP note into *D*, the description section.

Some settings use narrative reports as documentation and provide site-specific guidelines for expected content and format. Narrative documentation usually consists of written information in paragraph form, often with headings that show key assessment areas. Narrative documentation is common in many community settings, such as schools.

Some facilities use template-based documentation, such as a checklist or specially designed form. Often when a therapist completes the form, documentation is done. Each facility determines the appropriate documentation style to use. Because the intricacies of documentation style are beyond the purview of this chapter, readers should consult current documentation textbooks.

Regardless of the style used, a therapist is responsible for accurate and thorough reporting based on assessment outcomes, documented observations, and clinical reasoning. When a checklist does not permit sufficient description of individual evaluation outcomes, the therapist is responsible for ensuring complete documentation is recorded.

Design formats

Evaluation documentation also can be classified according to design format: paper based or electronic. In some facilities, practitioners continue to document services using the traditional paper-based method. However, the electronic format has become the rule, so many facilities are working to scan older paper-based documentation into client records.

Community occupational therapists have known for decades the benefits of the electronic format. Many community therapists have developed electronic report systems that make documentation efficient. In medical-model facilities, electronic health records have become mandatory because of the **Health Insurance Portability and Accountability Act of 1996 (HIPAA).**

To comply with federal regulations, many facilities use digital template formats that provide an outline of the required documentation. Therapists provide documentation by completing checklists, selecting appropriate choices from menus (e.g., drop-down), making connections to other parts of the electronic record, and inputting specific information. The electronic format has unique storage and retrieval opportunities as well as data mining capabilities. Data mining allows easy comparison of a single person to norm-referenced information

(a typical group) or criterion-referenced information (a standard) as well as ipsative-referenced data that allow comparison of a single person with his or her own information to track changes over time.

Electronic client records bring up other issues related to availability, access, and security. Availability of digital records can be a problem if the machine is down, the server is overloaded, the system has crashed, the router has difficulties, or the power has gone out. To provide continuity of care despite electronic glitches, some clients have started carrying printed versions of their basic electronic records. Access and security are addressed in the next section, and the section on general documentation recommendations (particularly the last four recommendations) provides further information about using the electronic format for documentation purposes and protecting privacy.

Information Confidentiality and Privacy

Information related to persons receiving health care services has had confidentiality protections for centuries. From the time of Hippocrates, professional codes of ethics have emphasized confidentiality as a basic tenet. In the occupational therapy profession, confidentiality is addressed in the *Occupational Therapy Code of Ethics and Ethics Standards* (AOTA, 2010). Failure to comply with the professional code of ethics can result in sanctions, including suspension for life.

When professional codes of ethics failed to adequately protect patient and client confidentiality, governmental entities enacted privacy laws. Many states have had privacy statutes for years, protecting various aspects of a person's life. The federal government also has enacted legislation related to privacy. Financial information was one of the first areas to receive federal privacy protections. Educational records are protected by the **Federal Educational Rights and Privacy Act of 1974 (FERPA).** HIPAA extends earlier privacy legislation to health care.

HIPAA's two main goals are reflected in its name: (1) health insurance portability and (2) accountability. The electronic health record is the key to complying with portability mandated by HIPAA. In theory, electronic records allow the capture and storage of all of a person's health-related information and permit that person to transfer to another insurance company. HIPAA also mandates accountability: explanation of costs in an effort to decrease waste and fraud. Electronic health records improve the efficiency of accountability.

HIPAA is composed of four standards (also called *rules*): (1) transactions, (2) identifiers, (3) security, and (4) privacy. Although the HIPAA standards corresponding to transactions, identifiers, and security cover only electronic information, the privacy rule protects personal health information delivered in any fashion. Many facilities require that a therapist be trained and certified in basic HIPAA regulations and processes.

The privacy rule was implemented first. Implementation of the other three electronic informa-[tion standards i]s having an interesting and stealthy [beginnin]g in a documentation evolution [out] of FERPA. In educational settings, [t]o open student records to parents [r]equest. As a result, evaluation re-[ports fo]r educational settings have evolved [documenta]tion that is understood by multiple [people] with diverse backgrounds and var-[...] Once the bastion of professional eyes only, medical-model facility documentation is now being accessed by patients and clients exercising their HIPAA rights to see and get copies of their personal health information.

Increased access affects information confidentiality and privacy. Access and security are indirectly related: as access increases, security decreases. The movement to wireless devices also decreases security and, by extension, privacy and confidentiality. Early wired electronic health systems were perhaps more secure than some newer web-based systems accessed with wireless devices. Earlier systems often were interfaced with a wired network with machines for input. In these closed systems, security risks were primarily with people who accessed the input devices.

More recently, some facilities and organizations have moved to electronic health care systems that are designed for access through secure websites on the Internet. Secure websites offer some safety in these open systems, but many of these Internet-based systems allow wireless access from any device (often unsecured) from any wireless hotspot. This can be problematic because on the Internet, hosting devices (sometimes called *nodes*), not the network, are responsible for transmitting information. Devices connected to different internal systems and routers to outside networks send information until the relay machine indicates the information has been received. Information is then sent to the next node of the network (and the next and the next) until the information gets to the secure website.

On the network of networks—the Internet— if something happens to one node, the network still functions. Even though the website accessed is secure, many access devices may not be secure. Additionally, having a secure device does not guarantee a safe device. *Malware* (a contraction of the words *malicious software*) is a reality. Started as pranks, early malware included viruses and worms that disabled system functions or shut down computers. The current generation of malware is more hostile. Newer malware applications (e.g., spyware, bots, keystroke loggers) are designed to steal data for profitable use. At any one time, the Internet is designed to function with several hosting devices that are infected with one or more forms of malware. To improve security, users can use various types of security applications (e.g., firewalls, encryption) to help improve security of personal access devices.

Using a secure access device and a secure website helps improve security, but the connection between the device and website is equally important. The safer hard-wired, closed system is often not an option when accessing the Internet. Although a computer terminal may be hardwired to a facility system, the facility system at some point will "open" when connected to an outside system to access the Internet.

Additionally, the movement to wireless connectivity presents new perils. Theoretically, if an access device is open, any file saved internally or by connection (through memory device or linking website) can be accessed and stolen. A secure wireless connection offers some safety, but many wireless hotspots are essentially radio based, which allows opportunities for stealthy electronic eavesdropping and robbery. Sometimes, access devices switch from one wireless connection to another without the user being aware that a change has occurred, resulting in unintentional piggybacking (connecting and using network services without explicit authorization).

It is important to know how and where access devices are connected at all times. To protect Internet-based electronic health records from danger, occupational therapists need to ensure security at four points: (1) access device, (2) transmission, (3) connection, and (4) website. With wireless connections, new security concerns arise daily.

To summarize, occupational therapists must adhere to the confidentiality standards set in the profession's code of ethics and comply with privacy rules or standards mandated by state and federal legislation. Because the complexity of privacy legislation is beyond the scope of this chapter, readers are referred to the online tutorials of the University of Miami's Privacy/Data Protection Project (2006).

General Documentation Recommendations

Solving the mystery of Morgan—reinterpreting the evaluation evidence to prove she qualified for direct occupational therapy services—was tantamount to justifying the early intervention services this child and her family needed. For the other therapists involved, however, this mystery represented a worst-case scenario, demonstrating what might happen when documentation is read by another health care professional. Still, one important takeaway is that Morgan, and her family, were able to receive an appropriately interpreted evaluation in part because the original results were documented in a way that Al could reevaluate and resolve the mystery.

Documenting occupational therapy services is as important as providing services in the first place. Long after services are provided, documentation remains as evidence of the occupational therapy services a client received. Occupational therapists display their public presence through their documentation. From documentation, another therapist can determine clinical reasoning skills, therapeutic abilities, and general competence of practitioners who originally wrote the documents. Documentation can be well-written or poorly developed and uninformative. Both writing styles have equal longevity.

Realize that recordable equals recoverable and discoverable

Occupational therapists are well aware that documentation becomes a legal document, but many practitioners are not equally cautious about creating other records that become permanent. One poorly written note could be damaging to a professional's reputation. Occupational therapists are trained to exercise caution when documenting for occupational therapy services. Some therapists are unaware, however, that other records are discoverable. Discoverable records include email, personal notes, texts, and voicemail. Therapists should keep in mind the legal ramifications whenever they make a permanent record. Professional reputations may be protected by adhering to the general recommendations below. With technology readily available, just about any kind of record is recoverable and discoverable; information can be subpoenaed and used in court cases. Digital information, which can last forever, leaves traces even after being "erased."

Time is likely to become a new issue related to service delivery. In the future, there may be challenges to billing for occupational therapy services because of multitasking. For example, a client who sees a therapist using a personal communication device during a treatment session may dispute whether occupational therapy services were delivered. The third-party payer could request phone records to determine whether the communication was professional in nature and related to the person being billed for the time period. Nonprofessional multitasking could result in reimbursement being denied.

Using time to look for discrepancies between professional and personal activities is becoming easier. Today's world includes automatic record-keeping of time, date, and location. Many people can be tracked throughout the day.

For example, an occupational therapist might be tracked on the way to work through transactions such as credit card purchases for fuel or using automated toll booths. She may be traced from one traffic light to the next with cameras mounted at intersections. If she stops at a store, security cameras in the parking lot and building may shadow her. Some credit cards (and some library books) are equipped with radio frequency devices that are recognized by equipment at multiple sites and time-stamped even without a transaction. Computer systems provide a record of all actions, including signing on, making records related to a client, using the Internet, and logging off. At home, the therapist leaves a record of phone, cable, satellite, and Internet access. These examples provide an indication of why occupational therapists need to make certain there is an accurate record of service delivery without nonprofessional multitasking.

Follow the guidelines for documentation of occupational therapy

The **Guidelines for Documentation of Occupational Therapy** (AOTA, 2013) is an official AOTA document that provides recommendations for report writing. This document offers suggested content with examples for various types of reports and a listing of fundamentals that should be present in all documents. An example of a fundamental is including the "client's full name and case number (if applicable), on each page of documentation" (AOTA, 2013, p. S37).

Request examples of best practice in documentation

Documentation varies from facility to facility. And certainly, as any occupational therapy student who is supervised by more than one fieldwork educator can attest, report writing within a single facility can vary from therapist to therapist. Although some variation is purely style, facilities often have specific requirements or regulations that documentation must meet.

One of the best ways to become proficient in the documentation of a new facility (or for more than one supervisor) is to request and study examples of previously written documentation the facility (or supervisor) considers best practice. Report examples need to be **deidentified** (a HIPAA term): stripped of all identifying personal health information.

Respect the reader

If the primary purpose of documentation is communication, respecting the reader is necessary. The first step in respecting the reader is determining who will read the occupational therapy report. The second step is writing the documentation for the readers, who may include clients receiving occupational therapy services, their families, referral sources, third-party payers, and other professionals. Occupational therapy evaluation findings need to be consolidated into one document that communicates to all readers.

Keeping report readers interested enough to finish an entire document is the third step of respecting the reader. If evaluation reports are lengthy, the occupational therapist can make reading easier by dividing information into short paragraphs, using various levels of headings, and designing tables to summarize data.

Do not make the reader work

Each evaluation report should stand alone and include all information a reader needs to come to the same conclusion as the report writer. Initial reports can provide information related to delay, decline, or dysfunction in terms of percentages for a client, justifying the need for occupational therapy services. Progress and discharge reports should include all necessary preliminary information so the report reader does not have to search for and read old documentation to make comparisons to determine clinical change.

Demonstrate effectiveness by showing improvement

To show effectiveness of services, occupational therapists need to show clinical change in the direction that shows improvement. Use the word *improvement,* not the terms *increase* or *decrease,* to respect the reader while not making the reader work. At minimum, the discharge report should include comparisons of current performance with performance documented in a previous report, with improvement percentages calculated. Exhibit 11.1 provides an easy way to calculate improvement percentage.

Determining direction of improvement is key. In many cases, the direction of improvement is a higher value. For example, Charlie, a 10-year-old boy with severe and profound disabilities, is working to improve head control, a measurement of duration of time. As intervention, his occupational therapist added a mercury switch to the headset of Charlie's personal listening device. The switch activates the device to play music when Charlie holds his head

> Use the word *improvement,* not the terms *increase* or *decrease,* to respect the reader while not making the reader work.

EXHIBIT 11.1. EASY CALCULATION FOR IMPROVEMENT PERCENTAGE

$$\text{Improvement percentage} = \frac{\text{New (evaluation)} - \text{Old (evaluation)}}{\text{Old (evaluation)}} \times 100$$

EXHIBIT 11.2. EASY CALCULATION FOR IMPROVEMENT PERCENTAGE: CHARLIE

$$\text{Improvement percentage} = \frac{113-61}{61} \times 100 = 87\%$$

Note. The direction of improvement can be a lower value. If a client is working on improving speed, then the desired improvement is less time.

up; the switch stops the music when his head is down.

During the initial evaluation, Charlie was able to control his head for an average of 61 seconds. For a progress note a week later, the occupational therapist found that Charlie controlled his head for an average of 113 seconds. Exhibit 11.2 shows the calculation for improvement percentage for Charlie. The occupational therapist was able to provide evidence of occupational therapy intervention effectiveness: Her documentation indicated that Charlie showed an 87% improvement in head control performance.

Electronic systems can be set up to provide automatic calculation of improvement and demonstrate effectiveness of service delivery. In fact, the sophistication of some electronic systems allows comparisons as part of the available data-mining capability.

When in doubt, leave it out

Documentation must include only information pertinent to the person receiving occupational therapy services. In some styles of documentation, the therapist can check whether a phrase or sentence is really necessary by removing it and seeing how the document reads. The phrase or sentence should be deleted if the document is stronger without it. Careful proofreading, coupled with checking spelling and grammar, can find other unnecessary or inaccurate information. If the therapist trips over a sentence or component during proofreading, chances are the intended reader will also stumble. The passage should be rewritten or deleted to protect the reading rhythm (Whitney, 2013).

Explain professional jargon

Using frequent parenthetical phrases often allows the option of using both professional jargon and words that a reader who is not a health care professional can understand. A combination of professional and explanatory styles helps readers at various educational levels understand the documentation. For example, rather than write "ATNR has already begun to integrate," the following description provides more information about this 6-month-old baby:

> Sam showed signs of the asymmetrical tonic neck reflex (ATNR), a primitive reflexive motor pattern, which is typical for infants of his age. He demonstrated the ATNR, primarily when supine (on his back), when he either (1) moved his head out of midline (the "invisible" middle of his body) toward his left or right side or (2) extended (straightened) an arm to the side. The stimulus of Sam turning his head sideways or extending his arm resulted in his exhibiting the typical ATNR pattern: His arm and leg on the "nose side" extended and his arm and leg on the side opposite the nose flexed (bent). Sam was able to move out of the ATNR pattern (especially in sitting positions), a sign that the influence of this primitive reflex is disappearing. As expected when the session progressed and he became more tired, Sam demonstrated increasingly more instances of the stimulus–response ATNR pattern.

Use descriptions as educational teaching assessments

By providing both professional jargon and parenthetical explanations, written documentation can help teach people outside the profession more about occupational therapy. Every report should include an occupational-therapy-to-English-dictionary that educates readers to be advocates of occupational therapy. In the case of Sam's ATNR, the reader learns the full name of the reflex, that the reflex is typical for him at his age, and the components of the reflex. Later, if another therapist mentions ATNR without explanation, the readers of Sam's report will already have the necessary background information. Consider creating a list of commonly used descriptors, qualifiers, and modifiers to refer to when writing notes. Organizing these writing tools by purpose (e.g., descriptors of affect, of movement patterns, of pain) can improve speed and fluency in documentation.

Use appropriate terminology

Occupational therapy students often overuse the word *patient*, using this term (especially the abbreviation *pt.*) when referring to any person receiving occupational therapy services. In many settings, particularly medical-model facilities, the word *patient* is most appropriate. Other settings, however, may have specific terminology that must be used when referring to the person receiving services. The term *client*, for instance, has been popular for several years. In school settings, the person receiving occupational therapy services is called a *student*, whereas in an industrial setting, the person may be known as a *worker* or *employee*, or as *a resident* in a skilled nursing facility. Before making any assumptions, the therapist should check with the facility to determine appropriate terms and use the terms consistently.

Use past tense

Proper use of linguistic convention promotes communication and reduces the risk for misinterpretation. An experienced occupational therapist learned the hard way to use past tense for documentation verbs. After hard questioning from parents, who heartily maintained that their child did not have a specific skill included in a formal report, the therapist had to admit she had seen the behavior only once. By using present tense, the therapist implied that the behavior is always present, either ongoing or happening all the time. Had the therapist used the past tense, however, she would have indicated that the action happened before the current time, either as a one-time occurrence or on an ongoing basis in the past. This example underscores the importance of selecting the appropriate verb tense when writing documentation.

Observations that signify ongoing behavior should be in the past tense, indicating that something happened at least once. For instance, the past-tense version—"Lee sat with a straight back"—indicates that the behavior was observed one time or more. The present-tense versions—"Lee sits with a straight back" or "Lee is sitting with a straight back"—indicates a behavior he accomplished 100% of the times he was sitting during the session.

Can and *able* (as in "Lee can sit with a straight back" or "Lee is able to sit with a straight back") deserve special note. Although some practitioners make liberal use of *can* and *is able to* in their notes,

use of these present-tense terms leaves doubt in the reader's mind about whether these behaviors were seen during an evaluation or whether the therapist may simply have believed that the client had the potential to exhibit the behaviors. If the phenomenon was observed, using the past tense—*was able to*—is more appropriate; for example, "Lee was able to sit with a straight back." Then, checking the modifier list for frequency and support, a full note might read "Lee was able to sit with a straight back with minimal assist and complete a 15-minute table top task."

Use active rather than passive verbs

You can significantly improve readability in your writing by simply reorganizing sentences and using active voice (Whitney, 2013). What is the difference between the following two observations: "Mandy moved from prone into sitting" and "Mandy was moved from prone into sitting"? In the first observation, which used an active verb (i.e., *move*), Mandy was an active participant, accomplishing the action herself. In the second observation, with the passive verb (*was moved*), Mandy did not actively participate in the action; she was passively manipulated from one position to another.

Written descriptions of observations should reflect what happened during an evaluation session. In most cases, the person observed is an active participant, so the observation should include an active verb. Expanding the active-verb example provides additional information: "Mandy moved from prone (on her stomach) into side-sitting by pushing down with her left arm, leaning to her left side, and swinging her legs around to the right side." If passive action is observed, use passive-voice verbs but include the identity of the active agent in the description.

For instance, in the expanded passive-verb documentation, the identity of the active agent is the therapist: "Mandy was moved into sitting from prone (on her stomach) through four-point (hands and knees) by the therapist." Although this advice may remind you a bit too much of English class, an "active voice" in writing is clearer to the reader. Start with the subject of your sentence, for example, starting the previous sentence with "Mandy moved" rather than "Leaning to her left side and swinging her legs around to the right side, Mandy moved from prone."

Use seem and appear judiciously

Although some facilities may allow the use of words seem and appear, administrators in other settings believe that professionals such as occupational therapists should have the expertise to make documentation-writing decisions that eliminate these words. The observation "Mr. Oberfeldt demonstrated difficulty seeing objects within 6 to 12 inches from his eyes when he held a newspaper at arm's length for reading" provides much more definitive information about his skills than the observation, "Mr. Oberfeldt appeared to have difficulty seeing objects nearby."

If the habit of using these two words is difficult to break when writing, the therapist can fix the results when proofreading. Using the find feature available in many applications can help the therapist search for *appear* and *seem*. If either word is present, the therapist should rewrite the section.

Eliminate will, would, should, *and* could

The words *will, would, should,* and *could* mean that the client may show the behavior if given the chance—in other words, the behavior did not happen during the evaluation session. Practitioners using these four words in documentation are predicting future behaviors on the basis of their observations. Occupational therapists should not document an observation that they did not specifically see; records of observation must be legally defensible.

In the example "Mollie would visually track an object," readers of the report have no idea whether Mollie showed visual tracking skills during the session; *would* may indicate only that this behavior was possible in the therapist's professional opinion. The observation is transformed by eliminating *would*, changing the verb to past tense, and expanding to provide additional information:

> As expected for her age, Mollie used whole-head movements (rather than moving her eyes only—as anticipated when she gets older) to track visual objects. At the starting point of Mollie looking straight forward, she tracked objects 4 inches to the left and right in the horizontal plane, 2 inches up and down in the vertical plane, and 1 inch in each direction in the diagonal planes.

Use articles and personal pronouns

Writers of evaluation reports should individualize descriptions of the client by using articles *a, an,* and *the* and personal pronouns (e.g., *she, him, her, his*). Reports should match what the facility considers best practice in documentation, taking shortcuts (e.g., approved abbreviations) as allowed. In narrative reports, particularly those that are read by the client or client's family, write full sentences with all appropriate parts of speech (e.g., "The mother reported that her son did . . ." instead of "mom said son did . . .").

Beware of nonreferenced pronouns, a common error in writing (Whitney & Davis, 2013). Ensure it is clear who the "he" or "she" is in your sentence. For example, in the sentence "Morgan's father asked Al to reevaluate the report of another therapist written about Morgan and he was distressed," who is the "he" that was distressed? Morgan's father? Al? The therapist?

Separate judgments from descriptions

The written description should describe exactly what the therapist observed during the session documented. By "painting a picture" that is clear, the occupational therapist will allow the reader to make a judgment or draw an appropriate conclusion. Judgmental language can be included in a separate interpretation section, a consecutive sentence, a separate table column, or clearly labeled as interpretation if included in the same location as the corresponding description. Strong documentation avoids judgments; rather than stating "Mr. Oberfeldt was unmotivated," simply state the facts: "Mr. Oberfeldt collected fewer nearby objects today than in the previous 3 sessions." Instead of writing, "Mrs. Martinez did a better job of walking today," the description and judgment are divided into separate sentences as follows:

> Mrs. Martinez walked 500 feet, from her room to the independent living kitchen, within 10 minutes without resting. Her functional mobility performance showed an improvement compared with a week ago, when she walked 100 feet toward the kitchen over a period of an hour and required four 5-minute rest breaks.

Justify professional opinions using behavioral examples. When a therapist makes an observation on the basis of his or her knowledge of the underlying aspects of the client's situation, the report should cite a specific example to justify a professional opinion. The following two descriptions provide examples of using the phrases *as evidenced by* and *as indicated by*, respectively:

1. Mr. Martin showed difficulty discriminating three-dimensional space, as evidenced by tripping on the 4-inch step at the entrance of his house.
2. In the classroom, Sarah continued disregarding her central vision (looking straight at a task or object), as indicated by her viewing tasks with her head at a 45-degree angle and using her peripheral vision to complete activities.

Use spell check if available

Typos happen. But errors in documentation can make the occupational therapist look careless and sloppy, and by extension, incompetent. If a spell check is available in the documentation system, the therapist should take advantage of the feature. Some spell-check programs permit adding practice-related, technical terms to the dictionary. Adding words commonly used in documentation can save time and increase accuracy.

Use readability statistics if available

For some types of documentation, reading level may become an issue. With the rise of client-centered care and improved client access to their own records, documentation may need to be written at a level that matches the educational background of the person receiving services.

Fortunately, many electronic applications have features that provide information on readability. To find and activate the readability statistics feature, the therapist can click on the application help menu and search for the term *readability*. When this feature is activated, a dialog box appears after every standard spelling and grammar check. The box includes counts of words, characters, sentences, and paragraphs; averages of sentences per paragraph, words per sentence, and characters per word; and readability, which includes passive sentences percentage, a reading ease score, and grade level score.

Flesch Reading Ease score (Thomas, Hartley, & Kincaid, 1975) has a 100-point scale; a score >60 is considered good reading ease, whereas lower scores indicate a document that is more difficult to read. The Flesch–Kincaid Grade Level (Cotugna, Vickery, & Carpenter-Haefele, 2005) corresponds to a grade in school. For example, a Flesch–Kincaid Grade Level of 13 corresponds to the reading level of college freshmen. If an occupational therapist knows she is working with a client with a Grade 7 reading level, she can adjust her writing to provide documentation that reaches that level.

The Flesch Reading Ease score and Flesch–Kincaid Grade Level are inversely related: As one increases, the other decreases. Strategies to improve reading ease and decrease grade level include decreasing the length of words, number of words, and number of words per sentence and increasing the number of sentences, paragraphs, and sentences per paragraph.

Use autocorrect if available

Some electronic applications offer an autocorrect feature that can improve quality and speed of writing. Autocorrect can be found by accessing the help menu and searching for the term *autocorrect*. When the feature is accessed, an autocorrect dialog box appears with a blank area called *Replace* and another blank area named *With*. To improve efficiency of writing, an occupational therapist can develop codes for frequently used words or phrases. For example, a therapist who has grown weary of typing *occupational therapy* can save time by accessing the autocorrect feature, inputting *ot1* into the Replace area and *occupational therapy* into the With area, clicking on the Add button, and then on the OK button. From that time (until the option is removed from autocorrect), the application will replace *ot1* with *occupational therapy*.

Autocorrect also can be used to fix unique writing difficulties. For instance, a person intends to write the word *assess* but instead types *asses*. Both words are included in standard spell check features. The person can use autocorrect to replace *asses* with *assess* and not have to worry about the problem.

Other recommended additions to autocorrect include replacing *posses* with *possess* and replacing *defiantly* with *definitely*. Once added to autocorrect, the old word cannot be used in writing. For instance, many people may not have a need to use the plural of the words *ass* and *posse*. Autocorrect comes loaded with a listing of replacement items and has a removal feature. For example, autocorrect converts (c) to the symbol ©. To stop the conversion, a person needs to access the autocorrect dialog box, click on the Replace (c) with © line in the autocorrect listing, click on the Delete button, and then on the OK button.

Collect descriptions in a database

Writing a description (e.g., of a behavior or performance) professionally sometimes takes more time than scoring a standardized assessment instrument. Rather than writing from scratch each time, therapists should think about gathering well-crafted descriptions into a central place for later use. The centralized descriptions, which serve as templates for customizing the information for each client, can be stored in an electronic master file. All identifying information related to a client should be carefully removed from the description before it is saved as a template.

An efficient therapist can develop two data bases based on gender. The male version (with *he, his, him, himself*) can be developed first, then converted to a female version (with *she, her, herself*) by using the replace feature, available in most applications, to replace both *his* and *him* with *her* and *he* with *she*. These replacements will also convert *himself* to *herself*. Making an error of "he" when you are reporting on a female client exposes your habit of reusing material from previous reports and undermines the individualization of your findings.

When writing a new report, the therapist can search the file for similar descriptions using key words in the find feature of most applications or add descriptions newly written for the current report. The descriptions also can be printed as a checklist, with a hard copy for use during the evaluation session. Over time, as the electronic master file grows, the descriptions can be rearranged and categorized by content, age, setting, and so on.

Protect the privacy of electronic information

Because personal health information is used and stored electronically, ensuring the security of electronic information is of utmost importance. Newspaper accounts contain horror stories of electronic health information inadvertently released to the general public through computers—with confidential reports still stored on hard drives—stolen, or given to charitable organizations. Less spectacular violations of confidentiality occur frequently with information available to multiple people who use a single computer station. Access devices containing client information get lost, stolen, or cloned. Unsecured digital information can be replicated more than once. Privacy is becoming increasingly problematic.

Many facilities have information technology specialists who can consult with a therapist regarding the process to secure transmission and documentation procedures to ensure confidentiality. Be sure to consider both employer and personal devices that may contain work-related references when determining how to secure confidential information.

If a computer is shared by other people, a simple way to secure electronic information is to make sure that confidential files are closed before leaving the computer station. Saving all work to a password-protected folder is a good option. Another method of protecting client records is to save electronic information to portable storage devices (e.g., USB memory drives) with appropriate password protection and encryption. The storage devices must be kept safe.

Interconnections and wireless capabilities increase security dangers exponentially. For Internet-based health records, occupational therapists need to ensure security of the four points discussed previously: (1) access device, (2) connection, (3) transmission, and (4) website. Any website used for client information must have security. Personal access devices also need security. Keeping current with the most recent versions of security applications such as encryption and firewalls may help.

Working from a secured access point may offer additional security. The connection also must be secured. Occupational therapists need to be cautious of how and where an access device is connected at all times. If a therapist is documenting while in transit, the personal access device may change connection sites many times without the occupational therapist knowing. One way to make certain of secured connections is to manually turn off automatic wireless capabilities and work offline. Later, the occupational therapist can make the connection manually with full knowledge of the wireless access point. Occupational therapists working on client records need to exercise extreme caution if using unsecured wireless access sites.

> For Internet-based health records, occupational therapists need to ensure security of four points: access device, connection, transmission, and website.

SUMMARY

The mystery of Morgan, threaded throughout this chapter, serves as a reminder of the importance of interpretation in occupational therapy and the lasting power of documentation. To show effectiveness, occupational therapists must solve the mystery of each person by becoming lifestyle detectives who profile clients, examine clues within contexts, and synthesize multiple data points to give order to the complexities of life.

Documenting occupational therapy is of equal importance to providing the original services. Because documentation remains as evidence of occupational therapy, occupational therapists must be cognizant that their writing is part of their public image. To ensure a legacy that shows the record of a competent therapist, this chapter offers general documentation recommendations.

QUESTIONS

1. How would you adapt your documentation for the specified audience?
   - Another rehabilitation team where the client will be transferred
   - A child's parent with a high school education
   - A referring physician
   - A child's parent with a 6th-grade education
   - A classroom teacher of a student with a disability
   - A third-party payer interested in function and functional outcomes

   - An older adult with mild cognitive difficulties
   - A Hispanic mother who speaks and understands minimal English.
2. How can you protect the security, confidentiality, and privacy of your evaluation reports, if you use a hard-wired computer or computer network for documentation? What steps would you take to protect this information? If you are using an access device that is wireless, what steps would you take to protect this information?
3. Occupational therapists frequently perform audits on documentation for fieldwork students, junior staff occupational therapists, occupational therapy assistants, and other non–occupational therapist team members. What characteristics of best practices discussed in this chapter would you include in a chart audit form that you could use to audit the quality of evaluation documentation?
4. You are at your desk at work and a person you do not know gives you a written letter from a lawyer requesting immediate release of all your documentation on a specific client for a legal issue being investigated. You do not know whether the lawyer represents your facility or someone else. What do you do?

References

American Occupational Therapy Association. (2010). Occupational therapy code of ethics and ethics standards. *American Journal of Occupational Therapy, 64*(Suppl.), S17–S26. http://dx.doi.org/10.514/ajot.2010.64517

American Occupational Therapy Association. (2013). Guidelines for documentation of occupational therapy. *American Journal of Occupational Therapy, 67*(Suppl.), S32–S38. http://dx.doi.org/10.5014/ajot.2013.67S32

Cotugna, N., Vickery, C. E., & Carpenter-Haefele, K. M. (2005). Evaluation of literacy level of patient education pages in health-related journals. *Journal of Community Health, 30*(3), 213–219. http://dx.doi.org/10.1007/s10900-004-1959-x

Federal Educational Rights and Privacy Act of 1974, Pub. L. 93–380, 20 U.S.C. § 1232g *et seq.*; 34 C.F.R. § 99.

Health Insurance Portability and Accountability Act of 1996, Pub. L. 104–191, 45 C. F. R. § 160, 164.

Smith, J. (2013). Documenting occupational therapy services. In R. V. Whitney & C. A. Davis (Eds.), *A writer's toolkit for occupational therapy and health care professionals: An insider's guide to writing and getting published* (pp. 207–226). Bethesda, MD: AOTA Press.

Thomas, G., Hartley, R. D., & Kincaid, J. P. (1975). Test–retest and inter-analyst reliability of the automated readability index, Flesch reading ease score, and the fog count. *Journal of Literacy Research, 7*(2), 149–154. http://dx.doi.org/10.1080/10862967509547131

University of Miami. (2006). *Privacy/data protection project*. http://privacy.med.miami.edu/hips/index.htm

Whitney, R. V. (2013). Refreshing, renewing, and re-mediating your writing: Back to the basics. In R. V. Whitney & C. A. Davis (Eds.), *A writer's toolkit for occupational therapy and health care professionals: An insider's guide to writing and getting published* (pp. 53–64). Bethesda, MD: AOTA Press.

Whitney, R. V., & Davis, C. A. (Eds.). (2013). *A writer's toolkit for occupational therapy and health care professionals: An insider's guide to writing and getting published*. Bethesda, MD: AOTA Press.

CHAPTER 12

Reassessment and Reevaluation

Fern Silverman, EdD, OTR/L

Highlights

- Need for reassessment and reevaluation
- Defining the difference between reassessment and reevaluation
- Inherent complexity of reevaluation
- Purposes of reevaluation
- Collaborative nature of reevaluation
- Reevaluation as a discrete activity
- Reevaluation as an iterative process
- Reasoning processes supporting reevaluation
- Therapist skills needed for reevaluation
- Reevaluation: Linked to intervention outcomes and evidence-based practice
- Reevaluation and the termination of services
- Documentation and the reevaluation report.

Key Terms

Client
Clinical reasoning
Collaboration
Continuous monitoring
Data collection
Decision making
Discharge planning
Evidence-based practice
Groups
Occupational Therapy Intervention
    Process Model
Outcomes
Persons

Populations
Pragmatic reasoning
Progress notes
Reassessment
Reevaluation
Reflection
Response to intervention
Self-reflection
Step-down approach
Student, Environments, Tasks, and Tools
    framework
Telehealth
Termination of services
Universal design

This chapter discusses reassessment and reevaluation as integral components of the evaluation process in occupational therapy and defined in terms of their purpose and client goals. Both processes are related to the *Occupational Therapy Practice Framework: Domain and Process* (3rd ed.; *Framework*, American Occupational Therapy Association [AOTA], 2014).

This chapter begins by exploring the differences between reassessment and reevaluation. It then explains the components of reassessment and discusses the continuous monitoring approach. The next section discusses approaches to reevaluation and addresses some of the factors that influence the selection and types of reevaluations: contextual factors, the reasoning processes supporting reevaluation, and the competencies and skills required to conduct a reevaluation. After briefly examining the relationships among reassessment, reevaluation, treatment outcomes, evidence-based practice, and the role of reevaluation in the termination of services, the chapter concludes with a brief overview of the writing of the reevaluation report.

NEED FOR REASSESSMENT AND REEVALUATION

Throughout the intervention process, the occupational therapist is constantly gathering data about the status of the client. These data provide ongoing reassessment that will give the therapist an understanding of the course of intervention and the client's responses to it. As a critical part of occupational therapy practice, reassessment and reevaluation align with initial evaluation and help an occupational therapist answer some of the essential questions that guide treatment planning, such as "Is this client making progress toward his or her goals?" and "Is the frequency, intensity, and duration of treatment still appropriate?"

Reevaluation parallels initial evaluation as a conceptual process of collecting reliable and relevant information to support making informed clinical decisions about the intervention process (Krishnamurthy et al., 2004; Spruill et al., 2004). Both reassessment and reevaluation involve complex problem solving as the therapist generates, interprets, and translates client data into decisions and actions. In each process, the therapist strives

to understand the client as an occupational being and to describe the "gap between capacity and performance" (World Health Organization [WHO], 2001, p. 20) that prevents full participation and engagement in the client's chosen occupations. In both situations, the therapist describes the client's current occupational performance status (either comprehensively or focused on a discrete aspect) and makes projections about future performance.

The common purposes of initial evaluation, reassessment, and reevaluation center on the need to have accurate and complete information about the client as a basis for intervention planning. Hocking (2001) described this need as a primary practice issue for a professional because the initial evaluation, reassessment, and reevaluation all serve as the "basis from which occupational therapists define . . . their clients' occupational performance challenges, determine clients' priorities, and negotiate the goals of interventions" (p. 468). The *Framework* (AOTA, 2014) reiterates the importance of data, along with the client's desired outcomes and evidence, as a means to direct the therapy process. Reassessment and reevaluation are ways to support the therapist's design of treatment interventions that promote meaningful occupation-based outcomes and meet the needs of the client.

DEFINING THE DIFFERENCE BETWEEN REASSESSMENT AND REEVALUATION

Reassessment occurs throughout the intervention process as a continuous part of treatment (Clark & Miller, 1996; Krishnamurthy et al., 2004). It may include observations, notes of periodic changes in function, and at times the use of specific assessments. *Reevaluation* is the periodic use of specific assessments to perform a comprehensive evaluation to determine progress and decide whether the therapist needs to adjust the goals or a client is ready for termination of services.

A therapist should acknowledge the need for both reassessment (ongoing monitoring of the client's status within intervention) and discrete, periodic reevaluations (Sames, 2004). Both approaches produce information used to continue, modify, or discontinue the intervention approach. Evaluation, intervention, reassessment, and reevaluation are all interdependent processes.

Reassessment allows the therapist to determine on an ongoing basis whether the client is making progress and whether the intervention process or current goals need to be modified. In contrast, reevaluation occurs at regular intervals during the intervention process to determine whether the client is making progress, whether and how the occupational therapist should modify intervention or change goals, and when the therapist should terminate intervention. Reassessment

- Occurs frequently and regularly throughout the course of intervention,
- Involves observation and clinical judgment,
- May or may not include the use of standardized assessments,
- Has its intensity and methods of data collection determined by the therapist, and
- Should use an occupation-based perspective.

Reevaluation provides information about the client so that the occupational therapist can determine in a more formal manner whether the client is making progress, the intervention process needs adjustments, goals need to be changed, or it is time to terminate the intervention. A therapist should approach reevaluation with an awareness of the interdependencies within each clinical situation and understand that reevaluation itself can produce change (Krishnamurthy et al., 2004). Reevaluation

- Is generally performed using standardized assessments,
- Is often done at particular intervals,
- Has its frequency and format possibly determined by legal parameters or third-party payers, and
- Usually uses an occupation-based perspective.

The *Framework* (AOTA, 2014) addresses reassessment and reevaluation specifically by including intervention review as a substep within the intervention phase of service delivery and also explicitly delineating outcomes assessment in the outcomes phase of service delivery. The intervention review, as described in the *Framework*, consists of three steps: (1) reevaluating the plan and its implementation, (2) modifying the plan as appropriate, and (3) considering the need for further treatment (AOTA, 2014). The *Framework* describes the review phase

of occupational therapy intervention as one that is continuous and collaborative in nature to address the current and future needs of the client.

Continuous Monitoring as a Means of Reassessment

One approach to reassessment is **continuous monitoring**. Spruill and colleagues (2004) described continuous monitoring as an approach to reassessment used in psychology: "As treatment progresses, the clinician's initial assessment of the problem may change; as the assessment changes, so should the intervention" (p. 746). Within occupational therapy literature, there is support for this approach to reassessment (Clark & Miller, 1996; Opacich, 1991). Ongoing reassessment is a necessary component of occupational therapy intervention between initial evaluation and discharge, where the therapist "modifies the intervention process to reflect changes in client status, desires, and response to intervention" (p. 868). Opacich (1991) described the continuous nature of reassessment by saying,

> But as we have seen, information-gathering and decision making do not stop with the initial assessment and establishment of treatment goals . . . . Data and clinical observations regarding changes in human performance are continuously collected in the course of therapy. The information serves to support, refute, or amend the treatment hypothesis and allows the clinician to make informed decisions. Furthermore, such evidence, systematically collected, can help determine the efficacy of treatment. If the therapy is not beneficial, the practitioner can decide to alter or terminate therapy. (p. 361)

Clark and Miller (1996) presented a systematic approach to continuous reassessment. The authors described occupational therapy participation in the Heartland Problem Solving Model, a four-level "problem-solving approach to special education service delivery" (p. 702). In the model, occupational therapy progress monitoring is a system of intertwined intervention and assessment of children with special needs in which comprehensive information about the children's functioning and instructional, curricular, and environmental accommodations is collected on an ongoing basis using multiple data collection methods and sources. As information is gathered, the therapist reflects on the information and makes immediate decisions to modify current intervention. Children are included in self-monitoring and contribute to the database, when they are ready. Progress monitoring, as presented by Clark and Miller, is an example of a highly developed formal system of continuous reevaluation.

Another example of progress monitoring is the **response to intervention (RtI)** approach that is part of the Individuals With Disabilities Education Improvement Act of 2004 (IDEA). RtI is a tiered approach to school-based intervention that uses targeted interventions with progress monitoring to help all students who are in general education succeed (Fairbanks, Sugai, Guardino, & Lathrop, 2007). Occupational therapy delivered as part of RtI services makes use of ongoing progress monitoring to document and assess change.

Frequency of Reassessment and Reevaluation

Progress monitoring, by its very nature, implies ongoing reassessment that yields data gathered on a regular basis about a client's occupational performance. The frequency of this reassessment process is straightforward because, by definition, it is ongoing and continuous. **Progress notes,** which a therapist can maintain in various ways, serve as a record of a client's change in occupational performance. Almost any type of reassessment requires the continuous gathering of information and can be documented through progress or SOAP (*s*ubjective, *o*bjective, *a*ssessment, and *p*lan) notes.

Legal and administrative policies set by the educational or health facility involved determine the frequency of the discrete reevaluation process. Funding sources sometimes predetermine therapy duration periods on the basis of diagnoses or of protocols established by institutional agencies. However, it is the responsibility of the occupational therapist to conduct a reevaluation at any time, independent of set policies and guidelines,

if he or she ethically believes that it is warranted to formally reexamine the changed needs or status of a client. For example, in the regulatory requirements in Medicare Home Health regarding reassessments:

- The Centers for Medicare and Medicaid Services has specific, strict schedules for the timing of functional reassessments to ensure therapy is provided only the appropriate number of times to meet the patient's needs and show progress in meeting goals.
- Use of a standardized assessment is not required.
- The instruments used must assess aspects of occupation that are relevant to the patient's needs and goals.
- A therapy reassessment is not a full evaluation or comprehensive assessment.

In practice, reassessment and reevaluation result in a comprehensive database for the therapist's reflection and use in decision making. Although either process can stand alone, ideally a therapist should periodically review reassessment and reevaluation together. Weaving together subjective and objective data provides a basis for the therapist to understand the client as an individual and evaluate both the client and the intervention plan.

An example of weaving together these data might be an occupational therapist working in an inclusive early intervention center. Reassessment in his or her practice would have formal and informal aspects and would be both continuous and discrete. This therapist uses a day-to-day comparison of current and past performance with initial goals as an informal means of reassessing children to make incremental modifications in daily treatment activities (i.e., reassessment as continuous monitoring). Formal reevaluation occurs on an annual basis when the interdisciplinary team, including the parents, reviews the results of standardized tests and conducts a structured and systematic review of the child's goal attainment status (i.e., reevaluation as a distinct step). Each therapist must develop an approach to reassessment and reevaluation in response to many factors affecting his or her practice and clinical setting.

INHERENT COMPLEXITY
OF REEVALUATION

Although initial evaluation and reevaluation share a basic procedure and overarching purpose, as well as many of the same skills and thought processes, they represent distinct components of the evaluation process with differing characteristics. Reevaluation is a distinct step along an evaluation–intervention–reevaluation continuum (Egan & Dubouloz, 2000; Fisher, 1998; Moyers & Dale, 2007).

There are fundamental differences between evaluation and reevaluation. The initial evaluation establishes an occupational performance baseline; the reevaluation seeks to describe a new occupational performance baseline and document change in the client's performance resulting from intervention. The therapist obtains an updated view of the client's occupational performance that must be compared retrospectively with the initial status to determine the degree and nature of change that has occurred and prospectively to the client's desired status to determine the occupational performance issues still to be addressed.

Simultaneously, the therapist reviews the intervention plan to determine whether change has occurred and whether the intervention should be changed or continued. That review requires **self-reflection** to consider whether and how effectively the appropriate theoretical constructs have been used. The therapist then integrates all of this information to determine if, how, and why occupational performance has improved, regressed, or stayed the same and to make the next set of decisions regarding the subsequent course of intervention (Moyers & Dale, 2007).

Both evaluation and reevaluation processes are holistic and client centered; both require a reflective, occupation-based perspective. They differ in that evaluation occurs at the onset of the therapy and reevaluation follows it, continuing at various intervals throughout the intervention phase as an essential part of clinical reasoning and intervention planning.

Environmental Perspective to Reevaluation

The reevaluation process's complexity relates to the changing context of a client's natural environment. Occupational therapists increasingly use a societal perspective to view the client during reevaluation, aligning with the philosophy of WHO (2001), which views disability as a normal part of life that affects everyone at various times during the course of his or her life. WHO recognizes that health and well-being can be affected by environmental barriers, as well as by body structure or body function problems.

Using the WHO philosophy as a guideline, an occupational therapist must examine a client's limitation in participation as it relates to factors in the environment. An older client who moves to a first-floor, senior-friendly new apartment, for example, might have different intervention needs than one on the third floor of an old building. The therapist must consider the barriers and supports in the environment to gauge the client's needs during any reevaluative process.

One intervention approach that addresses reducing barriers and enhancing environmental support uses universal design principles from architecture, product manufacturing, and interior design to enable a client to participate fully in his or her environment. These interventions can be effective even when reevaluation indicates that a client has continued limitation or a decline in skills.

Universal design, "the design of products and environments to be useable by all people to the greatest extent possible without the need for adaptation or specialized design" (Center for Universal Design, 1997), promotes full access, embracing the philosophy of inclusion (Darragh, 2007). Typically, universal design results in a more functional environment or product for everyone (McGuire, Scott, & Shaw, 2006). The availability or lack of availability of universally designed products or environments should therefore be considered when a client's status is reassessed, reflecting the focus on society's role and responsibilities in enhancing participation for all citizens. Although universal design may be helpful to a client, it is not always accessible for a variety of reasons, including availability, cost, and eligibility for reimbursement.

If a client uses assistive technology to carry out his or her daily occupations, then the therapist should use that technology in the evaluation to determine optimal occupational performance. Therefore, it also must be included in the reevaluative process.

One lens for considering assistive technology in schools as a component of evaluation and reevaluation is the **Student, Environments, Tasks, and Tools (SETT) framework** (Zabala & Korsten, 2005). SETT is a four-part model intended to promote collaborative decision making in all phases of assistive technology service decisions and delivery, including evaluation of effectiveness within the scope of reevaluation. The SETT model encourages the occupational therapist to consider not just what data are gathered during reevaluation but also how they are gathered.

There can be numerous challenges to the use of assistive technology in the occupational therapy reevaluative process. In pediatric school-based settings, for example, therapists may encounter difficulties procuring and managing equipment. Further, adequate assistive technology assessment and planning processes may not be in place (Copley & Ziviani, 2004). Copley and Ziviani proposed a team model with the explicit purpose of evaluating and reevaluating the need and use of assistive technology for children with multiple disabilities. With the older adult, third-party payers may not support the purchase of assistive technology as essential to client occupational performance. A therapist can only conduct an up-to-date, environmentally relevant reevaluation if he or she addresses any barriers that would interfere with the effectiveness of the assistive technology.

Reevaluation and the *Framework*

The *Framework* (AOTA, 2014) complements the WHO (2001) guidelines by using language that supports the focus on function and participation ahead of client factors and disabilities. The *Framework* states that "despite their importance, the presence or limitation of specific body functions and body structures does not necessarily ensure a client's success or difficulty with daily life occupations" (AOTA, 2014, p. S7). The overarching stated goal of occupational therapy is to support health and participation in life through engagement in occupation (AOTA, 2014). Participation and health therefore frame the reevaluation process. When conducting a reevaluation, the therapist must consider a client's skills alongside factors in the physical and social environment to determine the need for further intervention.

The *Framework* (AOTA, 2014) uses language similar to that used in the *International Classification of Functioning, Disability and Health* (ICF; WHO, 2001) in an effort to create a meaningful picture of health and functioning. The *ICF* is applied at the individual level, the service or institutional level, and the population or community and social policy level for service delivery. In occupational therapy, the *Framework* looks at performance patterns of the client across the same parameters. Using these categories, the occupational therapy reevaluation process should take into account the client's occupational performance and patterns of behavior on multiple levels and in multiple contexts.

Reevaluation From an Occupation Perspective

Like all occupational therapy processes, a reevaluation must be true to the roots of the profession and views of occupation (Gillen, 2013). Although reevaluation is a discreet activity intended to gather key information about changes in a client's occupational performance, it is incumbent upon the therapist to maintain a holistic view of the reevaluation process and a focus on the occupational value of the skills being reviewed. In this way, reevaluation reaffirms a commitment to each client as an "occupational being" (Yerxa, 1990, p. 6) and the importance of occupation for health and well-being.

An example of the importance of the occupational perspective in the reevaluative process was shown in a study of occupational therapists' use of information when making driver licensing recommendations for older and functionally impaired adults (Unsworth, 2007). The study revealed that four factors were most important when assessing driver competence: (1) driving instructor interventions, (2) driver behavior, (3) cognitive and perceptual skills, and (4) vehicle handling skills.

In Victoria, Australia, where the researchers conducted the study, the therapist may recommend a range of graded driving privileges, including on-road reassessment as needed. Reassessment of driving skills is a critical occupation-based activity that can determine whether a person who is older or disabled can have the freedom of community mobility as well as the associated sense of autonomy and well-being. Therefore, an occupational perspective must be incorporated in the reevaluation process when considering driving and community mobility skills.

Another study, by Jack and Estes (2010), demonstrated the benefit of an occupational perspective during the reevaluation process in an orthopedic outpatient clinic. In this study, participants who received biomechanical interventions that were holistic, client centered, and occupation based had improved outcomes. This was accomplished by using the Canadian Occupational Performance Measure (COPM; Law et al., 1999) as a reevaluation tool and as a way to introduce an occupational adaptation framework into treatment (Schkade & Schultz, 1992). The COPM verified performance-based changes and documented the clients' occupation-based perceptions and priorities as part of the reevaluation process.

PURPOSES OF REEVALUATION

Reevaluation serves multiple purposes, including evaluating client progress, exchanging feedback and information with the client or care provider and other professionals, establishing progressive goals, modifying intervention approaches and techniques, changing the intensity of service, and evaluating the efficacy of intervention (AOTA, 2010b; Egan & Dubouloz, 2000; Moyers & Dale, 2007; Polgar, 2003). Reevaluation provides the therapist with information to support a range of potential decisions, including continuation of the intervention plan, changes in the intervention plan, discharge or discontinuation of services, or referral to another service or therapist (AOTA, 2008). Reevaluation is a simultaneous review of the many client, therapist, and procedural factors of occupational therapy intervention that provide valuable insight into the dynamic relationship among the client's occupational performance status, the therapist's repertoire of skills, and the integrity of the intervention plan.

COLLABORATIVE NATURE OF REEVALUATION

The therapist is not the sole evaluator or decision maker in the reevaluation process. The importance of **collaboration** between client and therapist in reevaluation is clear (Egan & Dubouloz, 2000; Krishnamurthy et al., 2004; Tickle-Degnen, 2002; WHO, 2001). Although the therapist, client, and family or caregiver collaborate during the initial evaluation, the relationship strengthens and develops as intervention progresses and becomes even more intense during reevaluation. The client (or family or care provider when the client is unable to participate) is the expert in how he or she has experienced changes in capacity and how those changes have altered performance in activity and participation across contexts.

It is the client who feels the dynamic interactions between health conditions and contextual factors (WHO, 2001) and who can inform the reevaluation from that unique perspective. The therapist is the expert in understanding causal links and associations between health and context. Together, these coexperts make sense of the results of the reevaluation and construct a new plan. As Egan and Dubouloz (2000) described in the reevaluation stage of the Occupational Performance Process Model, a client-centered treatment planning model, "therapist and client determine whether or not the desired results have been obtained" (p. 99).

Using a systems lens, the therapist can consider a broader collaborative process of reevaluation. The viewpoint is supported by the *Framework's* (AOTA, 2014) suggestion that a therapist look at the client from multiple angles and viewpoints, emphasizing context and interrelationships. The term *client* means any entity that receives occupational therapy services (AOTA, 2014). Clients are thus categorized in the *Framework* (AOTA, 2014) as **persons,** including families, caregivers, teachers, employers, and relevant others; **groups,** such as three children in treatment together in a classroom; and **populations** within a community, such as refugees or veterans.

The emphasis on interrelationships means a reevaluation may require that the therapist collaborate with multiple persons involved in the well-being of the client. For example, spouses of patients with Alzheimer's disease or parents of students with autism may collaborate in the decision-making process that occurs during reevaluation. Communication among those who collaborate with the occupational therapist may occur during official contacts, such as individualized education plan meetings or discharge planning conferences, or informally, in hallway conversations or during an observation of treatment by a family member. Silverman's research (2007) suggested that both forms of communication may influence the final decision with regard to therapy duration and amount. Further, a therapist must be aware of the effect of all contacts and collaborations among those involved.

REEVALUATION AS A DISCRETE ACTIVITY

Occupational therapy literature describes reevaluation as a discrete activity (Egan & Dubouloz, 2000; Fisher, 1998). AOTA's (2013a) *Guidelines for Documentation of Occupational Therapy* names the reevaluation report as a specific type of documentation and provides guidelines for the content to be addressed in it. The **Occupational Therapy Intervention Process Model** (Fisher, 1998), a top-down approach to intervention planning, describes reevaluation as a specific step in intervention planning. The model labels the step "Reevaluate for Enhanced Occupational Performance" and describes it as a time when the therapist uses "performance analyses to verify whether the client has met his or her goals" (p. 518). The therapist identifies additional problems, redefines performance discrepancies, and cycles back through previous steps in the model to modify and implement new intervention strategies. Fisher also made the key point that focused reevaluation provides critical information about the effectiveness of occupational therapy services.

Although the therapist and the client are the evaluators and decision makers, numerous contextual factors influence the therapist's approach to reevaluation within a particular clinical setting. Schell (2013) frame these influences as part of **pragmatic reasoning** "used to fit therapy possibilities into the current realities of service delivery" (p. 389). Schell clarified that pragmatic reasoning is "not focused on the client or client's condition but rather on the physical and social 'stuff' that surrounds the therapy encounter" (p. 389). Included in the therapy encounter are the therapist's resources, energy, and perception of the client's capacity. Pragmatic reasoning creates practice

and personal contexts that shape decision making around the scope and timing of services, including reevaluation. Practice context and the choice of reevaluation assessments are two contextual factors particularly relevant to an understanding of the reevaluation process.

Practice Context

Characteristics of the practice context have a clearly identifiable effect on reevaluation. Krishnamurthy and colleagues (2004) made the case that within psychology, the volume and type of reevaluations vary within specialty areas of the profession. This same argument can be made for occupational therapy. Therapists in different practice areas respond to very different regulatory requirements for reevaluation, such as IDEA in school-based settings (AOTA, 2011; Clark & Miller, 1996; Frolek Clark & Chandler, 2013) or Medicare requirements in skilled nursing facilities (AOTA, 2008). For example, the short length of stay in acute care settings may force the rapid integration of evaluation, intervention, and reevaluation within one or two sessions, but the residential environment of a group home for people with developmental disabilities may allow annual reevaluations.

Relevant legislation, reflected in new case law, continually alters the contextual parameters of reevaluation. In school-based assessment in Pennsylvania, for example, the Gaskin settlement (*Gaskin v. the Commonwealth of Pennsylvania,* 1995) heightened the need for therapists to consider a child's ability to participate in an inclusive classroom context as part of the reevaluation. The Gaskin settlement resulted from a class action suit by parents of children with disabilities who felt that their children's right to an education with their typical peers was being denied.

Occupational therapists in different countries encounter different cultural and geopolitical factors that may influence the frequency and nature of reevaluation procedures. In Australia, for example, funding for occupational therapy services in schools must be applied for annually from a set amount provided by the government for each child with a qualifying disability (Disability Act 23/2006). The school principal allocates the amount awarded each year, and the Student Support Group determines which services (e.g., instructional aide, occupational therapy, speech therapy, physical therapy) should be supported. Therefore, an extensive formal occupational therapy reevaluation must occur each year to put forth a strong case for continued funding.

Reevaluation Assessments

A second factor influencing reevaluation is the availability of appropriate evaluation assessments. As Davies and Gavin (1999) put it, "The most common method used to demonstrate a change in clients' performance as a result of the treatment is to measure the client's abilities before and after treatment" (p. 363). Occupational therapists across specialty areas of practice have vastly different assessments available to them, contingent on the client's occupational performance problems, age, or diagnosis.

Assessments used by occupational therapists also vary greatly in the psychometric qualities that influence their appropriate use in reevaluation. Experts in evaluation (Davies & Gavin, 1999; Polgar, 2003) caution occupational therapists on the psychometric issues relevant to selecting appropriate reevaluation assessments.

Additionally, therapists must be cognizant of the fact that standardized assessments often focus on discrete underlying skills rather than performance of the activity and participation levels, thus giving limited information about the client's volitional aspects, integrated performance, or the environmental components of occupational performance (Fisher, 1992). If the client is accustomed to using assistive technology in his or her daily occupational performance, it should be used during the reevaluation. However, the therapist must recognize that the use of any device affects the reliability and validity of a standardized assessment.

Often, a therapist will use the same evaluative assessment for reevaluation that he or she used for the initial evaluation. The use of the same evaluation assessment at targeted points across the duration of intervention yields data that facilitate comparison with a baseline level of skill performance. For example, a therapist could evaluate the range of motion of a client with a joint problem using a goniometer. By measuring the range of motion of a specific joint the same way using the same tool at the same time of day (i.e., under the same conditions), the therapist can quantitatively assess any changes made.

Polgar (2003) directed attention to another form of reliability relevant to reevaluation. Alternate-form reliability is a concern when a therapist must repeatedly evaluate a specific area of client performance. As Polgar explained, client performance may artificially improve when given the same test at both evaluation and reevaluation because of a memory or practice effect. In this situation, rather than use the same test at reevaluation, the therapist identifies and uses a different test that measures the same performance area, computing the reliability coefficient to establish the equivalence of the two measures.

Fisher (1992) noted that the prevalent use of "home-grown evaluation tools" (p. 278) is problematic because validity and reliability are not adequately established, limiting the appropriateness of comparing pre- and posttreatment evaluation scores. Polgar (2003) explicitly addressed the need for an instrument to have strong test–retest reliability or stability over time, because "an estimate of the test's stability is necessary when the measurement is used as an outcome measure" (p. 304).

Although initial evaluation directs reevaluation and provides a clear baseline for determining progress, the narrow focus that results from some initial evaluations also can constrain the reevaluation process. A therapist might use the initial evaluation to qualify the client for therapy and to describe performance. Therefore, when the therapist selected the initial evaluation assessments, the full impact of occupational therapy was not established.

Reassessment data should influence the reevaluation process. A reevaluation using the same assessments as initially used might not capture the qualitative information gained through the collaborative relationship with the client, resulting in documentation of restricted outcomes and constricted views of intervention effectiveness. For this reason, the therapist may decide to change assessments on the basis of unique factors. The following scenarios describe situations in which the therapist might choose to select a different assessment than the one used during the initial evaluation or augment the to reevaluation by adding an additional assessment to the reevaluation:

- *The client progresses across the developmental continuum from one age category to the next, and the initial assessment is no longer appropriate.* For example, an occupational therapist administers the Peabody Developmental Motor Scales (PDMS–2; Folio & Fewell, 2000) to a 5-year, 8-month-old boy with a delay of approximately 2 years in developmental skills who is enrolled in a preschool for children with special needs. One year later, the child reaches a chronological age of 6 years and 8 months. The PDMS–2 is no longer appropriate, because it is not standardized for children older than age 6 years. The therapist decides to administer the Bruininks–Oseretsky Test of Motor Proficiency (Bruininks & Bruininks, 2005), which is normed for children aged 4 through 21.2 years.
- *The client transitions from one type of service delivery setting to another with a different focus and legal parameters, triggering a need for a different evaluation.* For example, a therapist administers the DeGangi Berk Test of Sensory Integration (Berk & DeGangi, 1983) to a girl who is age 4 years, 1 month as part of an assessment for occupational therapy services in a private clinic. One year later, the child enters kindergarten in a typical classroom, where occupational therapy is now a related service. As part of the reevaluation, the therapist may choose to administer the Sensory Profile School Companion (Dunn, 2006) instead of the previous assessment to assess sensory processing issues that might be particularly relevant to school-based practice.
- *The client's condition (i.e., client factors) changes since the last evaluation with regard to the extent of his or her disability or medical status.* For example, an occupational therapist evaluates a 65-year-old patient with diabetes and neuropathy for bilateral hand function. His medical condition worsens, and he undergoes an amputation 4 months later. At the point of his 6-month reevaluation, the therapist must include assessments that look at prosthesis use.
- *An additional performance area gains importance to the client's overall well-being, and the therapist needs to evaluate the client's sense of self.* For example, a 38-year-old client with a spinal cord injury and lower-extremity paralysis is initially evaluated in the acute care unit, with a focus on range of motion and activities of daily living. At the time of his 6-month reevaluation, he has improved to the extent that he is ready to resume his job as an accountant at a nearby accounting firm. The therapist adds a work site assessment in the reevaluation to assist the client in reentering his work environment with his disability.

The occupational therapist uses a holistic, flexible, and reflective therapeutic thought process when determining which assessments to use during the reevaluation. The therapist must understand the limits of each individual assessment and avoid the expectation that a single assessment can address all client performance issues with psychometric integrity.

The therapist also must consider the changing dynamics of client factors and context that may necessitate an alteration of assessments. As a client's needs or performance skills change, assistive technology may play an increasing role in the person's ability to function. In this situation, the therapist must allow the client to use the assistive technology during the reevaluation.

Assistive technology can act as an environmental adaptation by compensating for declining or diminished performance skills. For example, a female client with multiple sclerosis is frustrated with challenges in a new home living situation, and the therapist plans to administer another occupational profile as part of the reevaluation. However, because of muscle weakness and fatigue, the client is struggling with oral communication. Using an augmentative communication device during the reevaluation, the therapist might be able to gain a true assessment of the client's occupational needs and priorities.

REEVALUATION AS AN ITERATIVE PROCESS

The multiple purposes of reevaluation dictate an organized yet flexible integration of three steps: (1) data collection, (2) reflection, and (3) decision making. Each step is distinct, involving specific thought processes and actions and producing requisite data to inform the next step. The steps flow from one to another, but they are also iterative, allowing the therapist to revisit steps in any order to produce a concurrent picture of the client, the intervention process, and the therapist's role in the process.

The therapist gathers information about the client, the intervention, and his or her own reactions and responses to the client and the intervention. The therapist then considers all of this information to understand what has transpired in the intervention process and to gain an insight into why and how the intervention has had this effect. This process leads to well-informed decisions to modify, maintain, or discontinue discrete or comprehensive intervention strategies and actions.

Step 1: Data Collection

To initiate **data collection,** the therapist makes the key decision about how extensive the collecting of data will be and identifies the sources and methods to collect information about the client, the intervention, and the therapist self-review. This process begins with a retrospective review of what has occurred from the point of initial evaluation until the current time, including the evaluations performed initially, the client's initial status in all areas evaluated, any information gained from ongoing reassessment, and the client's current status on both short- and long-term goals.

Collaborative review of the client's status includes not only recognition of his or her measured progress toward goals but also recognition of the client's emotional and affective responses to intervention and views on how intervention has addressed what is important to him or her (Kielhofner, Hammel, Finlayson, Helfrich, & Taylor, 2004). The therapist also reviews the course of intervention to confirm what was done and to clarify how it was done (i.e., the therapist's skills in providing the services).

Data collection itself is a multistep process in which the therapist collects all readily available information about the client and the intervention and quickly analyzes that information to decide whether more focused or in-depth information is needed and how to acquire it. The therapist and client (where possible) decide which assessments

to repeat, if any, and how to obtain additional information from other sources. Actual testing may be more specific than that done at the time of initial evaluation, and the reevaluation may focus on discrete problems or functional areas. The therapist seeks to answer two interconnected questions: (1) How has the client's occupational performance status changed since the initial evaluation? and (2) Has therapy had an impact on this change?

In some cases, reevaluations or components of the reevaluation may need to take place when the therapist is not in the same physical location as the client. In this case, a therapist might use telehealth technologies to facilitate face-to-face interactions with web-based technologies. *Telehealth* is "the application of evaluative, consultative, preventative, and therapeutic services delivered through telecommunication and information technologies" (AOTA, 2013b, p. 21). Occupational therapists use telehealth to provide access to clients (Heilmerl & Rasch, 2009) who otherwise might not receive intervention. In some cases, a therapist might use telehealth technologies with a client who has returned to his or her natural environment outside of the area where intervention had taken place. Some nonstandardized assessments, such as clinical observations and an occupational profile, can be administered through telehealth web-based systems.

Telehealth technology as a vehicle for reevaluation can be particularly helpful for two purposes. First, telehealth technology can assist with ongoing data gathering, allowing the therapist to have frequent face-to-face interactions with the client without being in the same place, thereby making ongoing data collection feasible and cost-effective. For example, a therapist might be working with a child on a dressing skill at home. With the assistance of a proxy, such as a parent, telehealth technologies would permit the therapist to observe and time the minutes required for the child to complete the dressing task every morning for a week without having to travel to the child's home.

Second, telehealth technologies can facilitate a view into the client's natural environment that might not otherwise be readily available. Telehealth web-based communications can therefore aid the process of context-based reevaluation in the natural environment. A therapist can view the situational variables and factors that may be impeding a client's successful participation in his or her work, home, or school setting.

Step 2: Reflection

Learning to analyze and reflect on data gathered through reevaluation from an occupation-based perspective is key to supporting a client's priorities.

The second step in reevaluation is **reflection.** In this step, the therapist seeks to answer two additional interconnected questions:

1. Why has change occurred?
2. What does the change mean for the client's future?

The therapist considers all of the information obtained during data collection, including reports from other health care providers, educators, and other documented providers to better understand the client's current occupational performance status.

As Schell (2013) described, "more data are collected and the occupational therapy practitioner gains a sharper clinical image. The clinical image is the result of the interplay between what the occupational therapy practitioner expects to see (such as the usual course of the disease or disability) and the actual performance of the client" (p. 135). In this step, the therapist also seeks to understand why change has occurred. The therapist considers the overall effectiveness of the intervention plan. At this point, the therapist asks,

- Did change occur as expected?
- Is there evidence to explain the change or to direct therapy from this point?
- Are the changes in the client's status meaningful to him or her or family?
- Are the changes important for functioning within the client's environment?
- Will the client, family, or caregiver be able to maintain these changes after discharge from therapy?
- Are the changes occurring at an appropriate rate and amount relative to the frequency and duration of treatment?
- How much more change can be expected?
- How much time is needed for the client to achieve the changes?

- Do I have the knowledge and skills necessary to continue the intervention?
- Are there services in addition to occupational therapy that are needed?
- Is the client invested and engaged in the intervention?
- Do I as the therapist believe in the client's ability to reach his or her outcomes?

The therapist asks and answers questions like these alone and in conjunction with the client to move to decision making, the final step of the reevaluation process.

Step 3: Decision Making

In the **decision-making** step of reevaluation, the therapist faces a choice of three decisions regarding the client and the intervention plan:

1. Continue the intervention plan.
2. Modify the intervention plan.
3. Discontinue intervention, and discharge the client.

As with the other reevaluation steps, the therapist makes a decision in collaboration with the client, and his or her family or caregiver, whenever possible. This step appears straightforward, but it involves an analysis of the pros and cons and potential ramifications of each decision before a selection is made. The decision of what to do with the results of the reevaluation is an ethical decision as the therapist sorts through the options to determine what could be done, what should be done, and ultimately what is done (Schell, 2013). Questions generated during the reflection stage serve as the basis for evaluating the options in the decision-making step. The therapist arrives at a decision having considered all available information and can provide a rationale for the decision.

One decision is that the therapist can continue the intervention plan. The decision to continue the intervention without alteration indicates that the therapist and client agree that the client is progressing satisfactorily and that the plan can continue to provide the right challenge to achieve further progress.

The therapist also can decide to modify the intervention plan. When the therapist decides to modify the intervention plan, he or she and the client also must make subsequent decisions regarding the nature, timing, and implementation of the changes. The therapist may elect to adjust discrete treatment activities or approaches within the plan or may substantially alter the frequency, duration, and intensity of the entire plan, including goals and outcomes.

Another choice is for the therapist to discontinue intervention and discharge the client from services. Typically, the therapist and client make this decision in one of several situations. In one scenario, the therapist and client choose discharge when the client has achieved all intervention objectives and can sustain that progress outside of the treatment environment. A reevaluation can be key in establishing whether, in fact, a client continues to qualify for services or even continues to have the criteria for a clinical diagnosis.

In a study that looked at assigning an autism spectrum disorder diagnosis, children were evaluated between 16 and 35 months and then reevaluated between 42 and 82 months (Kleinman et al., 2008). At each juncture, the same three criteria were used: (1) clinical judgment, (2) performance on the Childhood Autism Rating Scale (Schopler, Reichler, & Renner, 1986), and (3) the Autism Diagnostic Observation Schedule (Lord, Rutter, DiLavore, & Risi, 2001). Researchers found that 19% of the children moved off the autism spectrum by the point of reevaluation. Upon this discovery, many of these children would no longer qualify to receive intervention, depending on the context and funding for their services.

In addition to using reevaluation findings to determine whether to end an intervention program for which a client no longer qualifies, there are two other scenarios in which a therapist may decide to terminate services. First, the therapist may choose to discontinue services when the client is not able to meet all of the objectives but has achieved maximum therapeutic benefit. Second, the therapist may discontinue services when the client's personal needs, goals, or context changes.

If the therapist continues or modifies an intervention plan, he or she then continues to cycle through the steps of reevaluation as needed. A decision to terminate services ends the process of reevaluation. Throughout the three steps of reevaluation, collaboration with the client and family or caregiver is fundamental to the success of the reevaluation. The therapist draws upon a mixture of thinking and reasoning processes during reevaluation to ensure that the client is an active collaborator and that all of the multiple factors are drawn together and considered.

REASONING PROCESSES SUPPORTING REEVALUATION

Occupational therapists use multiple reasoning styles during reevaluation to assess overall intervention effectiveness and make decisions while maintaining the client–therapist relationship and managing a large volume of diverse information. In their textbook on clinical reasoning, Mattingly and Fleming (1994) described the process of clinical reasoning in occupational therapy as "deliberation about what an appropriate action is in this particular case, with this particular patient, at this particular time" (p. 10). They also described procedural, interactive, conditional, and narrative reasoning.

Schell (2013) defined *clinical reasoning* as a complex and multifaceted "process used by practitioners to plan, direct, perform and reflect on patient care" (p. 131). (Readers are encouraged to read Schell's work for a discussion of scientific, narrative, and ethical reasoning.) Through the use and integration of all of these modes of reasoning, a therapist learns the particulars of each case as he or she implements the intervention plan and the relationship with the client unfolds. During reevaluation, the therapist shifts fluidly across all of the modes of reasoning.

In the data collection and reflection steps of reevaluation, the therapist uses scientific and procedural reasoning when comparing the client's current performance status to his or her initial level of performance to identify changes in the client's status and response to specific interventions. The therapist then shifts to interactive and conditional reasoning as he or she incorporates subjective information from the client about his or her response to intervention, personal goals, and situation. A final shift to narrative reasoning occurs as the therapist and client look ahead and compare the client's current status to the desired intervention outcome. If the therapist makes a decision at any point to readminister a formal standardized assessment, he or she again switches to procedural reasoning in parallel with the thinking process of the initial evaluation.

During the decision-making step in reevaluation, the occupational therapist again uses multiple modes of reasoning. In continuing an existing intervention plan or selecting new intervention strategies, the therapist once more uses scientific and procedural reasoning to match the plan and strategies to the problem or deficit. However, the therapist simultaneously moves to interactive reasoning as the intervention plan is modified for the client, who is involved in decisions of how and when to modify the plan.

When the therapist makes the decision to terminate services, a final switch to conditional and narrative reasoning occurs. The therapist and client together must consider the client's life beyond the treatment setting and determine how able the client is to meet the demands and challenges of his or her life.

Throughout the reevaluation process, the therapist uses pragmatic reasoning as he or she negotiates the service delivery system with the client. The therapist considers the ethical implications of each decision when deciding on the best option for the client.

THERAPIST SKILLS NEEDED FOR REEVALUATION

The skills involved in reevaluation parallel the skills needed in the initial evaluation phase, with specific emphasis on or unique application of specific competencies. One of the most obvious skills needed is that of selecting and interpreting formal assessments, with special consideration of the psychometric issues identified earlier in this text.

Given the nature of reevaluation in occupational therapy, in which the challenge is to understand and integrate the multiple physical, social, cultural, and emotional features of a person and translate that information into occupational

performance in various temporal and performance contexts, additional skill areas are equally vital to an efficient and effective reevaluation process (Coster, 1998). Spruill and colleagues (2004) described 6 foundational competencies of clinical psychologists, which also apply to the skill set needed by an occupational therapist in the reevaluation phase:

1. Scientific foundations
2. Relationship skills
3. Communication skills
4. Individual and cultural differences
5. Ethical and legal guidelines
6. Critical thinking.

The complexity of reevaluation, in which the client relationship has evolved and the amount of information available to be synthesized and used has multiplied, intensifies demands in all of these areas. Krishnamurthy and colleagues (2004) reinforced the notion of integrating technical assessment skills with the ability to synthesize information with inferences and communicate results and feedback in a way that is understandable and useful to the client. Both Spruill and colleagues (2004) and Krishnamurthy and colleagues stressed the importance of self-reflection and analysis as components of the skill set used in evaluation and reevaluation.

REEVALUATION: LINKED TO INTERVENTION OUTCOMES AND EVIDENCE-BASED PRACTICE

Reevaluation, through its reiterative nature, serves as a way to look at a client's needs in relation to his or her initial status when therapy commenced. The therapist collects information that informs clinical decision making through the reevaluative processes of ongoing reassessment and systematic reevaluation. These data also provide a way for the occupational therapist to demonstrate measurable treatment outcomes resulting from occupational therapy. Reevaluation therefore aligns with **evidence-based practice** principles as a process that collects and uses data to guide therapy decisions and interventions.

Connection to Outcomes

Reevaluation can serve the dual purposes of determining a client's progress toward therapy goals and contributing to the evaluation of the service program (Fisher, 1992; Krishnamurthy et al., 2004; Polgar, 2003). Due in part to fiscal issues, therapists may be under pressure to use reevaluations to document outcomes and demonstrate the efficacy of occupational therapy intervention (Unsworth, 2000). However, the occupational therapist also must recognize that change is not always the sole object of intervention (Fawcett, 2007). Moreover, the therapist must recognize that outcome measures need to be sensitive to protective and preventative effects, as well as to improvements (Heaton & Bamford, 2001).

Kielhofner and colleagues (2004) identified four interrelated components of outcomes research that demonstrate the overlap between reevaluation of the individual client and measurement of effectiveness at the programmatic level: "(1) identifying client needs, (2) creating the best possible services to address those needs, (3) generating evidence about the nature of specific services and their impact, and (4) accumulating and evaluating a body of evidence about specific occupational therapy services" (p. 16). They also included understanding the process of therapy as an important element of treatment effectiveness research. The client's perspective on how therapy has progressed and what the experience has meant can inform outcomes research in much the same way the inclusion of the client's subjective information enhances the reevaluation process.

Outcomes are also central in the *Framework* (AOTA, 2014), which states they are "the desired end result of the occupational therapy process" (p. S10). The *Framework* identifies two types of outcomes. First are outcomes that a therapist uses for intervention planning, monitoring, or planning for discharge. The second types are those of the client as he or she experiences the consequences of intervention and can engage in daily occupations.

In the *Framework* (AOTA, 2014), the authors observed that outcome measurements must be holistic in nature, considering the client's occupational profile, contextual factors, and needs and desires. The therapist may modify the measures chosen during the intervention process to reflect a change in priorities or needs, as necessary.

Connection to Evidence-Based Practice

Reassessment and reevaluation provide concrete evidence to guide decision making. Such evidence can help answer prognostic questions (Bennett & Bennett, 2000) such as "Was the treatment effective?" and "Should treatment be altered?" Despite the importance of evidence, evidence and data alone cannot lead to appropriate decision making without clinical judgment and reflexivity. Lee and Miller (2003) proposed that decision making for the occupational therapist must be contextualized, not just evidence based, to truly serve the needs of clients. A contextualized therapy decision takes into account the client's perspective and the values of occupational therapy. Lee and Miller (2003) suggested that therapy decisions emerge from a triad of data: (1) formal assessment or reassessment, (2) therapist clinical observations, and (3) client self-report.

The sources of evidence determine the effectiveness of reevaluation. Sources of evidence include the client as expert and research literature. These sources allow the therapist to judge whether his or her interpretations are accurate and whether decisions about intervention modifications or discharge reflect best practice.

Evidence-based practice requires an "approach that integrates the best external evidence with individual clinical expertise and patient's choice" (Sackett, Rosenberg, Gray, Haynes, & Richardson, 1996)—the same factors that frame the reevaluation process. Reevaluation also can contribute to the development of evidence-based practice as a therapist examines in aggregate the results of individual client reevaluations. Bennett and Bennett (2000) made this connection, commenting that "evaluating the effectiveness of the treatment of clinical practices implemented, in terms of improvement in relevant outcomes, makes it possible to determine if the evidence-based decision-making process has been successful.

Evaluation leads to more questions and so the cycle continues" (p. 178).

Although reevaluation at the client level is not synonymous with outcomes research or the generation of evidence-based practice, if the therapist conducts the reevaluation systematically and then collects and analyzes the results in aggregate, the processes clearly can be mutually informative.

REEVALUATION AND THE TERMINATION OF SERVICES

A therapist can use the reevaluation process to determine a client's continued eligibility, program planning, or discharge. However, there are no uniform eligibility criteria for occupational therapy services (Muhlenhaupt, 2000), and similarly, there is no single criterion to establish when to terminate services. A therapist should terminate direct services "when the goal has been met or when the means of achieving the goal is no longer best accomplished through our legitimate tools" (Nesbit, 1993, p. 846).

Although multiple attempts have been made to unify or standardize discharge decisions (Kaminker, Chiarello, O'Neil, & Dichter, 2004; Long, 2003; Lovell & Russell, 2005), success has been limited and setting specific. Therefore, the skills and expertise of the occupational therapist are critical to the reevaluation process, which often guides the pace and timing of service termination.

Termination of services is subject to relevant laws and the rules, regulations, policies, and practices of the institution. Termination of services, however, can also occur in a client centered manner. Communication is vital to ensure that the termination of services is client centered. It is incumbent on the therapist to be certain that he or she communicates effectively with all stakeholders about the purpose of the therapy at the beginning of the therapeutic relationship, when the initial evaluative process takes place. The client, close family members, and administrators should understand the scope and domain of occupational therapy practice as it relates to the needs of the client.

It is equally important to communicate the results of reevaluation and ongoing progress monitoring. Keeping the client and other stakeholders informed means that a change in amounts of service delivery will be more understandable and less of a surprise to those involved. For example, if multiple treatment notes for a client with a brain injury repeatedly show no further gains, and a thorough reevaluation verifies this trend, the client and his or her family members might be more likely to agree with a therapist's decision to terminate services. A clear delineation of therapy goals and progress toward these goals can preempt unrealistic expectations among stakeholders and facilitate a smoother transition when the therapist recommends discontinuing therapy.

In many cases, a therapist can gradually reduce therapy services while tracking the success of each reduction with progress monitoring. A therapist can slowly terminate services in several ways. A therapist might shift the delivery model for therapy services from direct services to consultation, cutting back on the hands-on nature of the interaction between the therapist and the client. Or, a therapist can change a service from individual sessions to group sessions, reducing the intensity of the client–therapist relationship. Frequency can also be changed. For example, services can be decreased from once per week to once every other week, with further reductions in frequency occurring until service termination is complete.

These examples show a **step-down approach,** in which the therapist, as part of a team, develops a plan where maximum intervention is systematically reduced to less intensive intervention that is consistent with strictly defined criteria. A step-down approach to service termination has several advantages. First, the therapist can use progress monitoring to assess the ability of the client to maintain his or her new performance level and goals reached as services are reduced. In this way, a gradual reduction in services acts as a vehicle for ongoing progress monitoring. Second, the client and family members can separate more easily from any dependence on the therapist, transitioning from relying on the supportive role of an occupational therapist to an increased state of independence. Third, the client can apply new skills to meaningful, functional activities, transferring these skills to the natural setting while still receiving some occupational therapy support. Therefore, the client is more likely to generalize outcomes appropriately, enhancing his or her sense of empowerment and facilitating a smoother transition to life beyond occupational therapy.

A therapist must use a moral compass when using reevaluation to terminate services. Ethical decision making directly relates to **discharge planning,** which is the end-product of the reevaluation processes (Atwal & Caldwell, 2003). Atwal and Caldwell identified the ethical breaches that occur when a therapist fails to heed the *Occupational Therapy Code of Ethics and Ethics Standards* (AOTA, 2010a). In their research, Atwal and Caldwell identified unintentional gaps in an occupational therapist's adherence to the values of autonomy, beneficence, nonmaleficence, and justice in treatment and discharge decisions. Careful reevaluation is essential for making treatment decisions regarding decreasing frequency of services or service termination while maintaining high ethical standards.

DOCUMENTATION AND THE REEVALUATION REPORT

Once the process of reevaluation concludes, the therapist documents the results. The therapist can record reevaluation results, if brief, in the regular progress note by recording the changes in client status and resulting adjustments in the intervention plan. Lengthy, comprehensive reports may entail a separate format. A facility or source of reimbursement may determine the specific formats of reports.

AOTA's (2013a) *Guidelines for Documentation of Occupational Therapy* include the reevaluation report as a specific form of clinical documentation. The guidelines suggest 6 content areas as part of the report:

1. *Client information:* Name; date of birth; gender; and applicable medical, educational, and developmental diagnoses, precautions, and contraindications.
2. *Updated occupational profile:* Identification of performance areas that have been resolved or that continue to be problematic, as well as changes in the client's priorities or desired outcomes.
3. *Reevaluation results:* Focus of reevaluation, specification of outcome measures and assessments used, and client's performance and subjective responses.

4. *Analysis of occupational performance:* Description of and judgment about performance skills, performance, patterns, context, and environments, activity demands, outcomes from assessments, client factors, and outcomes expected.
5. *Summary and analysis:* Interpretation of data, including comparison with previous evaluation results.
6. *Recommendations:* Changes to occupational therapy services; revision or continuation of interventions, goals, and objectives; frequency of occupational therapy services; and recommendations for referral to other professionals or agencies as applicable.

According to AOTA (2013a), the reevaluation report provides documentation of periodic reassessments that are readministered at intervals established by the practice setting.

SUMMARY

When treating an individual, group, or population, the therapist is constantly reassessing the clients through many means. The continuous observations and notes that the therapist makes during intervention are part of the reassessment process. Periodically, as the therapist notes progress and changes in the client, the therapist is reassessing both the client and the intervention to determine whether changes are required in the goals or approaches to intervention. At times, the therapist needs to use a specific assessment to determine whether and how the approach to intervention should be changed. The reassessment process requires the therapist to use clinical reasoning and is an essential component in the ongoing intervention process.

Reevaluation is another, more formalized, critical component of the occupational therapy process. Mattingly and Fleming (1994) repeatedly reinforced the notion that reevaluation is an essential component of occupational therapy intervention. They identified "a process of nearly continuous hypothesis generation, evaluation, and revision" (p. 336) in occupational therapy. This continuous process of revision is essential no matter how thorough the initial assessment.

The therapist, through reevaluation, is able to adjust the intervention to adapt to client improvement or regression or to the evolution of the therapeutic relationship.

Reevaluation requires that the therapist collaborate with the client to work through the steps of data collection, reflection, and decision making to incorporate multiple pieces of information into a cohesive and responsive decision to continue or update the intervention plan or terminate treatment. The data collection step includes gathering information from a variety of sources about the client, the intervention process, and the therapist. The therapist and client reflect on the client's initial status and desired future status and consider both the client's and the therapist's subjective responses in determining the effectiveness of the intervention plan.

The evaluation of intervention effectiveness leads to decisions about continuing, modifying, or discontinuing intervention. Through the three reiterative steps of reevaluation, the therapist is continually drawing on a blend of reasoning modes and evidence to make intervention decisions that are clinically sound, holistic, and responsive to the unique situation of the client. Both reassessment and reevaluation are essential parts of the intervention process. They are critical to the provision of quality occupational therapy services.

QUESTIONS

1. Explain the difference between reassessment and reevaluation. Are they independent processes?
2. Explain the purpose of reassessment and the role that it potentially can play in reevaluation.
3. When performing a reevaluation, the therapist may choose to use the same assessments used previously or different tools. Give some examples of why the therapist might use the same assessments and why he or she might use different tools.
4. Reflection is a complex process. Discuss the various elements of the reflection process during reassessment and reevaluation.
5. Describe the clinical reasoning modes that are often used in the reevaluation process.
6. Explain how the reevaluation process can be occupationally relevant.
7. This chapter mentions that meaning of the term *outcomes* may vary. What are different types of outcomes one may find from intervention?
8. Describe the relationship between reevaluation and evidence-based practice.
9. Explain how technological advances, such as assistive technology and telehealth service delivery models, can play a role in the reevaluation or reassessment process.

References

American Occupational Therapy Association. (2008). *Reimbursement and regulatory resources: Information you need to successfully advocate for your patients and your profession.* Retrieved from www.aota.org/Practitioners/Reimb/Resources/2008conf/2008C.aspx

American Occupational Therapy Association. (2010a). Occupational therapy code of ethics and ethics standards (2010). *American Journal of Occupational Therapy, 64*(Suppl.), S17–S26. http://dx.doi.org/10.5014/ajot.2010.64S17

American Occupational Therapy Association. (2010b). Standards of practice for occupational therapy. *American Journal of Occupational Therapy, 64*(Suppl.), S106–S111. http://dx.doi.org/10.5014/ajot.2010.64S106

American Occupational Therapy Association. (2011). Occupational therapy services in early childhood and school-based settings. *American Journal of Occupational Therapy, 65*(Suppl.), S46–S54. http://dx.doi.org/5014/ajot.2011.65S45

American Occupational Therapy Association. (2013a). Guidelines for documentation of occupational therapy. *American Journal of Occupational Therapy, 67*(Suppl.), S32–S38. http://dx.doi.org/10.5014/ajot.2013.67S32

American Occupational Therapy Association. (2013b). Telehealth. *American Journal of Occupational Therapy, 67*(Suppl.), S69–S90. http://dx.doi.org/10.5014/ajot.2013.67S69

American Occupational Therapy Association. (2014). Occupational therapy practice framework: Domain and process (3rd ed.). *American Journal of Occupational Therapy, 68*(Suppl. 1), S1–S48. http://dx.doi.org/10.5014/ajot.2014.682006

Atwal, A., & Caldwell, K. (2003). Ethics, occupational therapy, and discharge planning: Four broken principles.

Australian Occupational Therapy Journal, 50, 244–251. http://dx.doi.org/10.1046/j.1440-1630.2003.00374.x

Bennett, S., & Bennett, J. W. (2000). The process of evidence-based practice in occupational therapy: Informing clinical decisions. *Australian Occupational Therapy Journal, 47,* 171–180. http://dx.doi.org/10.1046/j.1440-1630.2000.00237.x.

Berk, R. A., & DeGangi, G. A. (1983). *DeGangi–Berk Test of Sensory Integration.* Los Angeles: Western Psychological Services.

Bruininks, R. H., & Bruininks, B. D. (2005). *BOT–2: Bruininks–Oseretsky Test of Motor Proficiency (2nd ed.) examiner's manual.* Circle Pines, MN: AGS.

Center for Universal Design. (1997). *The principles of universal design, version 2.0.* Raleigh: North Carolina State University. Retrieved from http://www.design.ncsu.edu/cud/about_ud/udprinciplestext.htm

Clark, G. F., & Miller, L. E. (1996). Providing effective occupational therapy services: Data-based decision making in school-based practice. *American Journal of Occupational Therapy, 50,* 701–708. http://dx.doi.org/10.5014/ajot.50.9.701

Copley, J., & Ziviani, J. (2004). Barriers to the use of assistive technology for children with multiple disabilities. *Occupational Therapy International, 11,* 229–243. http://dx.doi.org/ 10.1002/oti.213

Coster, W. (1998). Occupation-centered assessment of children. *American Journal of Occupational Therapy, 52,* 337–344. http://dx.doi.org/10.5014/ajot.52.5.337

Darragh, J. (2007). Universal design for early childhood education: Ensuring access and equity for all. *Early Childhood Education Journal, 35,* 167–175. http://dx.doi.org/10.1007/s10643-007-0177-4

Davies, P. L., & Gavin, W. J. (1999). Measurement issues in treatment effectiveness studies. *American Journal of Occupational Therapy, 53,* 363–372. http://dx.doi.org/ 10.5014/ajot.53.4.363

Disability Act of 2006, No. 23/2006. Victoria, Australia.

Dunn, W. (2006). *Sensory Profile school companion.* San Antonio: Psychological Corp.

Egan, M., & Dubouloz, C. J. (2000). Evaluating client performance related to targeted outcomes. In V. G. Fearing & J. Clark (Eds.), *Individuals in context: A practical guide to client centered practice* (pp. 99–107). Thorofare, NJ: Slack.

Fairbanks, S., Sugai, G., Guardino, D., & Lathrop, M. (2007). Response to intervention: Examining classroom behavioral support in second grade. *Exceptional Children, 73,* 288–310.

Fawcett, A. (2007). *Principles of assessment and outcome measurement for occupational therapists and physiotherapists.* New York: John Wiley & Sons.

Fisher, A. G. (1992). Functional measures, Part 2: Selecting the right test, minimizing the limitations. *American Journal of Occupational Therapy, 46,* 278–281. http://dx.doi.org/10.5014/ajot.46.3.278

Fisher, A. G. (1998). Uniting practice and theory in an occupational framework [1998 Eleanor Clarke Slagle Lecture]. *American Journal of Occupational Therapy, 52,* 509–521. http://dx.doi.org/10.5014/ajot.52.7.509

Folio, M. R., & Fewell, R. R. (2000). *Peabody Developmental Motor Scales* (2nd ed.). Austin, TX: Pro-Ed.

Frolek Clark, G., & Chandler, B. (Eds.). (2013). *Best practices for occupational therapy in schools.* Bethesda, MD: AOTA Press.

Gaskin v. Commonwealth of Pennsylvania, 23 IDELR 61 (Pa. 1995).

Gillen, G. (2013). A fork in the road: An occupational hazard. *American Journal of Occupational Therapy, 67,* 641–652. http://dx.doi.org/10.5014/ajot.2013.676002

Heaton, J., & Bamford, C. (2001). Assessing the outcomes of equipment and adaptations: Issues and approaches. *British Journal of Occupational Therapy, 64,* 346–356.

Heimerl, S., & Rasch, N. C. (2009). Delivering development occupational therapy consultation services through telehealth. *Developmental Disabilities Special Interest Section Quarterly, 32*(3), 1–4.

Hocking, C. (2001). Implementing occupation-based assessment. *American Journal of Occupational Therapy, 55,* 463–469. http://dx.doi.org/10.5014/ajot.55.4.463

Individuals With Disabilities Education Improvement Act of 2004, Pub. L. 108–446, 20 U.S.C. § 1400 *et seq.*

Jack, J., & Estes, R. I. (2010). Documenting progress: Hand therapy treatment shift from biomechanical to occupational adaptation. *American Journal of Occupational Therapy, 64,* 82–87. http://dx.doi.org/10.5014/ajot.64.1.82

Kaminker, M. K., Chiarello, L. A., O'Neil, M. E., & Dichter, C. G. (2004). Decision making for physical therapy service delivery in schools: A nationwide survey of pediatric physical therapists. *Physical Therapy, 84,* 919–933. http://dx.doi.org/10.1097/01.pep.0000229863.59688.77

Kielhofner, G., Hammel, J., Finlayson M., Helfrich, C., & Taylor, R. R. (2004). Documenting outcomes of occupational therapy: The center for outcomes research and education. *American Journal of Occupational Therapy, 58,* 15–23. http://dx.doi.org/10.5014/ajot.58.1.15

Kleinman, J. M., Robins, D. L., Ventola, P. E., Pandey, J., Boorstein, H. C., Esser, E. L., . . . & Fein, D. (2008). The Modified Checklist for Autism in Toddlers: A follow-up study investigating the early detection of autism spectrum disorders. *Journal of Autism and Developmental Disorders, 38*(5), 827–839. http://dx.doi.org/10.1007/s10803-007-0450-9

Krishnamurthy, R., VandeCreek, L., Kaslow, N. J., Tazeau, Y. N., Miville, M. L., Kerns, R., . . . Benton, S. A. (2004). Achieving competency in psychological assessment: Directions for education and training. *Journal of Clinical Psychology, 60,* 725–739. http://dx.doi.org/10.1002/jclp.20010

Law, M., Baptiste, S., Carswell, A., McColl, M. A., Polatajko, L., & Pollock, N. (1999). *Canadian Occupational Performance Measure.* Ontario: CAOT Publications.

Lee, C. J., & Miller, L. T. (2003). The process of evidence-based clinical decision making in occupational therapy. *American Journal of Occupational Therapy, 57,* 473–477. http://dx.doi.org/10.5014/ajot.57.4.473

Long, D. (2003). Predicting length of service provision in school-based occupational therapy. *Physical and Occupational Therapy in Pediatrics, 23,* 79–93. http://dx.doi.org/10.1080/J006v23n04_06

Lord, C., Rutter, M., DiLavore, P. C., & Risi, S. (2001). *Autism Diagnostic Observation Schedule.* Los Angeles: Western Psychological Services.

Lovell, K. R., & Russell, K. (2005). Developing referral and reassessment criteria for drivers with dementia. *Australian Occupational Therapy Journal, 52,* 26–33. http://dx.doi.org/10.1111/j.1440-1630.2005.00454.x

Mattingly, C., & Fleming, M. H. (1994). *Clinical reasoning.* Philadelphia: F. A. Davis.

McGuire, J., Scott, S., & Shaw, S. (2006). Universal design and its applications in educational environments. *Remedial and Special Education, 27,* 166–175. http://dx.doi.org/10.1177/07419325060270030501

Moyers, P., & Dale, L. (2007). *The guide to occupational therapy practice* (2nd ed.). Bethesda, MD: AOTA Press.

Muhlenhaupt, M. (2000). OT services under IDEA 97: Decision making challenges. *OT Practice, 5,* 10–13.

Nesbit, S. G. (1993). Direct occupational therapy in the school system: When should we terminate? *American Journal of Occupational Therapy, 47,* 845–847. http://dx.doi.org/10.5014/ajot.47.9.845

Opacich, K. J. (1991). Assessment and informed decision making. In C. Christiansen & C. Baum (Eds.), *Occupational therapy: Overcoming human performance deficits* (pp. 356–372). Thorofare, NJ: Slack.

Polgar, J. M. (2003). Critiquing assessments. In E. B. Crepeau, E. S. Cohn, & B. A. B. Schell (Eds.), *Willard and Spackman's occupational therapy* (10th ed., pp. 299–312). Philadelphia: Lippincott Williams & Wilkins.

Sackett, D. L., Rosenberg, W. M., Gray, J. A., Haynes, R. B., & Richardson, W. S. (1996). Evidence based medicine: What it is and what it isn't. *British Medical Journal, 312,* 71–72. http://dx.doi.org/10.1136/bmj.312.7023.71

Sames, K. M. (2004). *Documenting occupational therapy practice.* Upper Saddle River, NJ: Pearson Prentice Hall.

Schell, B. A. B. (2013). Professional reasoning in practice. In B. A. B. Schell, G. Gillen, & M. E. Scaffa (Eds.), *Willard and Spackman's occupational therapy* (12th ed., pp. 384–397). Philadelphia: Wolters Kluwer Health/Lippincott Williams & Wilkins.

Schkade, J. K., & Schultz, S. (1992). Occupational adaptation: Toward a holistic approach for contemporary practice, Part 1. *American Journal of Occupational Therapy, 46,* 829–837. http://dx.doi.org/10.5014/ajot.46.9.829

Schopler, E., Reichler, R, & Renner, B. R. (1986). *Childhood Autism Rating Scale.* Western Psychological Services.

Silverman, F. (2007). *A study of occupational therapy service negotiations in educational settings* [Doctoral dissertation]. Arcadia University, Philadelphia.

Spruill, J., Rozensky, R. H., Stigall, T. T., Vasquez, M., Bingham, R. P., & De Vaney Olvey, C. (2004). Becoming a competent clinician: Basic competencies in intervention. *Journal of Clinical Psychology, 60,* 741–754. http://dx.doi.org/10.1002/jclp.20011

Tickle-Degnen, L. (2002). Client-centered practice, therapeutic relationship, and the use of research evidence. *American Journal of Occupational Therapy, 56,* 470–474. http://dx.doi.org/10.5014/ajot.56.4.470

Unsworth, C. (2000). Measuring the outcome of occupational therapy: Tools and resources. *Australian Occupational Therapy Journal, 47,* 147–158. http://dx.doi.org/10.1046/j.1440-1630.2000.00239.x

Unsworth, C. A. (2007). Using social judgment theory to study occupational therapists' use of information when making driver licensing recommendations for older and functionally impaired adults. *American Journal of Occupational Therapy, 61,* 493–502. http://dx.doi.org/10.5014/ajot.61.5.493

World Health Organization. (2001). *International classification of functioning, disability and health.* Geneva: Author.

Yerxa, E. J. (1990). An introduction to occupational science, a foundation for occupational therapy in the 21st century. *Occupational Therapy in Health Care, 6,* 1–17. http://dx.doi.org/10.1300/J003v06n04_04

Zabala, J. S., & Korsten, J. E. (2005). *Activity-based implementation and evaluation plan summary (used as SETT scaffold for implementation and evaluation planning).* Retrieved from http://www.joyzabala.com/uploads/Zabala_SETT_Scaffold_Implementation.pdf

CHAPTER 13

Accommodating Diversity Issues in Assessment and Evaluation

Ted Brown, PhD, OT(C), OTR
Helen Bourke-Taylor, PhD, BAppScOT

Highlights

- Traits of standardized assessments
- Legal obligations and cultural necessities with standardized assessments
- Modified or adapted standardized assessments
- Nonstandardized assessments
- Overaccomodation
- Universal design applied to assessment development
- Accommodating diversity in assessment development, validation, and application to clients
- Evaluator-related issues.

Key Terms

Accommodations
Adapting an assessment
Americans With Disabilities Act of 1990
Canadian Charter of Rights and Freedoms
Descriptive assessments
Discriminative assessments
Diverse client groups
Ethnocentrism
Ethnorelativism
Evaluative assessments
Every Child Matters
Generalizability
Individuals With Disabilities Education
    Improvement Act of 2001

Modifications
No Child Left Behind Act of 2001
Normative sample
Overaccomodating
Plain-language strategies
Predictive assessments
Reliability
Special populations
Standardized assessment
Utility
Validity

Occupational therapists must be able to screen and assess clients with diverse capabilities and backgrounds. On any given day, occupational therapists select assessments to evaluate preschoolers in early intervention programs; children in classrooms at school; office staff returning to work after an injury at their place of employment; and adults with conditions as varied as stroke, traumatic brain injury, spinal cord injury, autism, depression, and dementia, to name a few.

Therapists select, administer, and interpret assessments for the diversity, type, and range of the clients who receive occupational therapy services. In its broadest sense, assessment results help a therapist to make sound, reasoned, and informed decisions about goal setting, therapy planning, intervention provision, and reevaluation. Evaluation is one of the most fundamental, yet most complex, aspects of what therapists do in their day-to-day practice.

In this chapter, we address the occupational therapy assessment of diverse client groups. Best practice in evaluation and assessment requires that a therapist establish what the client wants and needs to do, critically consider relevant daily living contexts, determine potential barriers, and facilitate occupational performance (Dunn, 2011). Best practice also requires that a therapist select valid, reliable, and responsive measures that fit the client and his or her context and occupations of importance. When evaluating clients, the therapist must be aware of the legal obligations and cultural necessities that influence assessment practices with diverse and special needs client groups.

We discuss the various issues involved in using assessments with diverse client groups, along with the possible ways of adapting and modifying assessments, tests, and measures to fit the needs of clients. Accommodations to the evaluation process will differ depending on the type of evaluation, standardized or nonstandardized. Issues that might affect the evaluation process include a client's age or developmental level, functional capacity, or sociocultural context. In the context of this chapter, *special populations* and *diverse client groups* refer to occupational therapy clients who require unique considerations when being assessed.

TRAITS OF STANDARDIZED ASSESSMENTS

Standardized assessments and scales all have a set of specific characteristics. Assessments measure a defined construct, ability, or attribute. The construct is operationalized in the form of specific items (and related subscales) that are rated, answered, or performed by the participants being assessed.

For example, a therapist can assess self-concept as the overarching construct and its subconstructs (such as academic self-concept, social self-concept, athletic self-concept, and family self-concept; Butler & Gasson, 2005; Piers, Harris, & Herzberg, 2002) by using items that are deemed to adequately represent the construct. Similarly, children's motor skills may be appraised by the completion of a series of standardized motor skill tasks (or items) that are rated using specific criteria by an experienced examiner.

A **standardized assessment** has a manual or set of instructions about how a therapist can use the assessment, interpret findings, and apply findings to describe the client's level of functioning. Details of how the assessment was developed, standardized, and validated are also reported in the test manual. Test authors complete various psychometric studies that confirm or report on reliability, validity, responsiveness, and utility features of the test.

Typically, authors of standardized assessments gather a large dataset of scores referred to as a **normative sample.** The normative sample often mirrors the traits (e.g., gender, age, ethnicity, socioeconomic status, geographical distribution) of a population based on census data. Test authors then use the normative sample to generate performance scores that therapists can use to compare their clients' performance on the assessment. Examples of these scores include stanines, z scores, standard scores, percentile ranks, and age equivalents (Kubiszyn & Borich, 2013).

By definition, in standardized testing, the evaluator administers and scores the assessment uniformly every time. This uniformity is a critical dimension of standardization. If instructions, time limits, the way items are presented, and the way test takers respond are all the same, then the evaluator can be confident that any differences in performance are differences in ability, not differences in the conditions of the assessment process

(Harniss, Amtmann, Cook, & Johnson, 2007). This uniformity helps a therapist, as an evaluator, maintain a high level of confidence in his or her findings regardless of the construct being measured.

The final trait of a standardized assessment is that its refinement and revision are ongoing, iterative processes. Typically, a body of empirical literature is established about the measurement properties of the assessment and its application in different contexts (e.g., with diverse client groups, applied in cross-cultural environments). The body of evidence about a specific assessment is dynamic, and researchers constantly use this information to refine the assessment. The Assessment of Motor and Process Skills (Fisher & Jones, 2012) and the Beery–Buktenica Developmental Test of Visual Motor Integration (VMI; Beery, Buktenica, & Beery, 2010) are examples of assessments used by occupational therapists that have a large body of empirical work published about their use and application as well as their measurement properties.

It is imperative that assessment trials include diverse client groups when they are being standardized and that this information be reported in the test manual and in peer-reviewed journal articles. However, many older assessments have not been standardized with a diverse clientele. Occupational therapists who use such tests with diverse populations need to be conversant with the body of empirical evidence about the suitability, applicability, reliability, validity, generalizability, sensitivity, and utility of these instruments with diverse client groups.

> Therapists using assessments with diverse populations need to be conversant with the body of empirical evidence about the suitability, applicability, reliability, validity, generalizability, sensitivity, and utility of these instruments with diverse client groups.

When using standardized assessments with clients from diverse backgrounds, therapists need to be aware of the suitability and applicability of the tests. For example, if the assessment was developed in a Western cultural context and was then administered to clients from an Asian or Middle Eastern background, there is a reasonable chance that the test will not have the appropriate "cultural fit." For example, the vocabulary of the test instructions and items may be not applicable or suitable for use with clients from these cultural groups.

Diverse Clients and Types of Standardized Assessments

Assessments can be grouped into various categories or classifications. Two primary types of assessments used are (1) formal (including standardized tests) and (2) informal (nonstandardized), such as observing a child at a local playground or an adult planning and preparing a meal at home (Brown, 2012). Occupational therapy formal assessments have four main purposes: (1) descriptive, (2) discriminative, (3) predictive, and (4) evaluative (Brown, 2012; Fawcett, 2007). The purpose of the assessment influences the ensuing need for psychometric development of the assessment, as well as providing crucial information about the assessment's usability with diverse client groups.

Descriptive assessments provide information about the person's current functional status, problems, and needs. They address whether the assessment is accurate for the standardized test circumstance (Fawcett, 2007). Descriptive assessments provide a baseline or a way of describing functional status to plan intervention. When the therapist cannot follow the standardized procedures because of the client's background or circumstances, these assessments may be adapted or modified. However, adapting or modifying an assessment invalidates the standardized scores so the therapist should not use them. Instead, the therapist should describe the adaptations and modifications used and only describe the client's performance.

Discriminative assessments are norm-based assessments that aim to distinguish between individuals or groups on some characteristic or underlying dimension (Fawcett, 2007). Discriminative assessments determine whether a client is performing or developing in the specified range of typical performance or development. Applying discriminative assessments to occupational therapy clients who were not represented within the group on which the assessment was normed is questionable and must be done only with careful consideration. Therapists must keep perusing validation and reliability studies on the use of different discriminant assessments in different populations to ensure that they are current with the most recent psychometric updates.

Predictive assessments "classify people onto predefined categories of interest in an attempt to predict an event or functional status in another situation" (Fawcett, 2007, p. 99). Just as with discriminative standardized assessments, occupational therapists must use predictive assessments with careful consideration of the suitability to their client.

Evaluative assessments detect the magnitude of change over time within one person or a group of people, following an intervention or event (Fawcett, 2007). Evaluative assessments may be designed with the purpose of measuring changes in performance, competence, or satisfaction over time from the client's perspective and are otherwise described as outcome measures.

Evaluative assessments require sound test–retest and interrater reliability to determine responsiveness to change over time. The initial and subsequent administration are formalized, requiring stringent administration to ensure that the occupational therapist can definitely assert that the same conditions were applied to test and retest administrations. Consequently, the therapist can confidently attribute changes in the client's status or performance to real change rather than error during adaptation of the assessment to accommodate diverse client need.

Formal standardized assessments are used by occupational therapists to gather baseline information about a client's diagnosis, functional skills, or current status. Such derived data provide information from which informed decisions about therapy goals and intervention planning can be generated. Therefore, it is imperative that occupational therapists understand how assessments might be modified, if at all, so that decisions may be made about whether aspects of the administration of an assessment, or the assessment itself, can be modified or made more accessible for the particular clients with whom they are working. In the latter part of this chapter, we address ways that assessments might be adapted to improve accessibility and participation of diverse client groups.

Reliability and Validity

As stated in previous chapters, therapists need to be familiar with the reliability and validity of a standardized assessment. ***Reliability*** refers to the ability of a test to collect data on a consistent basis, whereas ***validity*** refers to how well the items of an assessment represent the construct they purport to assess. If a standardized assessment claims to assess the level of self-reported occupational engagement of adults, then the test items need to be representative of features of the occupational engagement construct and measure that construct in a reliable and valid manner.

Specific subtypes of reliability include internal consistency, correlations between subscales and total scale score, test–retest reliability, intrarater reliability, interrater reliability, split-half reliability, and alternate-form reliability (Mertler, 2007). Important subtypes of validity include content validity, criterion-related validity, predictive validity, construct validity, discriminant validity, and factorial validity (Brown, 2010).

Usually a standardized assessment must have established validity before its reliability can be considered; however, preliminary reliability scores are frequently reported before formal construct validity evidence is published. In other words, the items of an assessment can appear to reliably measure a construct without having evidence that the items adequately represent the construct in question.

Having knowledge of the assessment's validity and reliability is critical when using standardized assessments with diverse populations that were not included in the standardized assessment sample. In these cases, the therapist cannot have confidence in the accuracy of the scores but can use the information to get a clinical perspective of the client's level of function. Such information may include how well the client will comprehend the instructions, whether the client appears to be able to perform the tasks required by the assessment, and whether the client's performance scores can be compared with the assessment's normative sample with assurance.

Generalizability

Generalizability refers to the therapist's confidence that the assessment results are applicable to the person being evaluated. Therapists determine generalizability by examining the traits of the normative sample on which an assessment is based. For example, if the norms for a newly developed assessment were based on a sample of girls ages 4 to 8 years from India, then the scores derived would not be generalizable to test takers who were not similar in their demographic traits (e.g., age, gender, ethnicity, language spoken). However, assessments developed in one country (e.g., the United States) are often used in other countries (e.g., New Zealand, Australia, South Africa, Hong Kong, Singapore, United Kingdom), with norms developed relative to that country to generate scores for occupational therapy clients in cross-cultural contexts.

When standardized scores are not available for the person being evaluated based on his or her demographic traits (e.g., age, gender, ethnicity, language spoken), standardized scores should not be used or reported. Although the standardized scores may not be applicable, the utility of the assessment is still valuable to gain clinical information, without reporting the specific scores. The *utility* of an assessment refers to its usefulness and user-friendliness and is based on several factors, including cost, time taken to complete, equipment required for administration, cultural appropriateness, and accuracy.

LEGAL OBLIGATIONS AND CULTURAL NECESSITIES WITH STANDARDIZED ASSESSMENTS

Within the United States and internationally, many laws, legislative mandates, and regulatory requirements, some discussed here, guide the assessment of diverse client groups. For example, the U.S. **No Child Left Behind (NCLB) Act of 2001** and **the Individuals With Disabilities Education Improvement Act (IDEA) of 2004** specify certain accountability requirements, including the use of standardized assessments.

NCLB, IDEA, and ADA

NCLB and IDEA require that children with diverse needs participate in assessments and that accommodations be made where necessary to enable students with special needs to access assessment. NCLB and IDEA also mandate that the performance standards of children with disabilities be publicly reported (Thurlow, Lazarus, Thompson, & Morse, 2005). In many ways, NCLB and IDEA are seen as complementing each other in relation to

the accommodations required for the assessment of clients from diverse groups.

Another key piece of U.S. legislation that influences the assessment of diverse client groups is the **Americans With Disabilities Act of 1990.** ADA emphasizes empowerment, independence, and inclusion of people with disabilities in all aspects of community life and was designed to prohibit discrimination based on physical or intellectual disability. ADA also mandates accessibility and involvement for people with disabilities, including assessment within occupational therapy.

Accommodations such as various visual, hearing, and other sensory aides, as well as recognition of the rights of people with disabilities to have choice and control and be consulted about occupational therapy assessment and interventions, are imperative. Although legally, IDEA requires accommodations for students with special needs, it is unclear how these accommodations for NCLB tests affect the standardization.

Canadian Charter of Rights and Freedoms

In Canada, the **Canadian Charter of Rights and Freedoms** (**Charter;** 1982; part of the Canadian Constitution) affects the assessment of clients from diverse backgrounds. The Charter protects the basic rights and freedoms of all Canadians and applies to all levels of government (i.e., federal, provincial, territorial, local). The Charter includes protection of fundamental freedoms, democratic rights, legal rights, equality rights for all citizens, minority language education rights, and Canada's multicultural heritage. In the context of assessment of clients from diverse backgrounds, therapists need to abide by the principles set out in the Charter such as respecting linguistic and cultural rights.

For example, if a client referred to an occupational therapist did not speak fluent English or French, then the client would be entitled to an interpreter. The Charter also ensures that clients cannot be discriminated against on the basis of gender, age, race, national or ethnic origin, religion, language, mental or physical disability, or sexual orientation. The Charter ensures that every individual is considered equal under Canadian law and that governments do not discriminate against certain groups in their policies and programs.

This prohibition against discrimination includes health, education, and social programs where occupational therapists work and assess clients from diverse backgrounds. Again, it is unclear how this diversity affects the standardization of assessments.

Every Child Matters

Every Child Matters (ECM; Treasury, 2003) is a government policy in the United Kingdom that covers children and young adults up to the age of 19, or 24 for those with disabilities (Barker, 2009). ECM's aim is that every child, regardless of background or circumstances, has the support needed to stay safe and healthy, enjoy and achieve, have economic well-being, and be able to make positive contributions.

The ECM framework requires agencies that provide services for children (e.g., early intervention centers, public schools, children's social services, primary and secondary health services) to work in partnership with each other. Therefore, an occupational therapist working with children in a preschool setting or primary school context must be informed about the implications for the standardized assessment of children based on the ECM. The ECM framework provides guidelines for the appropriate assessment and service delivery provision approaches for children in the United Kingdom. Similar human rights legislation for adults also exists in the United Kingdom.

Legislative Summary

A clear understanding of professional and legal regulations is particularly important when the results of an assessment may determine the presence or nature of a disability or when the results will be used to determine service eligibility or placement (often referred to as *high-stakes assessments*).

The national laws and regulations of the countries discussed here and many other countries are intended to guarantee the right of individuals of diverse backgrounds to be assessed fairly and justly without prejudice and discrimination. Thus, in the context of these national regulations and legislative acts, testing accommodations and adaptations are considered reasonable.

What is not clear is how the therapist should interpret and report standardized scores. A therapist has a responsibility to be familiar with local, state, and federal guidelines and legislation that might regulate the assessment of diverse client groups. National professional organizations and regulatory bodies have professional codes of practice or practice guidelines to which therapists must adhere. Therapists need to be aware of these codes and guidelines as they relate to their day-to-day assessment practices with clients from diverse backgrounds.

MODIFIED OR ADAPTED STANDARDIZED ASSESSMENTS

This section describes assessments that are standardized and designed for use with diverse populations (e.g., people with disabilities, minority cultures or ethnicities). Many standardized assessments reflect the cultural norms of the country's context or the "majority culture" of the jurisdiction where they were standardized. There are many instances, however, in which a therapist needs to administer an assessment to clients who do not fit the typical assessment mold for which the standardized test was originally designed (Thompson, Morse, Sharpe, & Hall, 2005).

Many assessments and scales are developed based on the socioeconomic norms of the middle class and the social expectations and values of specific "majority culture" groups (predominantly White). These assessments are particularly appropriate for use with White clients presenting with specific differences in relation to cognition, language, motor skills, cultural beliefs, and social behavior. However, if an assessment developed and standardized within the United States primarily on White people is administered to Black and Hispanic clients, it is possible that the assessment could be overtly or subtly biased against them. This bias becomes an increasingly important issue with the growing cultural and ethnic diversity in many countries.

Some standardized assessments are not appropriate to use with specific client groups for several reasons. Some assessments require that the client have a specified level of cognitive and language comprehension skills or developmental level to complete test items. Another perspective that requires consideration is cultural expectations and characteristics. Culturally sensitive occupational therapy practice recognizes, accommodates, and adapts to a client's beliefs, social rituals, customs, and habits. Points of difference may be gender roles, communication styles, and expectations for therapy, including a power relationship imbalanced toward the professional. Other issues that may present points of differences are religion and beliefs about health, disability, and recovery, among many others.

When the client cannot complete an assessment following the standardized instructions, the therapist, as a last resort, may modify or adapt the administration of the assessment. In this situation, the therapist cannot ethically report the standard scores because they are not valid for this client. Nevertheless, the therapist may obtain valuable information about the client's performance, abilities, and areas of difficulty through the use of the assessment. The evaluation report should include only what the therapist observed and learned from the client's performance on the assessment.

When selecting an assessment, the therapist should consider whether it is more important to know how a particular client's performance compares with others who have taken the same assessment or to be able to discuss the person's performance in terms of speed, precision, or number of items correct without referring to the performance of others. If comparison is more important, a norm-referenced test would be the best choice, but if individual performance is more important, the best choice is a criterion-referenced or descriptive assessment.

If the therapist selects a norm-referenced assessment (e.g., discriminant assessment), he or she must recognize that norm samples vary and can be drawn nationally, regionally, or locally. Therefore, the therapist must consider whether the norms for the selected assessment are relevant to the client. To make this determination, the therapist must examine the norm sample or norm tables in the assessment manual. The more closely the client approximates the traits of the assessment's normative group, the greater the confidence that the assessment is an appropriate choice and that the norms can provide a meaningful basis of comparison. Sometimes normative assessments may be used just to get a clinical picture of the client's performance rather than a normative score.

The School Functional Assessment (Coster, Deeney, Haltiwanger, & Haley, 1998) is an example of a criterion-referenced assessment that would be appropriate across a wide range of clients. In the manual, Coster and colleagues explicitly stated that "items were carefully worded to apply to students with a wide variety of functional disabilities and to recognize the capabilities of students who perform functional tasks in an alternative manner, either because of impairments or differences in cultural practices" (p. 46). They also reported demographic characteristics of the standardization sample selected from both urban and rural settings. The standardization sample also includes

- Children with a variety of disabling conditions,
- A gender distribution that matched the nationwide demographic of students with disabilities (i.e., more males), and
- A racial and ethnic distribution that mirrored the population demographics of the U.S. census.

A therapist can comfortably use this ipsative assessment with a wide variety of clients.

Assessment Adaption

If a therapist decides to use a standardized assessment in a cross-cultural context, he or she may decide to adapt the assessment so that the results are valid and reliable. The process of **adapting an assessment** is difficult and time-consuming. It begins with a review and analysis of the assessment by a panel of experts who are familiar with the aspects of the culture unique to the environment. These experts should develop a set of recommendations for adapting the assessment. Some recommendations may include how to adjust the administration of test items as well as revisions made to any wording or terminology that does not fit with that cultural context.

One adaptation frequently required is translation when an assessment was originally developed in one language and a therapist wishes to use it in another language. In this situation, the adaptation does not end with translation of the assessment but must continue through a formal process of back-translation involving bilingual content experts plus qualified translators (Beaton, Bombardier, Guillemin, & Ferraz, 2000). Doing so ensures that the semantic meaning and translation of the terminology is of a high quality. After this process is complete, it is essential that the assessment be standardized in the appropriate cross-cultural setting to generate appropriate norms or scores (Hambleton, Merenda, & Spielberger, 2005). The translation process must be rigorous and monitored for the assessment to be used with speakers and readers of other languages with confidence.

Several assessments that occupational therapists use have been translated into other languages for use with clients from different cultures than the original norm sample. Some ipsative assessments developed by occupational therapists that have been translated include the Canadian Occupational Performance Measure (COPM; Law et al., 2005), the Occupational Self Assessment (OSA; Baron, Kielhofner, Iyenger, Goldhammer, & Wolenskil, 2006), the Model of Human Occupation Screening Tool (MOHOST; Parkinson, Forsyth, & Kielhofner, 2006), and the Occupational Performance History Interview–II (OPHI–II; Kielhofner et al., 2004). The COPM has been used in more than 35 countries and has been translated into over 20 languages, including French, German, Dutch, Swedish, Japanese, and Spanish. The OSA, MOHOST, and OPHI–II have been translated into Danish, Dutch, Finnish, French, German, Icelandic, Japanese, and other languages.

Some other examples of assessments that occupational therapists use that have been translated are the Peabody Developmental Motor Scales (Folio & Fewel, 2000), Motor Assessment of the Developing Infant (Piper & Darrah, 1994), Parenting Stress Index (Abidin, 1995), Functional Evaluation: The Barthel Index (Mahoney & Barthel, 1965), Bayley Scales of Mental and Motor Development (2nd ed.; Bayley, 1993), and the SF–36 health survey (Ware, Kosinski, Dewey, & Gandek, 2000).

When administering and interpreting the results of an assessment that has been translated, it is important to keep in mind that the assessment may still contain items that can be misinterpreted because of a lack of equivalency in the translation process or to geographic variations in the language. For example, a test translated to Spanish could be interpreted differently by clients from Spain, Mexico, and Puerto Rico.

Accommodations

Accommodations include any change in the conditions under which a standardized assessment is administered (Bolt & Thurlow, 2004). They include any changes in the way the assessment is delivered (when, where, how long), changes in the way the test items are presented, and **modifications** in the way the person responds to test items, including the use of special equipment (Fuchs, Fuchs, Eaton, Hamlett, & Karns, 2000).

When choosing the most appropriate assessment, the therapist must consider the nature of the client's disability and the design of the assessment. The therapist must judge whether the client needs an accommodation, and, if so, the nature and extent of such an accommodation. For example, persons with limitations in dexterity, vision, or perception may be allowed extra time to complete an assessment. It is the evaluator's responsibility to tailor the accommodation to the person's need. The therapist must be knowledgeable about testing accommodations and, when appropriate, encourage the client to be part of the decision-making process about accommodations. The evaluation report must include a comprehensive description of all accommodations.

> Any change made to a standardized assessment that is not included in the test manual will affect the validity of the assessment, and the standardized scores cannot be used.

According to Thurlow, Lazarus, and Christensen (2008), *assessment accommodations* "are changes in materials and procedures that enable the student with disabilities to participate in an assessment in a way that allows the student's [or adult's] true knowledge and skills to be assessed rather than the student's disabilities" (p. 18). More specifically, accommodations refer to changes in the assessment context or procedures that eliminate irrelevant variance, thereby producing a more valid representation of knowledge, skills, and competencies of children and adults from diverse populations (Thurlow, Thompson, & Johnstone, 2007).

Accommodations for the assessment of diverse client groups can be categorized in several ways, including "accommodations for presentation (e.g., large print, read-aloud questions), response (e.g., scribe, write in test booklet), scheduling [or] timing (e.g., extended time, extra breaks), and setting (e.g., small group, in student's home), as well as special equipment or materials" (Thurlow et al., 2008, p. 18).

Lazarus, Thompson, and Thurlow (2005) completed a survey of 798 special education teachers in 6 school districts in 4 U.S. states about the use of student accommodations. Their findings indicated that the most commonly provided assessment accommodations for students with special needs were extended or extra time, small group or individual administration, test items read aloud, and test directions read aloud. Specific ways to accommodate assessment practices are detailed below under the following categories: cultural, environmental, special situations, presentation and administration, and temporal.

Cultural Accommodations

Clients from cultural, linguistic, or religious backgrounds that are different from the majority culture, whether their backgrounds are from outside or within the country where services are delivered, are examples of culturally diverse client groups. One common group that falls into this category is immigrants or refugees from other countries who come to live in a new country.

Cultural differences may influence a client's performance on an assessment in many ways. Cultural factors that might influence testing include the client's socioeconomic status, language, educational level, ethnicity, migration history, generational level, reading and health literacy level, and comfort level in an assessment or test-taking situation. A therapist needs to examine the cultural sensitivity and, more specifically, the appropriateness of test items and phrasing of questions when used with diverse clients. For example, an assessment that contains language that a gay, lesbian, bisexual, or transgender client may find offensive, exclusionary, or stigmatizing (Prince, 1997) could lead the client to offer constricted responses, particularly when engaged in interview and self-report instruments (Muñoz, 2010). Therapists should also consider the potential cultural bias of test items and assessment protocols.

Moreover, the vocabulary of assessment instructions and items should be examined to determine whether certain terms fit the cultural norms of the client's cultural group. One way to establish

whether a client may have trouble with vocabulary or test instructions is to ask family members before the assessment occurs. It may be necessary for a therapist to adjust the way he or she administers the assessment or specific test items.

> Cultural factors that might influence testing include the client's socioeconomic status, language, educational level, ethnicity, migration history, generational level, reading and health literacy level, and comfort level in a test-taking situation.

The therapist might need to phrase questions differently to accommodate the client's background, because the terminology used in test items may mean something completely different in cross-cultural contexts. If a client's dominant language is different from that used in the assessment, that difference needs to be taken into account when interpreting test results. A therapist who is not conversant in a client's dominant language and lacks cultural knowledge of its nuances or of nonverbal mannerisms is more likely to misinterpret the client's meaning.

Asking someone from a cultural background that does not value competitiveness to complete a timed assessment may in itself have important implications for the client's performance. Whereas the therapist may interpret the lack of a rapid response as poor motivation, it may be that the client's culture does not value responding rapidly and competing with others. Thus, the client's performance on a timed assessment may not provide accurate information about the client's knowledge and skills, or even whether the tasks are relevant to the client's real-life occupations (Miller, Linn, & Gronlund, 2009).

Environmental Accommodations

Environmental accommodations are changes in the way a therapist administers an assessment to a client so the client can respond to the test item. Some changes a therapist might make are altering the setting, scheduling, timing, presentation, or method of responding (Goh, 2004). When making accommodations, the therapist must keep in mind that the goal is the client's full and active participation in the assessment.

> The goal of assessment accommodations is not to make an assessment easier for the client; it is a process of improving access and participation.

Note that the purpose of assessment accommodations is not to make an assessment easier for the client. Rather, it is a process of improving access and participation, thus providing clients with an opportunity to demonstrate what they can and cannot do. A reasonable accommodation is to administer the assessment in a quiet room with minimal environmental noise and distractions.

Accommodations for Special Situations

Assessment authors and publishers usually outline the allowable or standard accommodations for special situations that will not affect the validity of the assessment. For standardized assessments, publishers limit the degree to which an evaluator may modify the administration of the assessment to ensure that the assessment accurately assesses and measures what it is intended to.

When the assessment author or publisher lists the accommodations needed for a client as being "nonstandard," the client may still be assessed using all the typical accommodations, but it will not be meaningful to compare those test scores to the normative group. The assessment provides some indication of the client's performance at a given time with documented accommodations, and such descriptive data may be useful for later reevaluation. The therapist should not compare findings to other persons or use the normative data.

Whenever a therapist makes an accommodation to a standardized assessment, issues of validity and reliability of the results become critical considerations in the interpretation of the results. A therapist must specify clearly in the evaluation report any changes made to the standardized protocol. Occupational therapists should use their clinical reasoning skills and professional judgment about what is considered "reasonable accommodation" in terms of assessing clients from diverse backgrounds, as well as whether it is "allowable" in the assessment manual.

For example, if a therapist administering a cognitive screening scale to an older client admitted to an acute hospital after a fall finds out that the client has very poor eyesight, the therapist would have to make accommodations to the assessment to obtain meaningful results. Modifications to administering the cognitive screening assessment could include visual accommodations such as size of font, light–dark contrast, or other low-vision assistance. Further, if the client speaks English as a second language, verbal accommodations such as a translator may be used to administer the assessment in the client's first language. The situation could be more complicated if the therapist discovers that the client has limited endurance. In this case, the therapist might administer the cognitive screening assessment in two or three shorter sessions spread over one day.

All of these examples are what would be considered "reasonable accommodations." When interpreting the findings of the cognitive screening assessment, the therapist needs to read the manual carefully to determine whether any of the accommodations are acceptable for the standardized procedures. If the manual does not specifically approve the accommodations in the standardization procedures, the therapist cannot use the standardized scores and must report findings based on observation and clinical judgment. The therapist also must note in his or her report any modifications made and the rationale for the modifications.

Presentation and Administration Accommodation

It may be necessary for the therapist to alter the mode of how he or she presents or administers an assessment to suit the special needs of a specific client. The therapist may need to administer a written assessment orally or electronically by computer. Data may need to be collected in person, face to face, or by written format, online communication, webcam, or audio recording. Accommodations can include enlarging test sheets, highlighting key instructions and test items, providing visually high-contrast fonts and other test items, or drawing boxes around individual test items to minimize problems with visual tracking.

Other strategies therapists might use include less formal or less technical terminology or applying plain-language strategies. A therapist could provide instructions orally and modulate the tone, speed, and volume of delivery to clients who may have hearing or word-processing difficulties. Accommodations in terms of mode of administration and presentation that move away from the prescribed standardized approach outlined in a test manual need to be documented in any resultant assessment reports, and the interpretation of scores in relation to the normative sample must be carefully considered.

Temporal Accommodations

The therapist can make temporal accommodations for clients with diverse backgrounds. Typical temporal accommodations include extending the test completion time, allowing frequent breaks, or selecting the best time of day for a client to complete an assessment. A client who presents with fibromyalgia or chronic fatigue syndrome, for example, may require rest breaks between assessment tasks. It might be necessary to vary the time of day when the client completes the assessment (e.g., ask clients during what part of the day they have the most energy or the least pain).

It is also possible to vary the length of time clients have to complete specific test items that may be timed tasks or have specific time limits linked to them (particularly in standardized performance-based tests). If accommodations are made in relation to the specified temporal components detailed in a standardized assessment, this alteration needs to be clearly reported in any resultant reports or professional documentation.

NONSTANDARDIZED ASSESSMENTS

The use of nonstandardized rather than standardized assessments with special populations presents considerably fewer problems. With nonstandardized assessments, the therapist is obtaining an understanding of the client's strengths and limitations by observing behaviors. Further, the therapist is using clinical judgment related to those observations and other data obtained to explain the client's behaviors and plan an intervention strategy. Because statistical concepts of validity and reliability are not used in nonstandardized assessments, the therapist can make accommodations to these assessments without affecting the outcomes.

Adaptations of assessment strategies with nonstandardized assessments are designed to accommodate a client's needs so he or she can demonstrate skills and abilities. Adaptations of assessment administration and scoring do not represent unfair advantages to clients in and of themselves. Instead, the opposite is true: If appropriate adaptations are not considered and implemented, clients from diverse groups could be unfairly penalized, creating negative effects on their achievement and generating an unrealistic portrait of their abilities and strengths (British Columbia Ministry of Education, 2009). Assessments can be adapted for diverse client groups in several ways:

- Present assessment instructions or items in various ways (e.g., audio recordings, electronic text, increased font size for written material, ability to repeat oral instructions, including a known person who may provide instruction under close supervision by the administering therapist);
- Provide access to a computer for written assignments (e.g., use of word prediction software, spell check, idea generator);
- Provide alternatives to written assignments to demonstrate knowledge and understanding;
- Extend time to complete assessments, give rest breaks (if required), administer an assessment over several sessions, or vary the pace of completing test items;
- Provide support to develop and practice skills and strategies; and
- Use computer software that provides text-to-speech and speech-to-text capabilities.

Similarly, a therapist can adapt assessments to support culturally fair testing. Some recommendations by Miller et al. (2009) include

- Using materials that are primarily nonverbal,
- Ensuring that pictures and diagrams used are familiar to the cultural group being tested,
- Selecting materials and methods that are interesting to the client and relevant to the client's daily occupations,
- Liberalizing time limits and deemphasizing speed, and
- Simplifying the test-taking procedures to accommodate clients who have less experience in test-taking situations.

Consider a high school student completing final exams that are considered "high-stakes" because the exam results will be part of his college admission application and affect competitiveness for scholarships. The student was recently diagnosed with juvenile arthritis (with involvement of his wrist joints, metacarpal phalangeal joints, and proximal interphalangeal joints) with concurrent symptoms of chronic fatigue syndrome. Several of this student's final exams involve writing long essays (e.g., English, history, psychology, philosophy) in a sitting position for sustained periods. However, given the student's clinical presentation of painful joints, morning stiffness, nonrestorative sleep, and resultant fatigue, writing answers to long essay questions within specified time limits would be a disadvantage to the student and not demonstrate his true knowledge of these academic subjects.

The occupational therapist might suggest to the student's teachers that reasonable accommodations be made for the student to complete his exams. These accommodations could be allowing the student to provide oral instead of written answers to some essay questions, allowing the student to answer questions orally using technology to convert his speech into written text, allowing the student to take rest breaks and stretch breaks, and providing the student with extra time to complete the exams. These are reasonable accommodations for the student's clinical conditions.

Because final exams are not generally standardized, such accommodations would be appropriate and would not affect the scores. However, in the case of standardized assessments such as the Scholastic Aptitude Tests (SATs), the College Board (the oversight agency for the SATs) must approve any accommodations so it can ensure that the accommodations will not affect the standardized scores.

OVERACCOMMODATION

A therapist cannot assume that a person with a physical limitation will automatically perform less well or that an assessment designed for a nondisabled population will elicit an inaccurate measure of performance for persons with disabilities. Accommodations are adaptations that allow clients from special needs groups to access and participate in test taking. Therapists individually modify or differentiate assessment materials for a client to create an appropriate assessment environment for the client.

However, therapists need to be careful not to "overaccommodate" for a client. **Overaccommodating** does not automatically improve a client's access to or performance on an assessment. Not every test taker with a special need requires an accommodation, and not all test takers presenting

with the same disability require the same accommodation. Accommodations are individualized in collaboration with the client and his or her family. However, note that once a therapist has made accommodations to a standardized assessment, the data and results are no longer standardized but become observations.

UNIVERSAL DESIGN APPLIED TO ASSESSMENT DEVELOPMENT

Thompson, Johnstone, and Thurlow (2002) from the National Center for Educational Outcome in the United States conducted a review of all empirical research relevant to the assessment development process and the principles of universal design. From this review, they produced a set of seven elements of universal design that can be applied to assessments. Test developers should consider these elements when developing new assessments and revising already established instruments. Doing so will promote the design, development, use, revision, and application of assessments that are the most appropriate, reliable, and valid for use with client groups with diverse needs.

However, revising an assessment to make it more accessible to one group of clients may actually make it less accessible to another group of clients. The principles of universal design can be a useful point of reference for developing better assessments, but these principles cannot magically make all assessments accessible to all test takers.

Step 1. Ensuring an Inclusive Assessment for Populations

The first element of universal test design suggested by Thompson and colleagues (2002) is ensuring an inclusive assessment population. In other words, when developers design assessments, it is essential that they include in the normative group, during both design and field testing, participants who are representative of the client group or sample for which the assessment will be used.

For example, if an early intervention service is going to assess all new referrals received using a standardized screening assessment of children's development, the screening assessment can be used with confidence only if it was designed and field-tested to suit the client group. An inclusive approach to participant recruitment is needed at each phase of the screening assessment's standardization process.

Step 2. Use Precisely Defined Concepts

The second step recommended by Thompson and colleagues (2002) is using precisely defined concepts. The assessment developers must clearly define the specific skills, traits, or constructs that the assessment will measure so that all irrelevant cognitive, sensory, emotional, social, and physical barriers can be removed. Continuing with the example of the early intervention service developmental screening assessment, the test developer would have to delineate clearly what specific skills the assessment will measure. For example, the screening assessment would include items about the children's sensory processing skills, gross and fine motor abilities, social skills, cognitive abilities, self-care skills, expressive and receptive language skills, and play behaviors.

Step 3. Develop Accessible, Nonbiased Items

The third step suggested by Thompson and colleagues (2002) is developing accessible, nonbiased items. They recommended that accessibility be built into test items from the start and bias review procedures be put in place to ensure that item quality is retained. Using the developmental screening assessment example, the test developers would need to ensure that the items included were accessible to targeted client groups and exhibited minimal bias, particularly related to gender, ethnicity, and socioeconomic status.

For example, a person with a hearing impairment may be greatly disadvantaged by an oral test, even when content is provided visually. An oral test can usually be easily adapted for a person with visual impairments, but an assessment requiring motor performance is likely to present some challenge (Pitoniak & Royer, 2001).

On the other hand, some considerations are less obvious. For example, the Nottingham Health Profile (McEwen & McKenna, 1996) is a well-known

and frequently used measure of quality of life, yet it includes several questions concerning mobility that are ill-suited for people in wheelchairs. When a therapist uses and scores this assessment in the standard way, the physical functioning scores for people who use wheelchairs are understated (Post, Gerritsen, van Leusen, Paping, & Prevo, 2001).

Step 4. Design the Assessment to Be Amenable to Accommodations

In the next step, Thompson and colleagues (2002) suggested developing an assessment that is amenable to accommodations or designed to facilitate the use of accommodations needed by test takers. For example, all test items could be administered using Braille, in another language such as Spanish, as a parent report format, or as an oral interview. Additionally, the assessment could be used with a variety of widely used adaptive equipment or assistive technology (e.g., online version of the screening assessment that parents could answer remotely or on their mobile phone).

Step 5. Provide Simple, Clear, and Intuitive Instructions and Procedures

For the next component, Thompson and colleagues (2002) recommended that all instructions and procedures should be simple, clear, and presented in understandable language regardless of a client's experience, knowledge, language skills, or current concentration level. The early intervention center's developmental screening assessment, for example, needs to ensure that the items asked of parents and caregivers are written using plain-language principles and are easily understood by people with a variety of reading and comprehension skill levels.

Step 6. Maximize Readability and Comprehensibility

The next step recommended by Thompson and colleagues (2002) was maximizing readability and comprehensibility. Readability and plain-language guidelines should be followed (e.g., sentence length

CASE EXAMPLE 13.1. ENGLISH AS A SECOND LANGUAGE

A **77-year-old man** referred to an outpatient rehabilitation center speaks conversational English, but his native language is Spanish. His son has brought copies of his father's previous hospitalization records, but these records are in Spanish. It appears the client suffered a cerebrovascular accident (CVA) in the left temporal lobe 6 years ago.

Several salient issues might influence the assessment process. The occupational therapist might consider whether the client's CVA resulted in an expressive aphasia that, combined with English being his second language, could result in poorer scores on assessments requiring verbal responses. The therapist also needs to consider whether the client experiences issues with visual acuity or hearing that could influence accurate evaluation of his performance.

A therapist who intentionally considers how culture might influence the assessment process would question whether the client has had any experience with standardized testing or whether this type of testing will represent a novel situation. The therapist might consider whether the assessments chosen have valid and reliable Spanish versions, or the therapist with a level of Spanish fluency might consider whether to administer those assessments in Spanish.

and number of difficult words are kept to a minimum) to produce readable and comprehensible text. Using **plain-language strategies,** such as using common words, avoiding ambiguous words, avoiding multiple names for the same concept, being consistent in the use of typeface, and providing obvious graphic signals (e.g., bullets, letters, numbers) to indicate separate test questions, when developing assessment items will promote clients' understanding and comprehension.

These are all strategies that the designers of the development screening assessment need to take into consideration. Occupational therapists could also use strategies to promote maximum readability and comprehensibility of test items completed by clients from diverse backgrounds (see Case Example 13.1).

Step 7. Maximize Legibility

The final factor to consider suggested by Thompson and colleagues (2002) was to maximize legibility. For example, characteristics that ensure easy decipherability (e.g., visual contrast, type size, spacing, typeface, justification, line length and width, blank spaces) should be applied to text, tables, figures, and illustrations as well as to response formats. The developers of the assessment need to use strategies to ensure adequate understanding by the test taker filling out the developmental screening assessment.

ACCOMMODATING DIVERSITY IN ASSESSMENT DEVELOPMENT, VALIDATION, AND APPLICATION TO CLIENTS

The occupational therapy profession views people within their environments and in relation to the occupations that they want, need, or are required to perform (American Occupational Therapy Association, 2014). The *International Classification of Functioning, Disability and Health* (ICF; World Health Organization [WHO], 2001) provides an international framework that transcends professional boundaries, cultures, and countries.

The *ICF* (WHO, 2001) acknowledges and conceptualizes the influence of environmental and personal factors (i.e., characteristics and background of the person's life) on the health, capabilities, and capacity of the person to engage in activities and participate in opportunities available in the home and community. Environmental factors such as physical and human resources as well as personal factors such as age, gender, culture, values, interests, life roles, habits, and self-efficacy provide a highly influential backdrop that affects what a person does and how a person interacts with the world.

The *ICF* (WHO, 2001) has had a substantial influence on the development of assessments both within the occupational therapy field and outside of the profession. Many assessments have been developed that evaluate all factors across the *ICF* framework. In relation to special populations such as occupational therapy clients, the *ICF* has enabled the development of some specific participation measures that guide both research and practice. Examples include the development of measures of participation such as the Children's Assessment of Participation and Enjoyment (King et al., 2004), Participation Environment Measure for Children and Youth (Coster et al., 2012), Child Participation

Questionnaire (Rosenberg, Jarus, & Bart, 2010a), and Environmental Restriction Questionnaire (Rosenberg, Ratzon, Jarus, & Bart, 2010b).

Assessments may be developed in two main ways (Figure 13.1). First, a more traditional approach results in assessments being developed on the basis of the needs, skills, and status of most people in any given demographic. A normative sample provides an opportunity to compare the needs, skills, and status of the vast majority of occupational therapy clients. The traditional approach to assessment development is to select items that represent increasing levels of difficulty or challenge for the trait, construct, skill, or ability being assessed.

For example, the VMI consists of a series of geometric shapes and designs that children are asked to copy. The specific VMI items start with designs that are relatively easy (e.g., vertical line, horizontal line) and gradually increase in level of difficulty (e.g., three-dimensional overlapping rings) because it is designed to cover the ability ranges of clients 2 to 18 years old.

The authors of the VMI initially gathered performance data from a large standardization sample of typically developing children and adolescents representing a broad cross-section of American society in relation to several variables, including socioeconomic status, geographical location, age, gender, grade level, and type of school attended (e.g., private, public, charter, parochial). The authors of the VMI were then able to ascertain that a typically developing child at certain age levels should achieve a certain average score.

In other words, the VMI authors gathered data on healthy participants to establish a representative normative sample. The assessment uses healthy, typically developing participants' performance scores on test items to build up a bank of normative scores, and these scores are used as the benchmark against which clients' skills are compared (see Figure 13.1).

Such an assessment might be considered on par with a reductionist medical model of assessment and intervention that tends to emphasize reducing impairments rather than improving function performance, activity engagement, or participation. The initial stages of development of this type of test focuses on quantifying typical skills. The assessment performance scores of participants with known disabilities or special needs are usually not included in such standardization data. Instead of using an inclusive standardization data collection approach and potentially considering the abilities and skills of all test takers, including those with special needs or from diverse groups, only typically developing participants' test scores are included.

In contrast, the second approach to developing assessments uses a framework, such as the ICF (WHO, 2001) or an

> Developing assessments using a framework, such as the *ICF*, that is based on client need or the needs of a particular client group would increase the appropriateness, utility, and client-centeredness of an assessment.

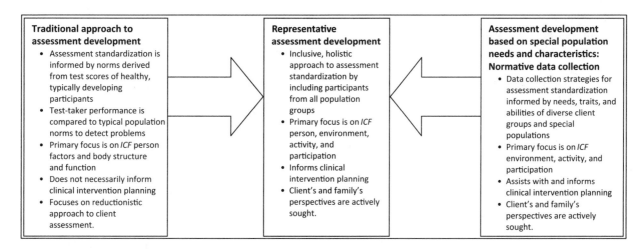

Traditional approach to assessment development	Representative assessment development	Assessment development based on special population needs and characteristics: Normative data collection
• Assessment standardization is informed by norms derived from test scores of healthy, typically developing participants • Test-taker performance is compared to typical population norms to detect problems • Primary focus is on *ICF* person factors and body structure and function • Does not necessarily inform clinical intervention planning • Focuses on reductionistic approach to client assessment.	• Inclusive, holistic approach to assessment standardization by including participants from all population groups • Primary focus is on *ICF* person, environment, activity, and participation • Informs clinical intervention planning • Client's and family's perspectives are actively sought.	• Data collection strategies for assessment standardization informed by needs, traits, and abilities of diverse client groups and special populations • Primary focus is on *ICF* environment, activity, and participation • Assists with and informs clinical intervention planning • Client's and family's perspectives are actively sought.

Figure 13.1. Approaches to normative data collection for assessment standardization.
Source. T. Brown and H. Bourke-Taylor. Used with permission.
Note. ICF = *International Classification of Functioning, Disability and Health* (WHO, 2001).

instrument design model, that is based on client need or the needs of a particular client group, which increases the appropriateness, utility, and client-centeredness of an assessment (see Figure 13.1). For example, the Participation and Environment Measure for Children and Youth (Coster et al., 2012) was developed using extensive interviews with parents about the extent to which their child participated in tasks at home, at school, and in the community. The Child's Challenging Behaviour Scale (Bourke-Taylor, Law, Howie, & Pallant, 2010) was designed around the need to identify and measure challenging behaviors associated with compromised maternal well-being and capacity to care for a child with a disability.

EVALUATOR-RELATED ISSUES

Beyond the assessments a therapist selects and administers to a client, the therapist needs to consider his or her own personal bias about culture, gender, and geographic and socioeconomic conditions. Personal bias may influence the therapist's choice of assessments. Further, and more important, a therapist's bias may influence how he or she interprets the client's performance. As discussed by Muñoz (2010), a therapist's clinical reasoning process can be influenced by the therapist's

- Perspective on the evaluation,
- Choice of assessment,
- Knowledge of and competence in administering the specific assessments,
- Interpretation of the data, and
- Openness to finding creative ways to understand the client and his or her family.

Ethnocentrism, a universal tendency of people to believe that their ways of thinking, acting, and believing are the right, proper, and normal ways (Andrews & Boyle, 2003), can influence how a therapist administers and interprets results. Ethnocentrism can become a serious problem in the evaluation process if a client's performance and responses are seen as a deficit, inferior, or bizarre. Ethnocentrism can lead to stereotyping, prejudice, and bias, which can be substantial impediments to accurate evaluation.

Therapist bias can be both conscious and unconscious, and an evaluator may make judgments or assumptions about the client based on the way the client dresses, talks, or presents him- or herself (Muñoz, 2010). Muñoz gives the example of a traditional Latino family where children are raised to show *respeto* (respect) to elders and authorities. During assessment, such a child may respond to the therapist with brief answers and look to the floor when the therapist is speaking. If these behaviors are not interpreted in a cultural context, the therapist may erroneously conclude that the child shows signs of depression or lacks interpersonal communication skills.

When evaluating clients, the therapist should strive to develop **ethnorelativism** (Muñoz, 2010), a multicultural ideology that reflects a therapist's ability to adapt his or her own cultural perspectives to accept a multicultural ideology (Brems, 1998). Ethnorelativism requires a therapist to realize and accept that the world is inherently multicultural and adapt his or her own cultural perspectives to accept a multicultural ideology (Wurzel, 2004). According to Muñoz (2010),

Adopting a multicultural ideology is particularly important to evaluation because it helps the therapist frame a client's occupational performance patterns within the context of the norms and expectations of the client's culture. A therapist often can hold values about health and healing that are at variance with the values held by persons from non-Western cultures (Iwama, 2006; Phipps, 1995). Practices based on Western, middle-class values, such as an emphasis on activism as a response to disability, routinely working toward autonomy in activities of daily living, and predicating intervention on future-oriented time perspectives often disregard non-Western cultural mores (Kinébanian & Stomph, 1992). Iwama (2006) has argued that occupational therapy models often present assumptions about occupational functioning that place considerable focus on the person; the person's social and physical environments are secondary or tertiary considerations. For individuals and groups who value interdependence over autonomy and who consider the collective needs before the needs of the person, evaluation processes focused on the latter may miss the mark (Iwama, 2006). (p. 287)

To be a competent evaluator, a therapist must avoid ethnocentrism and develop an ethnorelative perspective. Some strategies for developing an ethnorelative perspective are

- Develop a sound educational foundation about the worldviews of different cultures.
- Develop cultural literacy by actively constructing a personal knowledge base for culturally responsive caring (Muñoz, 2007).
- Develop an awareness of your own cultural identity and explore your own cultural heritage (Muñoz, 2007; Tervalon & Murray-García, 1998).
- Consciously examine your own biases and be committed to scrutinizing your prejudices.
- Recognize the client as the expert of his or her own experience, and respond with active listening and intentional respect.
- When assessing, judiciously use culture-specific knowledge, acknowledge within-group variations in cultural groups, and make a conscious effort to determine whether culture-specific information is applicable to this particular client (Muñoz, 2010).

SUMMARY

Occupational therapists work with many diverse clients who present with various needs and occupational performance challenges. Often, as part of the occupational therapy process, therapists need to complete assessments to establish a baseline of clients' occupational performance abilities to provide the basis for generating therapy goals and intervention planning.

Occupational therapists need to look at the unique needs of diverse clients when assessing them. Standardized assessments may not take into account a diverse population or particular challenges. Often assessments designed for use with majority culture, healthy, or typically developing participants require considerable

accommodations or are not suitable for clients presenting with special needs or from diverse backgrounds.

Accommodations need to be fair, valid, ethical, and realistic, yet they also need to adhere to the accommodations allowed in the test manual. Nonstandardized assessments allow for more accommodations but do not provide the standardized information that many laws require.

Therapists need to ensure that they maintain the validity and integrity of the assessments being used but also concurrently need to ensure that they are meeting the occupational performance needs of the diverse clients they serve. Because participation in meaningful and necessary occupations is the key basis of all occupational therapy services, the profession must continue to conceptualize, develop, evaluate, and use psychometrically sound assessments to this end. The special populations and diverse client groups to whom we provide services are relying on us to do so. Further, therapists need to be aware of their own potential biases so that they do not interfere with the evaluation process.

QUESTIONS

1. Describe 4 features of a standardized assessment.
2. Occupational therapy formal assessments have 4 main purposes. Identify and define what those 4 purposes are.
3. State 2 reasons why assessment adaptation is necessary. Identify 2 positive and 2 negative outcomes of assessment adaptation.
4. Identify 6 types of accommodations that can be made to the administration methods for clients from diverse groups.
5. Outline the universal design principles applied to the development of assessments for clients from diverse groups.
6. Think about a situation that you have observed during fieldwork. Can you identify potential areas of bias that occurred during an evaluation?
7. Choose 2 assessments. Review them to determine areas of the assessments that may exhibit cultural bias. Think about 2 ways the administration of the assessment could be adapted.

References

Abidin, R. R. (1995). *Parenting Stress Index: Professional manual* (3rd ed.). Lutz, FL: Psychological Assessment Resources.

American Occupational Therapy Association. (2014). Occupational therapy practice framework: Domain and process (3rd ed.). *American Journal of Occupational Therapy, 68*(Suppl. 1), S1–S48. http://dx.doi.org/10.5014/ajot.2014.682006

Americans With Disabilities Act of 1990, Pub. L. 101–336, 104 Stat. 328.

Andrews, M. A., & Boyle, J. S. (2003). *Transcultural concepts in nursing care* (4th ed.). Philadelphia: Lippincott Williams & Wilkins.

Barker, R. (2009). *Making sense of Every Child Matters: Multi-professional practice guidance.* Bristol, UK: Policy Press.

Baron, K., Kielhofner, G., Iyenger, A., Goldhammer, V., & Wolenskil, J. (2006). *Occupational Self Assessment (OSA) version 2.2 user's manual.* Chicago: MOHO Clearing House.

Bayley, N. (1993). *Bayley Scales of Mental and Motor Development* (2nd ed.). San Antonio, TX: Psychological Corporation.

Beaton, D. E., Bombardier, C., Guillemin, F., & Ferraz, M. B. (2000). Guidelines for the process of cross-cultural adaptation of self-report measures. *Spine, 25,* 3186–3191. http://dx.doi.org/10.1097/00007632-200012150-00014

Beery, K. E., Buktenica, N. A., & Beery, N. A. (2010). *Beery–Buktenica Developmental Test of Visual–Motor Integration* (6th ed.). Minneapolis: Pearson.

Bolt, S. E., & Thurlow, M. L. (2004). Five of the most frequently allowed testing accommodations in state policy. *Remedial and Special Education, 25,* 141–152. http://dx.doi.org/10.1177/07419325040250030201

Bourke-Taylor, H. M., Law, M., Howie, L., & Pallant, J. F. (2010). Development of the Child's Challenging Behaviour Scale (CCBS) for mothers of school-aged children with disabilities. *Child: Care, Health and Development, 36,* 491–498. http://dx.doi.org/10.1111/j.1365-2214.2009.01055.x

Brems, C. (1998). Cultural issues in psychological assessment: Problems and possible solutions. *Journal of Psychological Practice, 4,* 88–117.

British Columbia Ministry of Education. (2009). *A guide to adaptations and modifications.* Vancouver, BC: Author. Retrieved from http://www.bced.gov.bc.ca/specialed/docs/adaptations_and_modifications_guide.pdf

Brown, T. (2010). Construct validity: A unitary concept for occupational therapy assessment, evaluation, and measurement. *Hong Kong Journal of Occupational Therapy, 20,* 30–42. http://dx.doi.org/10.1016/S1569-1861(10)70056-5

Brown, T. (2012). Assessment, measurement, and evaluation/Why can't I do what everyone expects me to do? In S. J. Lane & A. C. Bundy (Eds.), *Kids can be kids: A childhood occupations approach* (pp. 320–348). Philadelphia: F. A. Davis.

Butler, R. J., & Gasson, S. L. (2005). Self esteem/self concept scales for children and adolescents: A review. *Child and Adolescent Mental Health, 10,* 190–201. http://dx.doi.org/10.1111/j.1475-3588.2005.00368.x

Canadian Charter of Rights and Freedoms. (1982). Part I of the *Constitution Act, 1982,* being Schedule B to the *Canada Act 1982* (UK), c 11.

Coster, W. J., Deeney, T., Haltiwanger, J., & Haley, S. M. (1998). *The School Functional Assessment: Standardized version.* Boston: Boston University.

Coster, W., Law, M., Bedell, G., Khetani, M. A., Cousins, M., & Teplicky, R. (2012). Development of the participation and environment measure for children and youth: Conceptual basis. *Disability and Rehabilitation, 34,* 238–246. http://dx.doi.org/10.3109/09638288.2011.603017

Dunn, W. (2011). *Best practice occupational therapy for children and families in community settings* (2nd ed.). Thorofare, NJ: Slack.

Fawcett, A. L. (2007). *Principles of assessment and outcome measurement for occupational therapists and physiotherapists.* West Wessex, UK: Wiley.

Fisher, A. G., & Jones, K. B. (2012). *Assessment of Motor and Process Skills* (7th ed., rev.). Fort Collins, CO: Three Star Press.

Folio, M. R., & Fewel, R. R. (2000). *Peabody Developmental Motor Scales.* Austin, TX: Pro-Ed.

Fuchs, L. S., Fuchs, D., Eaton, S. B., Hamlett, C., & Karns, K. (2000). Supplementing teacher judgments of mathematics about test accommodations with objective data sources. *School Psychology Review, 29,* 65–85.

Goh, D. S. (2004). *Assessment accommodations for diverse learners.* Boston: Pearson Education.

Hambleton, R. K., Merenda, P., & Spielberger, C. (2005). *Adapting educational and psychological tests for cross-cultural assessment.* Hillsdale, NJ: Erlbaum.

Harniss, M., Amtmann, D., Cook, D., & Johnson, K. (2007). Considerations for developing interfaces for collecting patient-reported outcomes that allow the inclusion of individuals with disabilities. *Medical Care, 45*(Suppl. 1), S48–S54. http://dx.doi.org/10.1097/01.mlr.0000250822.41093.ca

Individuals With Disabilities Education Improvement Act of 2004, Pub. L. 108–446, 20 U.S.C.

Iwama, M. (2006). *The Kawa Model: Culturally relevant occupational therapy.* Philadelphia: Elsevier/Churchill Livingstone.

Kielhofner, G., Mallinson, T., Crawford, C., Nowak, M., Rigby, M., Henry, A., & Walens, D. (2004). *Occupational Performance History Interview (OPHI–II) version 2.1*. Chicago: MOHO Clearing House.

Kinébanian, A., & Stomph, M. (1992). Cross-cultural occupational therapy: A critical reflection. *American Journal of Occupational Therapy, 46,* 751–757. http://dx.doi.org/10.5014/ajot.46.8.751

King, G., Law, M., King, S., Hurley, P., Hanna, S., Kertoy, M., & Young, N. (2004). *Children's Assessment of Participation and Enjoyment (CAPE) and Preferences for Activities for Children (PACS)*. San Antonio, TX: Harcourt Assessment.

Kubiszyn, T., & Borich, G. (2013). *Educational testing and measurement: Classroom application and practice* (10th ed.). New York: John Wiley & Sons.

Law, M., Baptiste, S., Carswell, A., McColl, M. A., Polatajko, H., & Pollock, N. (2005). *Canadian Occupational Performance Measure manual* (4th ed.). Ottawa, ON: CAOT Publications.

Lazarus, S. S., Thompson, S. J., & Thurlow, M. L. (2005). *How students access accommodations in assessment and instruction: Results of a survey of special education teachers (Issue Brief 7)*. College Park: University of Maryland, Educational Policy Reform Research Institute.

Mahoney, F. I., & Barthel, D. W. (1965). Functional evaluation: The Barthel Index. *Maryland State Medical Journal, 14,* 61–65.

McEwen, J., & McKenna, S. P. (1996). Nottingham Health Profile. In B. Spilker (Ed.), *Quality of life and pharmacoeconomics in clinical trials* (2nd ed., pp. 281–286). Philadelphia: Lippincott–Raven.

Mertler, C. A. (2007). *Interpreting standardized test scores: Strategies for data-driven instructional decision making*. Thousand Oaks, CA: Sage.

Miller, M. D., Linn, R. L., & Gronlund, N. E. (2009). *Measurement and assessment in teaching* (10th ed.). Upper Saddle River, NJ: Merrill/Pearson.

Muñoz, J. P. (2007). Culturally responsive caring in occupational therapy. *Occupational Therapy International, 14,* 256–280. http://dx.doi.org/10.1002/oti.238

Muñoz, J. P. (2010). Evaluating special populations. In J. Hinojosa, P. Kramer, & P. Crist (Eds.), *Evaluation: Obtaining and interpreting data* (pp. 275–293). Bethesda, MD: AOTA Press.

No Child Left Behind Act of 2001, Pub. L. No. 107–110, § 115. Stat. 1425, 107–110.

Parkinson, S., Forsyth, K., & Kielhofner, G. (2006). *The Model of Human Occupation Screening Tool (MOHOST) version 2.0 user's manual*. Chicago: MOHO Clearinghouse.

Phipps, D. (1995). Occupational therapy practice with clients from non–English speaking backgrounds: A survey. *Australian Occupational Therapy Journal, 42,* 151–160. http://dx.doi.org/10.1111/j.1440–1630.1995.tb01330.x

Piers, E. V., Harris, D. B., & Herzberg, D. S. (2002). *Piers–Harris Children's Self-Concept Scale* (2nd ed.). Los Angeles: Western Psychological Services.

Piper, M. C., & Darrah, J. (1994). *Motor Assessment of the Developing Infant*. Philadelphia: W. B. Saunders.

Pitoniak, M. J., & Royer, J. M. (2001). Testing accommodations for examinees with disabilities: A review of psychometric, legal and social policy issues. *Review of Educational Research, 71,* 53–104. http://dx.doi.org/10.3102/00346543071001053

Post, M. W. M., Gerritsen, J., van Leusen, N. D. M., Paping, M. A., & Prevo, A. J. (2001). Adapting the Nottingham Health Profile for use in people with severe physical disabilities. *Clinical Rehabilitation, 15,* 103–110. http://dx.doi.org/10.1191/026921501672698006

Prince, J. P. (1997). Assessment bias affecting lesbian, gay male, and bisexual individuals. *Measurement and Evaluation in Counseling and Development, 30,* 82–87.

Rosenberg, L., Jarus, T., & Bart, O. (2010a). Development and initial validation of the Children Participation Questionnaire (CPQ). *Disability and Rehabilitation, 32,* 1633–1644. http://dx.doi.org/10.3109/09638281003611086

Rosenberg, L., Ratzon, N. Z., Jarus, T., & Bart, O. (2010b). Development and initial validation of the Environmental Restriction Questionnaire (ERQ). *Research in Developmental Disabilities, 31,* 1323–1331. http://dx.doi.org/10.1016/j.ridd.2010.07.009

Tervalon, M., & Murray-García, J. (1998). Cultural humility versus cultural competence: A critical distinction in defining physician training outcomes in multicultural education. *Journal of Health Care for the Poor and Underserved, 9,* 117–125. http://dx.doi.org/10.1353/hpu.2010.0233

Thompson, S. J., Johnstone, C. J., & Thurlow, M. L. (2002). *Universal design applied to large scale assessments (Synthesis Report 44)*. Minneapolis: University of Minnesota, National Center on Educational Outcomes. Retrieved from http://education.umn.edu/NCEO/OnlinePubs/Synthesis44.html

Thompson, S. J., Morse, A. B., Sharpe, M., & Hall, S. (2005). *Accommodations manual: How to select, administer and evaluate use of accommodations and assessment for students with disabilities*. Washington, DC: Council for Chief State School Officers.

Thurlow, M. L., Lazarus, S. S., & Christensen, L. L. (2008). Role of assessment accommodations in accountability. *Perspectives on Language and Literacy, 34,* 17–20.

Thurlow, M. L., Lazarus, S. S., Thompson, S. J., & Morse, A. B. (2005). State policies on assessment participation and accommodations for students with disabilities. *Journal of Special Education, 38,* 232–240. http://dx.doi.org/10.1177/00224669050380040401

Thurlow, M., Thompson, S., & Johnstone, C. (2007). Policy, legal, and implementation issues surrounding assessment accommodations for students with disabilities. In L. Florian (Ed.), *The SAGE handbook of special education* (pp. 332–347). London: Sage.

Treasury, H. M. S. (2003). *Every Child Matters.* London: TSO (CM5860).

Ware, J. E., Kosinski, M., Dewey, J. E., & Gandek, B. (2000). *SF–36 Health Survey: Manual and interpretation guide.* Lincoln, RI: Quality Metric.

World Health Organization. (2001). *International classification of functioning, disability and health.* Geneva: Author.

Wurzel, J. (Ed.). (2004). *Toward multiculturalism: A reader in multicultural education* (2nd ed.). Newton, MA: Intercultural Resource Corporation.

CHAPTER 14

Ethical Issues in Evaluation

Penny L. Kyler, OT, ScD, FAOTA

Highlights

- Development of ethical decision making
- Principle-based ethics and the *Occupational Therapy Code of Ethics and Ethics Standards*
- Legal and ethical constructs
- Ethical decision making
- Special ethical issues in evaluation

Key Terms

Beneficence

Casuistry

Cultural dissidence

Cultural humility

Ethical dilemma

Ethical dissent

Ethics

Fidelity

Health Insurance Portability and
    Accountability Act of 1996

Health Information Technology for Economic
    and Clinical Health Act of 2009

Justice

Medicare Catastrophic Coverage Act of 1988

Metaethics

Morality

Nonmaleficence

Normative ethics

*Occupational Therapy Code of Ethics and
    Ethics Standards*

Patient Protection and Affordable Care
    Act of 2010

Principle-based ethics

Procedural justice

R.E.S.P.E.C.T Model of Cross-Cultural
    Communication

Social justice

Whistleblowing

This chapter discusses the ethical responsibilities of the occupational therapist as a professional who is an evaluator and assessor of occupational performance. The chapter begins with a discussion of **ethics,** personal values, and professional values, followed by a discussion of the professional code of ethics and current issues that may cause the therapist ethical distress. Guidelines to help determine ethical responsibilities are presented along with case examples to help readers consider their values and determine how these values coincide with or differ from the profession's core values and code of ethics. The chapter also covers some current trends associated with health care reform and social justice, as well as special concerns regarding electronic communication and copyright, and ends by outlining and analyzing some of the ethical issues and dilemmas that a therapist needs to consider when conducting an evaluation or assessment.

Occupational therapy curricula generally teach ethical concerns and ethical reasoning in a variety of classes. Some programs teach ethics and discernment of ethical issues and dilemmas as stand-alone classes, and others infuse ethics and ethical decision making within the context of other classes. This chapter assumes that occupational therapists administering evaluations will experience some ethical concerns and know how to detect ethical quandaries.

In the second edition of *Evaluation: Obtaining and Interpreting Data* (Hinojosa, Kramer, & Crist, 2005), Hansen (2005) discussed Joan Rogers's 1983 Eleanor Clarke Slagle Lecture. Hansen posed the following questions that a therapist needs to answer during the evaluation:

- What is the patient's status? (science)
- What are the available options? (art)
- What ought to be done? (ethics)

According to Hansen (2005), Rogers's focus on ethics was at the clinical reasoning stage of planning and implementing portions of the therapeutic process. Rogers' Slagle lecture is still relevant today, as is Hansen's critique of the application of the lecture. This chapter adds to that background by discussing the work of Catharyn Baird (2012).

DEVELOPMENT OF ETHICAL DECISION MAKING

Catharyn Baird (2012), founder of the EthicsGame™ online training tool for ethical decision making, indicated that based on Western philosophy our ethical decisions are made in the context of balancing four areas and viewing our decisions through four lenses. The four areas are (1) rationality (reason or head) and (2) sensibility (intuition or heart), which are at polar ends of one axis, and (3) autonomy (individuality) and (4) equality (community), at polar ends of the other axis. The four lenses are (1) relationships, (2) reputation, (3) rights and responsibilities, and (4) results.

Decisions may fall squarely into any of the lenses, or quadrants (Figure 14.1) or may be a mixture along a range of perspectives. Decisions are based on personal values and how they fall into the quadrants. According to Baird (2012), the following questions should be considered for each quadrant:

Rights and responsibilities
- What are your rights and responsibilities?
- What is your reason for acting?
- Are you willing to be on the receiving end of the action? For the reason given?

Results
- What results do you want?
- Will they make you happy?
- Will the results achieve the greatest good for the greatest number?

Relationships
- What relationships are important?
- What is a just system?
- Have you provided equal opportunities for each to succeed?

Reputation
- What do you want your reputation to be? (today and tomorrow)
- What are the requirements for your position? (education, social, emotional, employer, legal, insurer, yourself)
- What virtues do you have and what virtues should you cultivate?

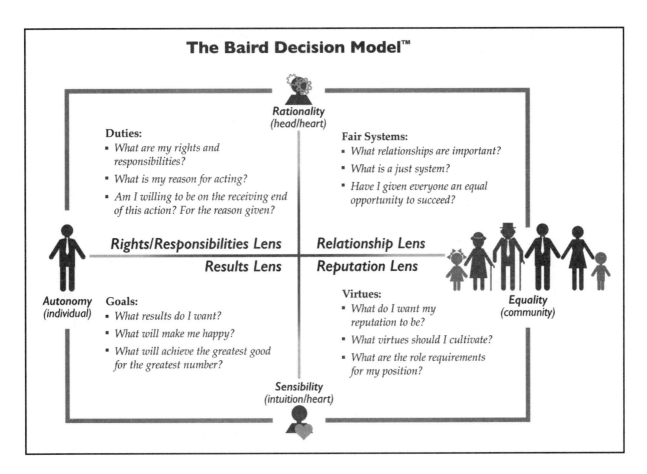

Figure 14.1. Ethical lens inventory.

Source. From "EthicsGame: Online Ethics Curriculum Tools," Copyright © 2012, by C. A. Baird. Used with permission.

Baird's four areas (Figure 14.1) provide a context for decision making. These areas are basic for making ethical decisions as a therapist evaluates a client. The four quadrants help the therapist analyze issues that may arise and decide on appropriate action. The process of doing so is very similar to an ethical case concept called *casuistry*, or case-based ethical discernment.

The term ***casuistry*** means "in flux" and has been in use since the early 1960s (Jonsen, 1986). Casuistry as a form of ethical discernment was used during the time of Aristotle and was based in religion as a way to determine who should receive penance. This method often brings forth diverse and divisive options and allows one to decide how to take action. During Aristotle's time, actions were based on religious beliefs. Casuistry has found resurgence in case-based teaching and discernment of ethical concerns because it provides the person using this method a clear paradigm for considering many facets within an ethical dilemma.

PRINCIPLE-BASED ETHICS AND THE *OCCUPATIONAL THERAPY CODE OF ETHICS AND ETHICS STANDARDS*

Over many years, health care ethics or bioethics has been associated with the Hippocratic tradition. Hippocrates (*ca.* 460 B.C.–*ca.* 370 B.C.), considered the father of medicine, is credited with advancing the systematic study of medicine and improving the prescribing practices for physicians. Traditionally, physicians swearing to practice ethical medicine take the Hippocratic Oath (Edelstein, 1943).

As members of the occupational therapy profession, our oath is more often symbolic and we pledge to abide by the ***Occupational Therapy Code of Ethics and Ethics Standards*** (***Code and Ethics***

Standards; American Occupational Therapy Association [AOTA], 2010a) for the profession. Chapter 1, "Evaluation: Where Do We Begin?" discusses three key ethical principles of the *Code and Ethics Standards* related to evaluation and assessment: (1) beneficence, (2) autonomy and confidentiality, and (3) nonmaleficence. The profession's *Code and Ethics Standards* stipulates certain kinds of conduct to which all occupational therapists and occupational therapy assistants must adhere and affirms that they are accountable for their actions.

AOTA has developed professional resources for occupational therapy practitioners that inform and guide all aspects of clinical and educational practice. In addition to the *Code and Ethics Standards* (AOTA, 2010a), several official documents, including *Guidelines to Documentation of Occupational Therapy* (AOTA, 2013), the *Occupational Therapy Practice Framework: Domain and Process* (3rd ed.; *Framework;* 2014), and the *Standards for Continuing Competence* (2010b), cover practice requirements and have direct application to evaluation.

The *Code and Ethics Standards* has evolved over the past 70-plus years. AOTA's 1994 *Occupational Therapy Code of Ethics* defined a principle-based ethics approach that we still use today. **Principle-based ethics,** a branch of applied philosophy, focuses on ethical theories and the importance of general principles such as respect for autonomy, nonmaleficence, and justice and has been the basis for all revisions to the occupational therapy ethical code (Beauchamp & Childress, 2009; Veatch & Flack, 1997). Over the course of years, the occupational therapy profession moved away from the ephemeral realm of theory and abstract speculation toward addressing practical questions and concerns raised by real problems and everyday practice that occupational therapists may see during evaluation.

The AOTA's first code of ethics, *Draft Principles of Occupational Therapy Ethics* proposed in 1976, specifically addressed evaluation and research. Principle VIII noted, "Occupational therapists shall accept the responsibility for evaluating; developing and refining services…at all times protect[ing] the rights of subjects, clients, institutions and collaborators. The work of others shall be acknowledged" (AOTA, 1976, p. 4).

This 1976 version of the code of ethics provided guidelines for each of the principles. For example, Principle VIII focused on evaluation and the guidelines stated that the "clients' families have the right to have and occupational therapists have the responsibility to provide, explanations of the nature, the purpose and results of the occupational therapy services" (AOTA, 1976, p. 4). The guidelines further stated that when the occupational therapist reported test results, he or she had the obligation to indicate any reservations regarding validity or reliability of testing as well as circumstances or inappropriateness of the test norms for the person who was tested.

The *Occupational Therapy Code of Ethics* was revised in 1988, 1994, and 2005, and after several versions without a focus on evaluation, the duties regarding evaluation reemerged in 2010 in the *Code and Ethics Standards*, which provides the individual occupational therapist with specific guidelines regarding evaluation (see Chapter 1, "Evaluation: Where Do We Begin?"). The current *Standards of Practice for Occupational Therapy* (AOTA, 2010c), another AOTA official document, specifies in the section on professional standing and responsibility:

> An occupational therapy practitioner is knowledgeable about and delivers occupational therapy services in accordance with AOTA standards, policies, and guidelines and state, federal, and other regulatory and payer requirements relevant to practice and service delivery. (p. S107)

As noted in Chapter 1, "Evaluation: Where Do We Begin?" AOTA's official documents treat the concept of evaluation inconsistently. For example, the current AOTA *Standards of Practice for Occupational Therapy* (2010c) has one standard related to screening, evaluation, and reevaluation, and the *2011 Accreditation Council for Occupational Therapy Education (ACOTE®) Standards* (ACOTE, 2012) defines separate standards for screening and evaluation. This difference is important because educational programs rely on accreditation standards for curricula and course development.

Clinical reasoning is fundamental to the ethics of evaluation and is essential to ethical discernment and decision making (Schell, 2014; Schell & Schell, 2008). Ethical reasoning was initially a form of clinical reasoning (Schell, 2014; Schell & Schell, 2008) and, therefore, the focus is on what should be done rather than what could be done for the client.

Ethical reasoning is not just about right and wrong or good and bad; it is about value systems

Table 14.1. U.S. Census Statistics

Race	% of Population
White	78.1
Black	13.1
American Indian or Alaska Native	1.2
Asian	5.0
Native Hawaiian or Other Pacific Islander	0.2
Two or more races	2.3
Hispanic or Latino Ethnicity	**% of Population**
Hispanic or Latino origin	16.7
White, not Hispanic	63.4

Note. From "2010 Census Data," 2010, by U.S. Census Bureau. Persons of Hispanic origin may be of any race. The racial categories included in the census questionnaire reflect a social definition of race recognized in this country and not an attempt to define race biologically, anthropologically, or genetically. The U.S. Office of Management and Budget requires the census to collect five categories: White, Black or African American, American Indian or Alaska Native, Asian, and Native Hawaiian or Other Pacific Islander.

and perception of care and caring. Think back to what drove you to enter the occupational therapy profession with the hope of helping individuals and communities. What do you care about, and how did you come to that level of caring? Such personal motivations drive the person you are or the person you want to become. The technical concept is called *normative ethics,* which attempts to guide us in understanding our actions, attitudes, and behaviors from a morally praiseworthy approach.

The *Code and Ethics Standards* (AOTA, 2010a) is a principle-based code of normative ethics that articulates principles, provides a general approach to terminology, and proposes a framework for a systematic ethical stance. The *Code and Ethics Standards* also educates members and the general public and helps occupational therapists and occupational therapy assistants recognize and resolve ethical distress or dilemmas. The *Code and Ethics Standards* continues to use principle-based ethics of beneficence, nonmaleficence, autonomy and veracity, and fidelity. In addition to these internationally recognized Judeo-Christian principles, the *Code and Ethics Standards* also covers confidentiality, social justice, and procedural justice. Exhibit 14.1 explains and defines ethics terminology.

Changing Demographics

The latest U.S. census indicates that previous majority groups are becoming the minority and that the average age of citizens is rising (U.S. Census Bureau,

2010). National policies have enabled many cultures to come to the United States. They come with different perspectives on concepts of health and health care. Table 14.1 shows race and ethnicity data.

Between 2000 and 2010, the population under the age of 18 years grew at a rate of 2.6%. The growth rate was even slower for ages 18 to 44 years (0.6%). These rates contrast with the substantially faster growth rates seen at older ages. The population aged 45 to 64 years grew at a rate of 31.5%. The large growth in this age group is primarily caused by the aging of the Baby Boom generation. Finally, the population aged 65 years or older also grew at a faster rate (15.1%) than the population age 45 years or younger.

Social Justice

The concept of *social justice* has its roots in Aristotle and most notably, the work of John Rawls (1999). Today, the social justice movement is focused on social and economic inequities and distribution of wealth and access to services as we witness what

Reich (1991a) called the "secession of the successful" (p. 16), that is, increased poverty, an economically insecure middle class, and a small group of very wealthy. This situation has resulted in economic and moral detriment to our society, a condition that calls for social justice (Reich, 1991b).

Brief history of social justice and health care in the United States

In U.S. health care legislative history, a social justice concept was first put forth by Theodore Roosevelt in 1912 when he advocated for a national health insurance. Other U.S. presidents who followed his lead included but were not limited to F. D. Roosevelt, Truman, Johnson, Nixon, and Clinton. In 1971, President Nixon backed a proposal requiring employers to provide a minimum level of health insurance for their workers while also maintaining competition among private insurance companies. In 1976, President Carter promptly called for "a comprehensive national health insurance system with universal and mandatory coverage." However, he never sent a bill to Congress to address a national system of health care.

In July 1988, Congress passed the **Medicare Catastrophic Coverage Act (MCCA),** the most important health legislation since President Johnson signed the Medicare bill in 1965. It was overturned by Congress in 1989 after many hundreds of thousands of affluent senior citizens grew resentful over having to pay a surtax to help finance a program that merely duplicated benefits that many of them had already been receiving before MCCA's enactment.

In 1993, President Clinton launched an effort to provide universal health care coverage on the basis of the idea of "managed competition," wherein private insurers would compete in a tightly regulated market. It too failed to win Congressional approval. In 1997, President Clinton signed legislation to create the State Children's Health Insurance Program (as part of the Balanced Budget Act), an initiative designed to provide federal matching funds to states for health insurance covering children whose family incomes were modest but too high to qualify for Medicaid.

In 2010, President Obama signed the **Patient Protection and Affordable Care Act of 2010 (ACA; 2010)** that provides an avenue toward attaining social justice regarding health care for more than 20 million uninsured or underinsured Americans. The ACA includes occupational therapy services under the habilitation and rehabilitation definition and other sections. According to the ACA, no one except patients covered by grandfathered individual plans can be refused health care coverage for any preexisting condition, an important stipulation for practices dealing with juvenile rheumatoid arthritis, autism, mixed metabolic disorder, or early onset diabetes. Occupational therapy practitioners may be employed in community health centers for prenatal care, general primary care, and specialized care for more serious conditions, including mental health, substance abuse, and HIV/AIDS. Community health centers are open to everyone regardless of their health insurance status.

How does social justice affect occupational therapy practice?

The concept of **justice** is much broader and nuanced than what appears in the *Code and Ethics Standards* (AOTA, 2010a) and has two concepts: (1) social and (2) procedural. Both apply to the occupational therapy community and in the context of evaluation apply to both the evaluator and the recipient of care. The principle of *justice* is concerned about the ways good and harm are distributed. Many use the terms *common good* or *distributive justice*. The ethics of justice, or distribution of resources, must deal with the fact that some clients need health care because their voluntary lifestyle choices create medical problems.

Social justice comes into play when working with all people, but it is of particular importance when working with people who depend upon the existence of social and economic programs to live, work, and thrive. Consider for a minute the immigrant, migrant, and refugee communities where the work they do for subsistence wages and need for health care challenge our concept of common good or social justice.

As a professional, an occupational therapist must understand *social justice* to mean "the fair, equitable, and appropriate distribution of resources" (AOTA, 2010a, p. S21). Underlying the fair distribution of goods (e.g., food, shelter, pay, access to care) is the clear expectation for the occupational therapist to provide just services. Although there may be differences in lifestyle and concepts of health and wellness, the concept of providing just services is how the therapist embraces the value of social justice.

Some justice issues deal with commitments that create inconsistency and pull the occupational therapist into conflict between justice and fidelity. For example, the commitment to justice would mean that the therapist sees each person, regardless of his or her socioeconomic standing, at his or her appointment time, thereby showing equal respect. The concept of fidelity, however, may come into play when a client has an emergency that requires immediate attention. The *Code and Ethics Standards* (AOTA, 2010a) currently describes **fidelity** in terms of meeting the client's reasonable expectations and the contractual relationship formed between the occupational therapist and the client. Therefore, someone with an emergency should take precedence over someone with a routine situation.

In evaluation, the ethical principle of fidelity refers to the obligation (or duty) to the client based on a real or implied promise. Fidelity, from the Latin *fides,* meaning faithful, includes both the expectations that the recipient of service brings to the encounter and the obligations that the therapist brings to the encounter (Purtilo & Doherty, 2011). This real or implied promise is part of the therapeutic relationship that occupational therapists develop with their clients.

Fidelity directs the therapist to balance duties and conflicts on a case-by-case basis to maximize the possible benefits to clients receiving intervention. Fidelity means keeping promises, which is inherent in scheduling appointments, agreeing to fee schedules, and keeping records. Fidelity is also reciprocal in that each party offers something to another and is bound by the mutual agreement, hence the fundamental relationship between a therapist and client is based on fidelity (Lohman, Gabriel, & Furlong, 2004; Peloquin, 2007).

The *Code and Ethics Standards* (AOTA, 2010a) also identifies concerns regarding conflict of interest, safeguarding information, and refraining from exploiting resources for personal gain. These concepts are very important in relationship to evaluation. A client and a therapist must base their relationship on fidelity. The evaluation may expose a vulnerable side of the client, and the therapist shares evaluation information with payers and other team members. How does the therapist establish a relationship and safeguard information gained during the evaluation as the clinical relationship moves forward? Consideration of these areas is the backdrop of competent clinical and ethical practice.

Procedural justice is giving people what they deserve under laws, contracts, policies, and procedures. As a licensed employee of an organization, the therapist is governed by the national certification, state practice act, and institutional or employer policies and procedures. The *Code and Ethics Standards* (AOTA, 2010a) provides enough information to enable the occupational therapist, the occupational therapy assistant, and the public to understand professional values.

Further, the *Code and Ethics Standards* (AOTA, 2010a) states the duties, rights, and responsibilities of all parties engaged in the occupational therapy process. Sometimes the language is expressed in terms that are not necessarily direct (i.e., **nonmaleficence** is to refrain from any undue influences that may compromise delivery of service), and sometimes the language is very direct (i.e., **beneficence** is to provide services that benefit the client). Nonmaleficence and beneficence deal with preventing harm and doing good, respectively.

The *Code and Ethics Standards* (AOTA, 2010a) is also a rule-based code, indicating that occupational therapists and occupational therapy assistants must comply with laws, hence the clear statements in Principle 5 regarding procedural justice. The *Code and Ethics Standards* is the basis for many state practice acts, thus the *Code and Ethics Standards* is both an aspirational document and a guideline for legally expected clinical practice behaviors.

The *Code and Ethics Standards* (AOTA, 2010a) primarily covers evaluation in Principles 1 and 3. Each principle, which follow, indicates the need for appropriate training and use of tools within the scope of occupational therapy practice

Principle 1. Occupational therapy personnel shall . . .
- Provide appropriate evaluation and a plan of intervention for all recipients of occupational therapy services specific to their needs.
- Reevaluate and reassess recipients of service in a timely manner to determine if goals are being achieved and whether intervention plans should be revised.
- Avoid the inappropriate use of outdated or obsolete tests/assessments or data obtained from such tests in making intervention decisions or recommendations.
- Provide occupational therapy services that are within each practitioner's level of competence

and scope of practice (e.g., qualifications, experience, and the law).

- Use, to the extent possible, evaluation, planning, intervention techniques, and therapeutic equipment that are evidence-based and within the recognized scope of occupational therapy practice.
- Take responsible steps (e.g., continuing education, research, supervision, and training) and use careful judgment to ensure their own competence and weigh potential for client harm when generally recognized standards do not exist in emerging technology or areas of practice. (AOTA, 2010a, pp. S19)

Principle 3. Occupational therapy personnel shall...

A. Establish a collaborative relationship with recipients of service including families, significant others, and caregivers in setting goals and priorities throughout the intervention process. This includes full disclosure of the benefits, risks, and potential outcomes of any intervention; the personnel who will be providing the intervention(s); and/or any reasonable alternatives to the proposed intervention.

B. Obtain consent before administering any occupational therapy service, including evaluation, and ensure that recipients of service (or their legal representatives) are kept informed of the progress in meeting goals specified in the plan of intervention/care. If the service recipient cannot give consent, the practitioner must be sure that consent has been obtained from the person who is legally responsible for that recipient.

C. Respect the recipient of service's right to refuse occupational therapy services temporarily or permanently without negative consequences.

D. Provide students with access to accurate information regarding educational requirements and academic policies and procedures relative to the occupational therapy program/educational institution.

E. Obtain informed consent from participants involved in research activities, and ensure that they understand the benefits, risks, and potential outcomes as a result of their participation as research subjects. (AOTA, 2010a, pp. S21.)

Case Examples 14.1 and 14.2 illustrate Principle 1 and Principle 3 of the *Code and Ethics Standards* (AOTA, 2010a). After reading each case example, answer the questions included with each case and also answer the following two questions:

1. How does the *Code and Ethics Standards* apply to this case?
2. Which principle and subarea applies?

CASE EXAMPLE 14.1. EVALUATION AND RESEARCH ETHICS

During routine monitoring of a **therapist with less than 5 years' experience** within a research practice, the **occupational therapy supervisor** observes the therapist during a consent process for several participants in a study. The supervisor finds that the therapist administering the informed consent does not explain all of the information on the consent form, as was planned at the staff training. The therapist paraphrased most of the information on the consent form and did not cover some essential elements. All participants sign the consent form.

When the supervisor questions the therapist about this situation, she states that the women at this site are not capable of understanding everything in the consent form, so the therapist decided to emphasize only the most important aspects. The supervisor speaks to the investigator about this issue. The investigator tells her that she encourages therapists to review and modify consent forms as necessary to account for local conditions. The investigator feels that the occupational therapist was correctly following the informed consent process. The supervisor feels that she has a duty to report her findings to the hospital's Research Ethics Committee (REC), which includes a representative from the department of occupational therapy. In this case, the REC should

- Recommend termination of the study (not allowed to continue),
- Retrain the site investigator and the study staff in the informed-consent process,
- Rely on the site investigator's knowledge of the study population, or
- Take no action; signed consent forms for each participant are on file.

Explain your choice and why. As in most ethical situations, the answer depends on values, context, and factors that influence your decision, and there can be more than one appropriate response.

CASE EXAMPLE 14.2. COMMUNITY PROGRAM

A **health and wellness program for teenagers** is being conducted in a minority community. The study, part of a grant, requires quarterly evaluations and targets previously identified at-risk teen groups, including drug and alcohol users. The focus will also be on wellness, along with building habits to overcome the stigma associated with poverty.

The research team of occupational therapists, music therapist, and exercise physiology staff plans to enroll intravenous drug users at city-run rehabilitation centers and a local church. Most drug users in the rehabilitation centers have been sent there by the local legal system. Teens who agree to participate in the research will receive an identification card with a participant number and contact information for questions or problems.

In preparation for the study, the researchers met with rehabilitation center management, church staff, and police to discuss the study and ask for their cooperation, because during the course of treatment each participant will need a quarterly evaluation. The authorities who run the rehabilitation centers are optimistic that most of the drug users will agree to participate. In addition, the police request that participant identification cards include the police department's official seal. Further, the police request that the names of participants recruited on the street be provided to them so that they are not arrested and thus denied access to the study. The local church decided that it would also like the participants at its site to have a similar form of identification. Answer the following questions:

- What measures can the staff take to ensure that informed consent is given freely by all participants?
- Are there special considerations for working with a vulnerable underage population that may participate in illegal activities?
- What part of the *Framework* (AOTA, 2014) should be considered as the researchers design their therapeutic interventions?
- If the researchers believe that the potential participants will not be able to give voluntary informed consent, what could be done to change the informed-consent process?
- What measures should the researchers take to ensure that evaluations are done in a timely fashion?

LEGAL AND ETHICAL CONSTRUCTS

AOTA's official documents are meant to be guidelines and standards for practice. Additionally, federal, state, and local regulations directly influence the occupational therapist's evaluation of clients. Regulations may determine when a client is evaluated, what assessments a therapist is qualified to use, and what information is provided and to whom.

The ethical concept of *justice* is based on the legal sense of fairness and following rules. Legal issues are interwoven with ethical considerations. For example, the right to due process (a legal construct) is a basic consideration behind the ethical principles associated with autonomy and informed-consent procedures. Laws and ensuing regulations are one type of consideration or perspective that a therapist must follow when providing any occupational therapy service.

An occupational therapist must also follow the *Code and Ethics Standards* (AOTA, 2010a) and the profession's other official documents, including *Standards of Practice for Occupational Therapy* (AOTA, 2010c), *Standards for Continuing Competence* (AOTA, 2010b), and practice guidelines. These documents provide a therapist with a framework for clinical reasoning and an approach to practice. When conflicts occur between what is legal and what is ethical, the therapist faces an ethical dilemma that must be resolved before proceeding with the evaluation process.

Legal precedents for a client's civil rights stem from legislation and resulting government regulations. Following federal law, a therapist must not use evaluations or assessments that discriminate on the basis of age, race, gender, economic status, medical condition, or behavioral or physical disability. For example, federal laws and regulations such as the Education of the Handicapped Act Amendments of 1983 and the Individuals With Disabilities Education Act of 1990 (IDEA), reauthorized as the Individuals With Disabilities Education Improvement Act of 2004, govern the practice of occupational therapy in educational settings.

Other federal laws that must be adhered to include the **Health Insurance Portability and Accountability Act of 1996 (HIPAA)** and the Family Educational Rights and Privacy Act of 1974 (FERPA). Federal regulations such as Title VI of the Civil Rights Act of 1964 for persons with limited English proficiency and the U.S. Office of Minority Health's Cultural and Linguistically Appropriate

Standards for health facilities have been embraced by The Joint Commission. Courts' legal positions (i.e., interpretations of laws) and decisions must also be followed by therapists.

ETHICAL DECISION MAKING

How are evaluation dilemmas different from other types of ethical dilemmas characteristic of providing intervention? A simple response to the question is that there is no difference. Competing issues that may not have clear right or wrong answers characterize an ethical dilemma.

By definition, an *ethical dilemma* involves the need to choose among two or more morally acceptable courses of action. At times, a therapist's choices may be mutually exclusive, or all available alternatives may be equally unacceptable (Hansen, 2005; Purtilo & Doherty, 2011). As a therapist works with other clinicians to care for a client with complex needs, he or she may come face to face with varying expectations and values from coworkers, employers, health care industry representatives, and even the client. These events will challenge the therapist's personal sense of ethical correctness and may cause him or her to rethink the chosen approach.

An evaluation begins the occupational therapy intervention process. As noted in Chapter 1, "Evaluation: Where Do We Begin?" ethical considerations are extremely important during the evaluation and decisions about what is the "right" action in a given situation are an integral part of the occupational therapist's daily life. The *Code and Ethics Standards* (AOTA, 2010a) clearly states, in Beneficence (Principle 1), that a therapist should select an appropriate evaluation related to the specific goals and needs of the recipient of service. The planning and implementation of the evaluation must be congruent with the client's or surrogate's interests and goals.

Once the therapist completes the evaluation, his or her recommendations and goals must be congruent with any goals that the client or surrogate has identified (AOTA, 2010a). No matter the venue—education, clinical practice, or research—the therapist must give the recipient of service or his or her surrogate the opportunity to decide whether the goals are both acceptable and desirable.

A therapist makes decisions on the basis of what he or she learned in school, what ethnocultural

traditions he or she may have absorbed, and general life experiences. These areas constitute the basis of ethical decision making because they reflect a person's values and beliefs.

Aside from religious and spiritual beliefs, familiar patterns may serve as the root of what a person believes about right and wrong. Therefore, the foundations of ethical behavior include

- Family traditions, standards, and interactions;
- Culture and norms of the society in which people live;
- Influence of friends, colleagues, and teachers;
- Professional culture of occupational therapy;
- Writings and speeches (teachings or conveyed beliefs) of people who are important or influential in our lives (e.g., grandparents, friends);
- Avocational activities (e.g., reading, social groups, sports); and
- Wild-card events that we do not control but change the dynamics of our lives and our civilization (e.g., war, technology, economy, sociological changes).

Exhibit 14.2 includes questions that practitioners can ask themselves. It is important that the occupational therapist know and understand his or her own values to be aware of the values he or she brings to the interaction with a client. In addition, the therapist must examine interactions to assess whether what he or she believes is ethically right and wrong is reflected in the interaction.

**EXHIBIT 14.2. REFLECTION:
I AM ETHICAL BECAUSE...**

Consider your background and your family's background. If you can, go back 3 generations to your grandparents:
- Where were you born?
- Where were your parents and grandparents born?
- Who in your family has influenced your moral beliefs?
- Think about a seminal event in your life that helped crystallize your moral underpinnings. What was it? When did it occur?
- How have you used that experience?
- What else has influenced your concept of morality or right and wrong?
- Have your morals changed?

The determination of right action in a given situation is complex and multidimensional. In some cases, there are no good choices or clear winners and losers. Not all ethical determinations end in a win–win outcome. Deciding the best solution under specific circumstances is not simple.

An occupational therapist makes determinations of right and wrong based on his or her personal and professional values. Ethical dilemmas exist because there are no clear-cut answers in many practice situations. Two or more options that a therapist could consider acceptable may be available, but in most cases, there should be one resolution that is the best solution. Although decision making can be approached in many ways, it is personal, with each person bringing to the thought process his or her own biases. Each person is a mixture of some good qualities (i.e., strengths) and some not-so-good qualities (i.e., weaknesses), which makes a person unique and is part of how he or she approaches making decisions.

There is no right or wrong approach to making a decision as long as the person makes the decision based on facts. A therapist responds to facts at his or her personal core. Do the facts bring forth anger, disbelief, calmness, and so on? A therapist must be aware of facts that create emotional or perceptional responses to a situation. With each fact involved in the ethical concern, a therapist must decide whether to explore or overlook the emotional reaction.

An analogy to approaching an ethical decision is making a meal for friends. A person must first consider the mixture of menu, place, time, and people. This mixture can change depending on the circumstances. A person must make sure the food is cooked and presented in such a way as to be pleasing to the eye, taste buds, and digestion. Throwing in too much spice or salt, or a bad glass of wine, or dining with an overly perfumed or demanding person will disrupt the meal and lead to indigestion. In planning the meal, a person considers the many forces involved.

Similarly, in considering an ethical decision, a therapist thinks of the parts that may go together to find a resolution to the dilemma. In the process, the therapist asks questions and considers several options. The mixture of choices and the characteristics of ethical evaluation require the integration of all aspects of decision making.

When administering an assessment, the occupational therapist has to begin at the personal level and ask whether he or she is competent to administer and interpret the assessment. This basic question derives from the *Code and Ethics Standards* (AOTA, 2010a) Principle 2, Nonmaleficence. Without competence to perform the assessment, the therapist may cause harm. Beyond competence as an evaluator, two critical questions to ask include

1. To whom does the occupational therapist have a primary duty when making decisions about which evaluations to use?
2. How should these data be reported, and to whom?

Most occupational therapists view the client as their first priority. When the therapist is evaluating a child, *client* also can mean the client's family or caregiver. The occupational therapist has to consider the client's family and significant others, along with his or her own employer and the facility for which he or she works, his or her fellow professionals, and the agency or person who is paying for the evaluation. Conflicts can and do arise when others believe that they are on solid ground regarding priorities, goals, and values. Thoughtful ethical reasoning and the moral agency of each group come into play when different people and groups clash or, at least, do not function in a harmonious manner (Purtilo & Doherty, 2011).

A therapist asks questions to discern the facts before resolving an ethical dilemma. What are the facts and what do the facts mean to the outcome of the evaluation? Aside from the first question of "Am I competent to perform the evaluation?," other questions to consider include

- Has there been collaboration between the client and me?
- Have I considered occupational performance areas from the client's perspective of participation?
- Have I considered the ethnocultural components of the client?
- Have I considered the client within a family-centered context?
- Have I considered the subjective (i.e., emotional, psychological) and objective (i.e., physically observable) aspects of performance?

EXHIBIT 14.3. DISSECTING AN ETHICS CASE

Before identifying potential conflicts, think about the need for information. Facts help clarify how you decide on an intervention. Reviewing your approach to analyzing an ethical quandary involves the following steps:

- Gather relevant information.
- Identify whether there is a problem.
- Decide which ethics approach to use.
- Reflect.
- Explore practical alternatives.
- Complete the decision-making process and action.
- Evaluate by reflecting on the process and outcomes of your actions.

Note. Adapted from Purtilo & Doherty (2011).

When dissecting an ethics case, therapists need to explore and identify potential conflicts. Exhibit 14.3 details the steps that one should use to effectively dissect an ethics case.

Steps in Ethical Decision Making

A therapist might take simple steps in discerning ethical issues. However, once a therapist begins with simple steps, he or she may find himself or herself led down a path of further quandary. To mitigate larger quandaries, the occupational therapist needs to develop some basic ethical analysis skills: finding the facts; understanding the circumstances; listening to the therapist's own voice; and, as needed, using other resources. The thought processes used in resolving ethical issues are the same as those used in selecting an assessment and developing an intervention approach. Exhibit 14.4 shows the specific questions that the practitioner should ask himself or herself to identify potential conflicts in assessment.

- Have I accurately performed and documented the assessment?
- Most importantly, is the summary a true reflection of what I have seen and heard from the client and his or her family?

EXHIBIT 14.4. QUESTIONS FOR IDENTIFYING POTENTIAL CONFLICTS IN ASSESSMENT

Occupational therapist
- Am I competent enough to do this assessment?
- Do I have the necessary knowledge, skills, and attitudes to select, administer, and interpret the results of each evaluation?
- Am I competent enough to supervise other occupational therapy personnel in the collection of data for this assessment? Am I sure that competent people are carrying out all delegated tasks properly?
- Have I accurately documented the services provided? Is the summary assessment an accurate reflection of the separate evaluations?

Occupational therapy assistant
- Am I competent enough to carry out the data collection and evaluations that I am expected to perform?
- Am I receiving adequate training and supervision to carry out the assigned portions of the assessment process?
- Have I accurately reported the data and contributed to the overall assessment process?

Client (family, significant others, guardian)
- Has the client been informed about the purpose of the assessment, how it will be administered, and by whom?
- Does the client understand how the results of the assessment will be used?
- Has the client been informed how this service will be billed?
- Has the client been given the opportunity to decide whether the assessment should be done?
- Are the client's goals the basis for developing and carrying out the assessment process?

Employer (facility, agency, company)
- Is the assessment consistent with the mission of the facility?
- Will there be accurate billing for services?
- How will the interpretations and recommendations of the occupational therapist be used?

(Continued)

EXHIBIT 14.4. QUESTIONS FOR IDENTIFYING POTENTIAL CONFLICTS IN ASSESSMENT *(Cont.)*

Payer
- Is the assessment a necessary and billable service?
- If there is no third-party reimbursement, does the client know this? Has the client given consent before the initiation of the evaluation?
- Will the occupational therapist and the billing office request fair compensation for the services and request payment only for services provided?

Professional colleagues
- Is the referral consistent with the client's goals and needs?
- Is this assessment necessary?
- Has the occupational therapist communicated the results of the assessment clearly, so that other members of the service delivery team have useful information?
- Have copyrighted evaluation materials been used according to the laws regulating their use?
- Is it necessary to pay fees to use the assessment tool? If so, have the fees been paid?
- Must the occupational therapist obtain permission to use the materials?
- Are specific training and supervision required to conduct the evaluation?
- Does the evaluator hold the appropriate credentials to conduct the evaluation?
- Has the occupational therapist used the correct forms and procedures in conducting the evaluation and reporting the results?
- If it is a standardized evaluation, has the evaluator followed the procedures exactly?

Community and society
- Is this assessment consistent with the concepts of due process, reparation for wrongs that have been done (physical or emotional), and the fair and equitable distribution of occupational therapy services to persons needing those services?

Note. Adapted from "Ethical Implications in Evaluation," by R. Hanson, 2005. In J. Hinojosa, P. Kramer, and P. Crist (Eds.), *Occupational Therapy Evaluation: Obtaining and Interpreting Data* (2nd ed., pp. 249–250). Bethesda, MD: AOTA Press. Copyright © 2005 by the American Occupational Therapy Association. Adapted with permission.

Conceptual frameworks influence how the therapist explores ethical dilemmas and client problems. Conceptual frameworks also influence the types of assessments and interventions a therapist decides to use (Neistadt, 2000). The therapist may resolve an ethical concern by looking at the profession's *Code and Ethics Standards* (AOTA, 2010a) and practice guidelines in conjunction with his or her background and sense of ethics. The therapist might determine the appropriate assessment based on the frame of reference he or she selects to use.

Just as ethical discernment may be based on a lifetime of experiences and formal education, an occupational therapist has approaches to evaluation that are drawn from a frame of reference not explicitly articulated but based on clinical practice experience (Rogers, 1983). Table 14.2 outlines some areas to review to help resolve ethical issues dealing with choosing evaluations and interventions.

Case Example 14.3 shows how to deal with ethical issues when the therapist is working with an evaluation that has been done by another therapist. It describes a situation and provides a seven-step process to review the situation.

When considering the steps portrayed in Case Example 14.3, there are two ways of approaching the issue. One way is to claim that acts are right to the extent that they produce good consequences and wrong to the extent that they produce bad consequences. The key terms here are *good* and *bad*. When thinking about good and bad, one must consider the benefits and harms of particular actions.

Another way to view the situation is to consider ethical decision making from the societal perspective. What are the norms of the society? This perspective recognizes that different societies reach different conclusions regarding the rightness or wrongness or the goodness or badness of an action (Purtilo & Doherty, 2011; Veatch & Haddad, 2008). The occupational therapist must choose from several alternative actions, delineated in Table 14.3.

Table 14.2. Six Steps to Resolving Ethical Issues When Choosing Evaluations and Interventions

Step	Resolving an Ethical Issue	Choosing Evaluation Assessments
1.	Identify ethical concern or problem.	Identify client problems or assets.
2.	Develop questions about the ethical concern.	Develop questions regarding client problems or assets.
3.	Choose an approach to resolve the ethical concern.	Choose an assessment or evaluation tool.
4.	Ask the questions; get the facts.	Gather data to develop intervention approach.
5.	Analyze answers.	Project (predict) outcomes after intervention and monitor client progress.
6.	Make decision.	Make recommendations about further services.

CASE EXAMPLE 14.3. INTERVENTION ON THE BASIS OF EVALUATIONS DONE BY OTHERS

Sue, an occupational therapist, has been seeing **Franklin, age 8 years,** in her private practice for more than a month. He comes twice a week. His mother tells Sue that her major concern is that Franklin has motor deficits. Previously, Franklin's mother had him evaluated at a well-respected multidisciplinary clinic that includes an occupational therapist, a psychiatrist, a developmental psychologist, a social worker, and others. The psychiatrist told Franklin's mother that Franklin has an attention deficit hyperactivity disorder.

Franklin's mother has come to Sue's clinic because she likes Sue's philosophy: "Just collaborate with the parents and do what the parents want to work on." At this time, Sue does not have a formal treatment plan and did not do an evaluation because the parents did not want to pay for it. Using the results of the copy of the evaluation from the clinic, Sue is focusing only on motor performance problems because that is what Franklin's mother wants. Sue, however, has noticed several behavioral issues that the multidisciplinary clinic had addressed in the information she received from them. Sue follows the 7 steps listed here in an ethical decision-making process.

1. Decide what the central question is and what the known facts are. Gather information.
2. Seek additional information if needed to answer these questions:
   • Are there some financial concerns driving the family?
   • Is Sue observing something that needs further evaluation?
   • Is Sue seeking further evaluation to increase her reimbursement?
   • Does Sue have the expertise to do an evaluation battery?
   • What does Franklin's mother say are her goals for her child?
   • What does Franklin say are his goals for himself?
3. Decide on an action, and understand your justification of the selected action. Use your moral guides; consider the clinical reasoning of your action. What ethics approach will you use?
4. If needed, decide on alternative actions.
5. Reflect on the thought process, on concepts of care, and on law and institutional guidelines.
6. Implement the decision while thinking of these questions:
   • Is the action legal? (Has Sue reflected on the legal consequences?)
   • Is it balanced? Is it fair to all concerned? (Not all actions have to result in a win–win situation.)
   • Does it set up a situation that produces the most good or provides the least harmful outcome for all involved? (Does Sue's response help create a positive environment?)
   • How does the decision make Sue feel about her moral self?
7. Evaluate and reflect on your actions.

Note. Adapted from Hansen, Kyler-Hutchison, and Trompetter (1994) and Purtilo and Doherty (2011).

Table 14.3. Sue's Alternative Actions to Decide What to Do Next

Action	Consequence	Ethical Principle Involved (*Occupational Therapy Code of Ethics and Ethics Standards* [AOTA, 2010a])
Decide to approach the mother about the need for an evaluation	Child continues in occupational therapy without proper evaluation Mom feels uncomfortable	Fidelity to client Obligation of competence—concept of justice by adherence to the *Framework* (2014) Concept of autonomy Family vs. individual power Informed consent Beneficence and nonmaleficence
Decide not to do a formal evaluation and go with the assessment done by the clinic	Goes against the *Framework* (AOTA, 2014) because an occupational therapist must observe and analyze performance skills personally (could or should this step be done without formal evaluation?)	Procedural justice—possible violation of state regulations Possible violation of *Code of Ethics and Ethics Standards* (AOTA, 2010a)
Meet with the family and child to explain the limitations imposed on her because of the lack of formal evaluation on site	Family has reasons for selecting current program and does not wish to discuss their finances	Duty of veracity to client, professional code of ethics Possible violation of occupational therapy practice act and regulations about service delivery
Decide not to continue treating the child	Child does not get needed services Missed opportunity for family education about the scope of occupational therapy services Family gets turned off regarding occupational therapy and does not seek further services	Duty of veracity Duty of fidelity

Note. AOTA = American Occupational Therapy Association.

Case Example 14.3 illustrates how to review a case. The primary ethical principles involved are beneficence, Principle 1.B, with a particular focus on 1.A, B, and C; nonmaleficence, Principle 2, with a focus on 2.A and I; and fidelity, Principle 7 (AOTA, 2010a). However, remember that there can be differences in judgment about the actions in this case example. Differences are the result of dissimilar views of the facts, matters of personal preference, and differences in the view of rightness or wrongness. Should veracity, Principle 6, come into the discussion of this case example?

Case Example 14.4 provides a very different scenario, which concerns how a therapist is using (or not using) standardized assessments.

Lessons From Others

The process of evaluating is not the sole domain of occupational therapy. Many health professionals focused on emphasizing evaluation as a specific clinical area before occupational therapy. Evaluation emphasizes building relationships and partnerships among clients and professionals and providing a clear view to the provider of what needs to be done.

In fields such as psychology, medicine, nursing, social work, education, and mental health, professionals have established critical definitions and expectations of evaluations. One example, developed by the American Psychological Association (APA; 2010), defines *evaluation* by the evaluation

---

CASE EXAMPLE 14.4. HARRY AND STANDARDIZED EVALUATIONS

Harry, an occupational therapist, has been in practice for more than 20 years and has always worked with the same client population. Other therapists consider him an expert clinician with this population. He has seen formal assessments come and go and has watched as the profession has contributed to and championed various assessments. During these years, Harry has developed excellent clinical intuition for knowing in which areas his clients will have demonstrated occupational performance deficits and on what areas of health and participation through occupational engagement the clients should focus.

Over the years, Harry has taken parts of multiple formal standardized assessments and made up his own. For example, Harry's homemade assessment provides an understanding of the client's occupational history and experiences, including their interests, values, and needs. His assessment provides a clear picture of the client's physical, emotional, and cognitive strengths and deficits. Harry says, "Why pay money for these formal assessments when I have taken the best from each of them and constructed a quicker and more comprehensive, economical, and useful tool? In this day and age, money saved from the purchase of these evaluations has allowed me to hire an additional occupational therapy assistant." Consider the following questions:

- What are the rights of the clients receiving these evaluations?
- What are the implications for borrowing from other sources?
- What are the potential concerns when a client moves to another facility and it requests a copy of Harry's occupational therapy evaluation?
- If the therapist believes that outcomes from the assessment are excellent, is it appropriate for the therapist to take certain liberties?
- What are the legal concerns? What about copyright laws?

---

format used. The organization notes in its code of ethics that services should be provided regardless of age, gender, gender identity, race, ethnicity, culture, national origin, religion, sexual orientation, disability, language, or socioeconomic status.

The APA's current code, developed in 2002 and amended in 2010, devotes an entire section to assessment and evaluation (APA, 2010). APA's code of ethics addresses the use of current and obsolete evaluative tools, cost, training in administering the assessments, and explaining the test results.

As occupational therapy moves toward more involvement with research, the occupational therapist should be concerned with fairness, veracity, and equity when collecting data. Other matters touched upon by the APA (2010) code that directly translate to occupational therapy are responsible data collection, retention, and sharing and interpretation of data that bear on the integrity of data.

APA and other professional organizations also clearly discuss fair treatment of collaborators, including fair apportionment of funds and preservation of confidentiality of research subjects or proprietary knowledge of sponsors and collaborators. It is interesting to note that the current *Code and Ethics Standards* (AOTA, 2010a) does not explicitly discuss either assessment or evaluation, or how issues of ownership of or fabrication of data may relate to evaluation and assessment.

As more occupational therapists become involved in research, they need to consider several areas of ethical concern. Principle 6 in the *Code and Ethics Standards* (AOTA, 2010a) discusses veracity, fabrication, falsification of data, and borrowing from others without explicitly stating that these topics are part of truth telling. Fabrication is lying, and our moral system usually treats lying as wrong. The *Code and Ethics Standards* clearly indicates that a member should "refrain from using or participating in the use of any form of communication that contains false, fraudulent, deceptive, or unfair statements or claims" (p. 641).

SPECIAL ETHICAL ISSUES IN EVALUATION

This section covers ethical issues related to electronic health records, culture, language, copyright, ethical dissent, and confidentiality.

Electronic Health Records

A situation that many occupational therapists are facing more often is working with an electronic format for data keeping. Electronic health records are being promoted in the belief that they will

Table 14.4. American Medical Informatics Association Ethical Concerns Regarding Use of Information

Protecting Private Information	Ethical Dilemmas Created by the Use of Health Information Technologies	Patient Safety	Ethics of Good Design and Data Displays
User involvement	System implementation	Liability	Risk assessments
Training adequacy	Secondary data use	Research ethics	Autonomy and empowerment (especially in light of new health regulations and telehealth)
Social networking	Policy and regulation	N/A	N/A

Note. N/A = not applicable. Adapted from American Medical Informatics Association (2013).

improve record keeping, facilitate communication among professionals, drive down health care costs, and decrease medical errors. The **Health Information Technology for Economic and Clinical Health (HITECH) Act,** part of the 2009 economic stimulus package (American Recovery and Reinvestment Act, 2009), was developed to give physicians more incentive to adopt electronic health records. Since 2009, several regulations have been promulgated for implementing the HITECH Act. The rule most applicable to occupational therapy is the requirement for due diligence by the provider in protecting information. The American Medical Informatics Association (2013) has championed the concern regarding protecting information (Table 14.4).

The move toward electronic record keeping and fully integrated electronic health records raises concerns about data sets, registries for research, and electronic evaluations. As an example, the Federal Communications Commission chairman noted that the ubiquitous use of tablet data devices and smart phones and frequent theft of these items containing sensitive information have posed a unique problem for law enforcement (Genachowski, 2012). They may also pose a concern for professionals using these devices to input sensitive information associated with clinical care, education, or research. Exhibit 14.5 describes who and what is covered by the HIPAA privacy rules.

An occupational therapist, as an employee of a covered entity, must know how to protect confidential information. Does the employer use a form of encryption that is included on the therapist's

---

EXHIBIT 14.5. COVERED ENTITY DEFINITION: WHO AND WHAT IS COVERED?

HIPAA privacy rules pertain to the following covered entities:
- Health plans (e.g., insurers, managed care organizations, federal health programs);
- Health clearinghouses that unify data in standardized formats; and
- Health care providers who engage, directly or through contractual arrangements, in HIPAA standard electronic transactions (e.g., computer-to-computer transmission of health care claims, payment and remittance, benefit information, health plan eligibility information).

HIPAA rules pertain to *personal health information,* defined as individually identifiable health information, transmitted in any format (electronic, paper, or oral) by covered entities (U.S. Department of Health and Human Services, 2013).

Note. HIPAA = Health Insurance Portability and Accountability Act.

---

data devices? Is the therapist using these devices properly? Should a therapist use a personal tablet or smart phone to input evaluation information or notes for future use? These questions raise ethical and legal concerns for the therapist and for those whom the therapist treats.

Although electronic health records may represent beneficence (as outlined in Principle 1 [AOTA, 2010a]) to many because of the associated increased access to health care information and potential improvement of the quality of care and health, such records may also represent a threat. Disadvantaged people may not have equal access to health information because of their socioeconomic class or age. A disadvantaged person's justice may be breached because he or she lacks access to health information resources.

Electronic health records also may jeopardize a person's autonomy when a client's health data are shared or linked without the client's knowledge. A therapist needs to be aware of who has access to assessment data. A client's fidelity may be breached by the exposure of health data through mistakes or theft, which violates Principle 2, Nonmaleficence, particularly the concept of infliction of harm and not imposing the risk of harm to the client. Lack of trust in the security of health data may persuade a client to conceal critical health information, thus compromising his or her treatment. Therapists need to protect the confidentiality of a client's record by password-protecting files and using procedures and programs that thwart identity theft and protect private information from computer hackers.

In December 1995, the American Nursing Association (ANA) Board of Directors approved the establishment of the Nursing Information and Data Set Evaluation Center (NIDSEC; Marek, 1997). NIDSEC defined review criteria to evaluate and recognize information systems from developers and manufacturers that support documentation of nursing care within automated nursing information systems or within computer-based patient record systems. Since then, ANA has created a sustained focus on standardizing nursing terminology (Thede & Schwiran, 2011). The benefits of using standardized terminology include

- Better communication among nurses and other health care providers,
- Increased visibility of nursing interventions,
- Improved patient care,
- Enhanced data collection to evaluate nursing care outcomes,
- Greater adherence to standards of care, and
- Facilitation of assessment of nursing competency (Rutherford, 2008).

Similar benefits could be obtained in occupational therapy from these practice guidelines and uniform terminology.

Culture

Evaluating a person from a different culture also may have an ethical component. Many of the evaluations occupational therapists use are based on Western medicine and American norms. Because dysfunction is culturally specific, an evaluation may falsely identify a disability in a person from a different culture. The *Code and Ethics Standards* (AOTA, 2010a) obliquely addresses culture under the concept of Beneficence (Principle 1) by discussing the need to provide an evaluation specific to the client's needs that is within the therapist's level of competence.

The *Code and Ethics Standards* (AOTA, 2010a) notes that the occupational therapist recognizes and appreciates a variety of cultural components and provides services in a fair and equitable manner. In Principle 3, Autonomy and Confidentiality, the *Code and Ethics Standards* indicates that to have meaningful communication, the therapist must be cognizant of language, literacy, and culture. This awareness is a form of **cultural humility** (defined in Exhibit 14.6). Knowing what you do not know and recognizing it are important in working with clients, families, and communities of other cultures.

An occupational therapist must be aware of and concerned with the real or perceived coercion inherent in the imbalance of power between the occupational therapist and the client. Occupational

---

EXHIBIT 14.6. WHAT IS CULTURAL HUMILITY?

Cultural humility includes

- Pride for one's own culture coupled with the knowledge that the clinician's world view is not universal;
- Acknowledging that a patient's culture can only be appreciated by learning from the patient; and
- Knowing that attributing certain traits or attitudes to people who belong to a certain group is an act of generalization that may not be accurate or helpful in understanding an individual client.

"To be sensitive to a patient's culture, clinicians must possess cultural humility."

Note. From "What Is Cultural Humility," 2010, by the University of California–San Francisco, Department of Psychiatry's Cultural Humility Task Force at San Francisco General Hospital. Used with permission.

therapy can look to the American Medical Association (AMA) for guidance in the area of culture and evaluation. Berlin and Fowkes (1983) and Welsh (2003) suggested a mnemonic, LEARN, for remembering how to engage people from other cultures:

- **L**isten with sympathy and understanding to the patient's perception of the problem.
- **E**xplain your perceptions of the problem and your strategy for treatment.
- **A**cknowledge and discuss the differences and similarities between these perceptions.
- **R**ecommend treatment while remembering the patient's cultural parameters.
- **N**egotiate agreement.

Welch (1998) suggested the **R.E.S.P.E.C.T. Model of Cross-Cultural Communication,** a mnemonic that can be helpful in everyday practice not only during treatment but also during the evaluation process:

- *Rapport.* Establish rapport with the client without judgment and preconceived ideas.
- *Empathy.* Develop empathy for the client who needs your assistance by recognizing the client's feelings and understanding his or her behaviors of illness.
- *Support.* Support the client by understanding and helping him or her resolve barriers to his or her care.
- *Partnership.* Partner with the client by being flexible and addressing stress that may emerge as you work together.
- *Explanations.* Clearly explain information to the client and check for understanding.
- *Cultural competence.* Respect and seek to understand the client's culture and its influence on the client's health and decisions.
- *Trust.* Trust the client's willingness to disclose information and take the time to develop an effective working relationship.

The American College of Physicians provides some enlightening discussion of the pulls of ethics and culture, noting ethical barriers to culturally competent evaluation (Forrow, 2008). Forrow observed that an ethical conundrum requires the person to do something that may violate his or her fundamental personal values to maintain standards of scientific practice. AMA (2002) approached this topic by what it called *cultural dissidence.* **Cultural dissidence** may be a misunderstood concept

---

CASE EXAMPLE 14.5. CULTURAL SENSITIVITY: WAR OF FEELINGS

As a new graduate, **Sally** sees **Mr. Yujiro, a 24-year-old** male outpatient of Japanese descent with a concussive traumatic brain injury (TBI) suffered during military service in the Iraq war. Not only has Sally been an advocate against the war, but she has also never treated a person of Japanese descent. Mr. Yujiro arrived in the United States at the age of 11. His family's memories of World War II have influenced his view of war and being a warrior. Although educated and trained in the United States, Mr. Yujiro has a distinctly Japanese perspective on life, health care, and his status as a patient. This case is Sally's first of a person with a TBI and her first chance to talk with an Iraq war veteran. Mr. Yujiro's mood swings as Sally talks to him and his emotions frighten her.

It is the protocol of the facility to always perform an occupational profile for each person during the first appointment and to provide a completed evaluation by the end of the second meeting. The occupational profile answers who, what, and why questions about the person.

Questions to consider:
- What obstacles could stand in the way of Sally's completing this task?
- What are some feelings Sally might have regarding treating a warrior?
- What happens when Sally's values are in conflict with Mr. Yujiro's values?
- How would Sally go about developing a collaborative relationship with this client?
- What would be Sally's concerns regarding not completing the task in the required timeline?
- How would Sally ascertain Mr. Yujiro's reason for seeking services and assess his current concerns relative to engaging in occupations and daily life activities?
- Does Sally have enough experience to treat Mr. Yujiro?
- How would Sally determine Mr. Yujiro's priorities and desired outcomes?
- What is Sally's duty? To whom or what? What is in conflict?

CASE EXAMPLE 14.6. CULTURAL SENSITIVITY: RELIGIOUS SYMBOLISM

John is seeing a **52-year-old Sikh man, Hardeep,** employed as a cab driver, who was in an auto accident. Hardeep has been a driver for 6 months and has been in the United States for 6 years. He is referred to occupational therapy with a variety of arm fractures. John has evaluated him using a standardized assessment for motor function and is working with him on his activities of daily living (ADLs) and his instrumental activities of daily living.

Hardeep currently has the use of only one arm and is very concerned about his inability to wrap his hair and beard and his ability to sit and work for his 60- to 80-hour work week. John learned that the traditional head wrap is a sign of piety. Wrapping the head involves using several meters of material and having one's arms above the head for more than 15 minutes. John feels that there is a language barrier because he finds it hard to understand Hardeep's English. In addition, Hardeep does not appear to be able to follow John's ADL instructions and is not progressing as quickly as John thinks he should. John is hoping that Hardeep's son, who is acting as the translator, will bring in the materials needed for the head wrap.

Questions to consider:
- To whom should John should provide primary information, Hardeep or Hardeep's son?
- To whom should John should provide information regarding Hardeep's progress?
- What is John's role and obligation to Hardeep's son?
- Are there any laws or regulations that John should consider?
- What hospital and health insurance information should John obtain?
- What is John's duty?
- How can John respect Hardeep's autonomy?
- Can Hardeep's son be the proxy for his father?

---

because it involves personal feelings and prejudices that have the potential for misuse of power by professionals.

As an example, issues of racial or ethnic profiling have been in the news frequently because of the issue of cultural dissidence. In occupational therapy, a therapist may have developed some preconceptions and values about persons of Middle Eastern descent without ever meeting such a person. A therapist must be aware of his or her prejudices, consider what he or she does to ensure that he or she does not misuse power, and provide intervention within the values and cultural framework of the client.

In some cases, it may be difficult to resolve an ethical dilemma. For example, a therapist attempts to evaluate an Indo-Asian female client who seeks approval from her spouse for everything she says or does. The therapist may consider this behavior incorrect and inappropriate. This behavior, however, may be the cultural imperative within an ethnic group. A therapist can resolve these feelings by remembering that he or she must regard the client and his or her spouse as having equally important ethical concerns in making decisions. Case Examples 14.5 and 14.6 explore the ethical issues involved in a situation requiring cultural sensitivity.

Language

One specific aspect of culture is language. People communicate with each other through language. Language reflects people's culture, revealing where they live and their education level, ethnic group, and cultural affiliations. Case Example 14.7 illustrates ethical concerns a therapist must address when confronted with a language barrier.

Copyright

With the rapid advancement of information technology, copyright has become more complex and challenging. The current *Code and Ethics Standards* (AOTA, 2010a), the *Framework* (AOTA, 2014), and the *2011 Accreditation Council for Occupational Therapy Education (ACOTE®) Standards* (ACOTE, 2012) do not address copyright in sufficient detail. Copyright law poses a series of concerns for ethical professional behaviors.

As noted in the *Framework* (AOTA, 2014), evaluation includes information about the client and the client's needs, problems, and concerns about performance in areas of occupation. The analysis of occupational performance focuses on

---

CASE EXAMPLE 14.7. LANGUAGE BARRIER

An occupational therapist evaluated a previously healthy 10-year-old girl because of a fractured radius and generalized weakness. The girl and her parents spoke only Russian, and the facility did not have any Russian-speaking staff or interpreters. One of the housekeeping staff spoke broken Russian and was able to explain to the parents that the occupational therapist wanted to do an evaluation of their child.

The occupational therapist did an evaluation, including active and passive range of motion, muscle tone, and eye–hand coordination. The girl used scissors, tied her shoe, and played a variety of games. The parents were thankful for the attention and nodded in understanding. The therapist provided a written home program in English with expectations that the parents would actively engage their daughter in play. Three weeks later, the family returned and the girl had lost considerable function in all areas of occupational performance. Consider the following ethical questions:

- What would be proper preparation for working with this family?
- Are there any issues of autonomy that the therapist needs to consider?
- When a client is using an interpreter or translator, can a therapist make sound clinical judgments and reach conclusions with the same degree of certainty or effectiveness as when an interpreter is not needed?
- Was informed consent for treatment given?
- Is there a difference between working with clients of limited English proficiency and working with non-English speakers?
- Does the therapist have appropriate language skills for administering the evaluation in another language?

---

collecting and interpreting information using assessments designed to observe, measure, and inquire about factors that support or hinder occupational performance. Many occupational therapy professionals use copyrighted assessments, and occupational therapy educators use these same assessments in teaching students how to perform a particular assessment. Copyright guidelines address how frequently a therapist can use a photocopy of the evaluation booklet or score sheet, and for what purposes, without paying for the original assessment and score sheets.

According to R. Kifer (personal communication, dean, San Jose State University Library, July 2, 2013), a work is copyrighted when that work has been created in a tangible form, such as writing or recording. In the case of a single creator for a work created after January 1978, it is protected for the creator's life plus 70 years. If the work is created as a work-for-hire or in conjunction with one or more persons, the work is copyrighted for 95 years after the first publication or 120 years from creation, whichever expires first (U.S. Copyright Office, 2012).

The copyright law allows libraries and archives to reproduce and distribute one copy of a work under certain circumstances ("Limitations on Exclusive Rights: Reproduction by Libraries and Archives" of the Digital Millennium Copyright Act of 1998). For example, libraries may photocopy journal articles, book chapters, and so on, and send these copies to other libraries through interlibrary loan.

Copies of materials from libraries given to faculty, therapists, or students should have clearly printed on them "Notice: This material may be protected by Copyright Law (Title 17 U.S.C.)." Faculty and students have the ethical and legal duty to abide by the copyright laws. Therefore, faculty and others who reproduce several pages of a copy of a book may be in violation of the copyright laws (R. Kifer, personal communication, July 2, 2013). Guidelines for what a person can and cannot copy are widely available and should be sought out and reviewed before copying information for clients and other professionals. Answer the following questions to determine whether a person can use copyrighted material:

- Are there fees that the therapist must pay to use this assessment? If so, has the therapist paid the fees?
- Does the therapist need additional permission to use the assessment materials? Some assessments are available without charge (e.g., Behavioral and Emotional Screening System [Kamphaus & Reynolds, 2007]), but a therapist must obtain permission from the author before using them.

- Does use of the assessment require the evaluator to undergo any training and supervision to administer the evaluation? For example, a therapist should not use the Assessment of Motor Performance (Fisher & Jones, 2012) unless he or she has received training from the publisher or an approved representative of the publisher.
- Does the therapist who is administering the evaluation hold the appropriate credentials to do this evaluation? For example, some evaluations, such as the Vineland Adaptive Behavior Scales (Sparrow, Cichetti, & Balla, 2005), require that the evaluator be a licensed psychologist.
- In addition, the occupational therapist must be sure to use the correct forms and procedures when conducting the assessment and reporting the results. If the assessment is standardized, the therapist must follow the administration procedures as stipulated in the assessment manual.

Many assessments that occupational therapists use are not copyrighted. Evaluators must properly acknowledge the developer or publisher of any assessment used whenever writing an evaluation report; otherwise, readers of the report assume that the assessment is original to the occupational therapist doing the evaluation, which is rarely the case. Although there is a great deal of information about copyright available from the Library of Congress Copyright Office, an occupational therapist must seek out and ask an expert such as a librarian about copyright. Lack of knowledge is not an acceptable excuse for copyright infringement and is not ethical behavior. However, copyright obligations are not always clear-cut (see Case Example 14.8).

Ethical Dissent

There are situations in which an occupational therapist will follow his or her ethical decision, but in doing so, clashes with employer rules or legal regulations. These ethical judgments stem from the therapist's concern for others. In addition to personal moral philosophies, contextual factors such as rewards, rules, and codes also influence ethical decisions. In these cases, ethical distress occurs. The focus in resolving dilemmas cannot be only on the therapist's subjective ethical convictions; instead, the therapist must focus on the context of the ethical dilemmas.

Ethical dissent is a multistep process that involves feeling apart from one's organization and is driven by the following four factors: (1) the recognition of wrongdoing, (2) the need for intervention, (3) perceived responsibility, and (4) the screening of alternatives. ***Ethical dissent*** is essentially a person's expression of disagreement with an organization's practices, policies, and operations (Kassing, 1998). ***Whistleblowing***

CASE EXAMPLE 14.8. ETHICS OF COPYRIGHT

Harry and Louise are a husband-and-wife occupational therapy team and own a large practice in a metropolitan area. Their clinic rent has increased. Because of privacy laws and other regulations governing their practice, they have to complete and store extra paperwork. Some of their client records include drug tests, radiographic notes, physician notes, and physician's certifications for leaves of absence.

Lately, Harry and Louise have been discussing how to lower their overhead costs. Louise said that they should photocopy the evaluation booklet and score sheet for the copyrighted assessment they frequently use. They had been purchasing these sheets from the evaluation company at a cost of $50 per booklet and $50 for a packet of 25 score sheets. Harry is willing to try it. His primary concern is that the photocopying cost will not lower their expenditures, because he thinks it will exceed the rate negotiated with their photocopy company for number of copies and thus increase costs. Consider the following questions:

- What are the benefits and burdens associated with this case? How should they be assessed?
- What patient information do Harry and Louise have that they might not need?
- Is there any culpability involved with Harry and Louise having such extensive records?
- Are there any rules, regulations, guidelines, or laws that come into play in this situation?
- What copying of the evaluation does U.S. copyright law permit?
- Is there any harm associated with the actions of Harry and Louise?

is an extreme case of ethical dissent involving the disclosure of unethical practices to people both inside and outside of the organization who possess the ability to initiate a change in the outcome of a dilemma (Kassing, 1998). Ethical dissent in the form of whistleblowing may present a threat to the formal chain of command but can improve long-term organizational effectiveness.

Ethical dissent is broader than whistleblowing. Ethical dissent is considered an antecedent to whistleblowing because whistleblowers tend to express disagreements within the organizations initially and only turn to public, external sources when organizations are unresponsive to their concerns (Stewart, 1980). External sources are people outside of the normal departmental chain of command, such as the human resources department of a facility or the agency administrator. An occupational therapist should assess available strategies for expressing ethical dissent in response to personal, relational, and organizational influences that other people will not perceive as adversarial or unconstructive.

Confidentiality

Last, but certainly not least, are issues associated with evaluation and confidentiality. Principle 3 of the *Code and Ethics Standards* (AOTA, 2010a) addresses confidentiality; however, the concept is also embedded in beneficence, nonmaleficence, and veracity. Since the passage of HIPAA, an occupational therapist has to consider how, with whom, and when to share information regarding client care, including evaluations.

The purpose of HIPAA was to give clients control of their medical information when moving between locations. In essence, HIPAA states that professionals must maintain high levels of privacy and confidentiality and must handle information with the utmost care and security. Only people or groups with a clear need to have the information should receive it, and all privileged information—oral, written, and electronic—must be protected from unnecessary or casual access. Under HIPAA, a client:

- Must be told (in writing) how his or her personal health information (PHI) may be used,

- Has a right to see his or her medical records,
- Has a right to amend (change) incorrect or incomplete information in the records,
- Must give authorization before information is released (with a few exceptions), and
- Has a right to complain formally if he or she feels his or her privacy was not protected.

The privacy rule applies only to covered entities, which include individuals such as occupational therapists, health care organizations, health insurers, and clearinghouses that store or transmit PHI. These groups must comply with the privacy rule's requirements to protect the privacy of health information and provide people with access to and other rights regarding their health information. If an entity is not a covered entity—for example, another patient in a semiprivate hospital room who overhears a conversation between doctor and patient—it does not have to comply with the privacy rule. (More information about HIPAA is available from the official government website at http://www.hhs.gov/ocr/privacy/index.htm.)

The issue of confidentiality and evaluation is also important in the educational arena. **FERPA** provides parents the right to inspect and review education records, the right to make amendments to education records, and the right to have some degree of control over information that can be disclosed from education records. This statute extends to the records maintained by an educational agency of all children who receive services under Part B of IDEA.

Additionally, any student's medical or health records maintained in an educational agency or institution are viewed as "education records" and are subject to FERPA. It is the responsibility of therapists practicing in school systems to be aware of FERPA regulations and provide opportunities for parents to review evaluation reports. If the student is younger than 18 years of age, his or her parents have the right to make amendments to reports. Finally, therapists have to abide by the parents' wishes as to what information the school can share from the child's evaluation records. If the student is older than 18 years of age, the parents do not have the right to review the student's education records without the student's permission.

SUMMARY

As with other aspects of the intervention process, evaluation requires attention to professional requirements and the ethical and legal guidelines for good practice. An occupational therapist should be familiar with the list of ethical considerations regarding evaluation and assessment from the perspective of the key players in the process. Using the analysis system provided in this chapter and remaining cognizant of the differences and similarities between ethics and the law will help an occupational therapist resolve the ethical dilemmas encountered in practice.

QUESTIONS

1. Create a list of your own personal values. Identify ways that each value might influence your practice decisions regarding evaluation or assessment. Provide examples.
2. List how core values and attitudes may influence your professional behavior in regard to how you conduct an assessment.
3. We make decisions based on what we learned at home and in school, our ethnocultural traditions, and life experiences. Wild cards are events that we do not control that change the dynamics of our lives. Give an example of a wild card and how it has changed your life. How have the wild cards of technology changed how you view evaluation?
4. Today, technologies using very small, relatively inexpensive, wireless-enabled computers have resulted in the near omnipresence of information-gathering devices that can analyze, store, and share data via the Internet. Some of these technologies will also be autonomous, making decisions about what data to gather and share and what actions to take. Given these circumstances, how should an occupational therapist protect patient confidentiality?
5. You receive a referral from another professional for an evaluation. You do not think that this evaluation is necessary or beneficial to the client. How can you handle this situation? Are you obligated to perform this evaluation?
6. The facility where you work copies all assessment forms rather than purchasing this copyrighted material. What should you do in this situation?
7. An occupational therapist has evaluated a client and, on the basis of clinical observations, documents that this client needs services even though the assessment data do not support the need for intervention. If you were the treating therapist, what action would be appropriate?

ACKNOWLEDGMENTS

The author acknowledges Dr. Pamela Richardson, Dr. Al Copolillo, and the Occupational Therapy faculties at San Jose State University Occupational Therapy Program and Virginia Commonwealth University, Occupational Therapy Program; Dr. Marcie Weinstein, Associate Dean, College of Health Professions, Towson University; and Ruth E. Kifer, Dean, San Jose State Martin Luther King, Jr. Library, for their review and feedback on this chapter.

DISCLAIMER

The views expressed in this publication are solely the opinions of the author and do not necessarily reflect the official policies of the U.S. Department of Health and Human Services or the Health Resources and Services Administration, nor does mention of the department or agency names imply endorsement by the U.S. government.

References

Accreditation Council for Occupational Therapy Education. (2012). 2011 Accreditation Council for Occupational Therapy Education (ACOTE®) standards. *American Journal of Occupational Therapy, 66*(Suppl.), S6–S74. http://dx.doi.org/10.5014/ajot.2012.66S6

American Medical Association. (2002). *Racial and ethnic disparities in health care. Report from the council on scientific affairs.* Retrieved from http://www. ama-assn.org//ama/pub/about-ama/our-people/ member-groups-sections/minority-affairs-section/

news-resources/racialethnic-health-care-disparities. page

American Medical Informatics Association. (2013). *Ethical, legal, and social issues.* Retrieved from http://www.amia.org/programs/working-groups/ethical-legal-social-issues

American Occupational Therapy Association. (1976). Draft principles of occupational therapy ethics. *OT News, 30,* 4.

American Occupational Therapy Association. (1988). Occupational therapy code of ethics. *American Journal of Occupational Therapy, 42,* 795–796. http://dx.doi 10.5014/ajot.42.12.795

American Occupational Therapy Association. (1994). Occupational therapy code of ethics. *American Journal of Occupational Therapy, 48,* 1037–1038. http://dx.doi.org/10.5014/ajot.48.11.1037

American Occupational Therapy Association. (2005). Occupational therapy code of ethics. *American Journal of Occupational Therapy, 59,* 639–342. http://dx.doi.org/10.5014/ajot.59.6.639

American Occupational Therapy Association. (2010a). Occupational therapy code of ethics and ethics standards. *American Journal of Occupational Therapy, 64*(Suppl.), S17–S26. http://dx.doi.org/10.5014/ajot.2010.64S17

American Occupational Therapy Association. (2010b). Standards for continuing competence. *American Journal of Occupational Therapy, 64*(Suppl.), S103–S105. http://dx.doi.org/10.5014/ajot.2010.64S103me

American Occupational Therapy Association. (2010c). Standards of practice for occupational therapy. *American Journal of Occupational Therapy, 64*(Suppl.), S106–S111. http://dx.doi.org/10.5014/ajot.2010.64S106

American Occupational Therapy Association. (2013). Guidelines for documentation of occupational therapy. *American Journal of Occupational Therapy, 67*(Suppl.), S32–S38. http://dx.doi.org/10.5014/ajot.2013.67S32

American Occupational Therapy Association. (2014). Occupational therapy practice framework: Domain and process (3rd ed.). *American Journal of Occupational Therapy, 68*(Suppl. 1), S1–S48. http://dx.doi.org/10.5014/ajot.2014.682006

American Psychological Association. (2002). Ethical principles of psychologists and code of conduct. *American Psychologist, 57,* 1060–1073. http://dx.doi.org/10.1037/0003-066X.57.12.1060

American Psychological Association. (2010). *Ethical principles of psychologists and code of conduct with the 2010 amendments.* Washington, DC: Author. Retrieved from http://www.apa.org/ethics/code/index.aspx

American Recovery and Reinvestment Act of 2009, Pub. L. 111–5, 123 Stat. 115.

Balanced Budget Act of 1997, Pub. L. 105–33, 111 Stat. 251.

Baird, C. A. (2012). *EthicsGame: Online ethics curriculum tools.* http://www.ethicsgame.com/exec/site/index.html

Beauchamp, T. L., & Childress, J. F. (2009). *Principles of biomedical ethics* (6th ed.). New York: Oxford University Press.

Berlin, E. A., & Fowkes, W. C., Jr. (1983). A teaching framework for cross-cultural health care—Application in family practice. *Western Journal of Medicine, 139,* 934–938.

Civil Rights Act of 1964, Pub. L. 88–352, 78 Stat. 241.

Clinton, B. (1995, September 22). Address to Joint Session of Congress as delivered.

Digital Millennium Copyright Act of 1998, Pub. L. 105–304, 17 U.S.C. § 108.

Edelstein, L. (1943). *The Hippocratic oath: Text, translation, and interpretation.* Baltimore: Johns Hopkins Press.

Education of the Handicapped Act Amendments of 1983, Pub. L. 98–199, 97 Stat. 1357.

Family Educational Rights and Privacy Act of 1974, Pub. L. 93–380, 20 U.S.C. § 513.

Fisher, A. G., & Jones, K. B. (2012). *Assessment of Motor And Process Skills* (7th ed., rev.). Fort Collins, CO: Three Star Press.

Forrow, L. (March, 2008). Cultural differences complicate a terminal cancer diagnosis. *ACP Internist.* Retrieved from http://www.acpinternist.org/archives/2008/03/four.htm

Genachowski, J.; Federal Communications Commission. (2012, April). *Chairman remarks on stolen cell phones initiative.* Retrieved from http://www.fcc.gov/document/chairman-remarks-stolen-cell-phones-initiative

Gert, B. (2012). The definition of morality. In E. N. Zalta (Ed.), *The Stanford encyclopedia of philosophy.* Stanford, CA: Metaphysics Research Lab, Center for the Study of Language and Information. Retrieved from http://plato.stanford.edu/entries/morality-definition/

Hansen, R. A. (2005). Ethical implications in evaluation. In J. Hinojosa, P. Kramer, & P. Crist (Eds.), *Evaluation: Obtaining and interpreting data* (2nd ed., pp. 245–261). Bethesda, MD: AOTA Press.

Hansen, R. A., Kyler-Hutchison, P. L., & Trompetter, L. (1994, October). Ethical issues and the health professions. In *1994 Special Lecture Series.* Dallas, PA: College Misericordia.

Health Insurance Portability and Accountability Act of 1996, Pub. L. 104–19, 100 Stat. 2548.

Hinojosa, J., Kramer, P., & Crist, P. (Eds.). (2005). *Evaluation: Obtaining and interpreting data* (2nd ed.). Bethesda, MD: AOTA Press.

Individuals With Disabilities Education Act of 1990, Pub. L. 101–476, 20 U.S.C., Ch 33.

Individuals With Disabilities Education Improvement Act of 2004, Pub. L. 108–446, 20 U.S.C. § 1400 *et seq.*

Jonsen, A. R. (1986). Casuistry and clinical ethics. *Theoretical Medicine, 7,* 65–74. http://dx.doi.org/10.1007/BF00489424

Kamphaus, R. W., & Reynolds, C. R. (2007). *Behavior Assessment System for Children–Second edition (BASC–2): Behavioral and Emotional Screening System (BESS).* Bloomington, MN: Pearson.

Kassing, J. W. (1998). Development and validation of the organizational dissent scale. *Management Communication Quarterly, 12,* 183–229. http://dx.doi.org/10.1177/0893318998122002

Lohman, H., Gabriel, L., & Furlong, B. (2004). The bridge from ethics to public policy: Implications for occupational therapy practitioners. *American Journal of Occupational Therapy, 58,* 109–112. http://dx.doi.org/10.5014/ajot.58.1.109

Marek, K. (1997). Studies in health technology and informatics. *Studies in Health Technology and Informatics, 46,* 257–262.

Medicare Catastrophic Coverage Act of 1988, Pub. L. 100–360, 102 Stat. 683.

Neistadt, M. E. (2000). *Occupational therapy evaluation for adults: A pocket guide.* Baltimore: Lippincott Williams & Wilkins.

Patient Protection and Affordable Care Act of 2010, Pub. L. 111–148 124 § 119.

Peloquin, S. M. (2007). A reconsideration of occupational therapy's core values. *American Journal of Occupational Therapy, 61,* 474–478. http://dx.doi.org/10.5014/ajot.61.4.474

Purtilo, R. B., & Doherty, R. F. (2011). *Ethical dimensions in the health professions* (5th ed.). St. Louis: Elsevier/Saunders.

Rawls, J. (1999). *Theory of justice.* Boston: Harvard University Press.

Reich, R. (1991a). Secession of the successful. *New York Times Magazine,* 16–17.

Reich, R. B. (1991b). *The work of nations: Preparing ourselves for 21st-century capitalism.* New York: Alfred A. Knopf.

Rogers, J. C. (1983). Clinical reasoning: The ethics, science, and art [Eleanor Clarke Slagle Lecture]. *American Journal of Occupational Therapy, 37,* 601–616. http://dx.doi.org/10.5014/ajot.37.9.601

Rutherford, M. A. (2008). Standardized nursing language: What does it mean for nursing practice? *Online Journal of Issues in Nursing, 13*(1).

Sayre-McCord, G. (2012). Metaethics. *The Stanford encyclopedia of philosophy.* Stanford, CA: Metaphysics Research Lab, Center for the Study of Language and Information. Retrieved from http://plato.stanford.edu/entries/metaethics/

Schell, B. A. B. (2014). Professional reasoning in practice. In B. A. B. Schell, G. Gillen, & M. E. Scaffa (Eds.), *Willard and Spackman's occupational therapy* (12th ed., pp. 384–397). Philadelphia: Wolters Kluwer Health/Lippincott Williams & Wilkins.

Schell, B. B., & Schell, J. (2008). *Clinical and professional reasoning in occupational therapy.* Baltimore: Lippincott & Williams.

Sparrow, S., Cichetti, D., & Balla, D. (2005). *Vineland Adaptive Behavior Scale* (2nd ed.). Circle Pines, MN: American Guidance Services.

Stewart, L. P. (1980). Whistle blowing: Implications for organizational communication. *Journal of Communication, 30,* 90–101. http://dx.doi.org/10.1111/j.1460-2466.1980.tb02020.x

Thede, L., & Schwiran, P. (2011). Informatics: The standardized nursing terminologies: A national Survey of nurses' experiences and attitudes—Survey I. *Online Journal of Issues in Nursing, 16*(2), 12. http://dx.doi.org/10.3912/OJIN.Vol16No02InfoCol01

University of California–San Francisco, Department of Psychiatry. (2010). *What is cultural humility?* Retrieved from http://psych.ucsf.edu/sfgh/chtf/

U.S. Census Bureau. (2010). *2010 Census data.* Retrieved from http://www.census.gov/2010census/data/

U.S. Department of Health and Human Services. (2013). *Heath information privacy.* Retrieved from http://www.hhs.gov/ocr/privacy/hipaa/understanding/index.html

Veatch, R. M., & Flack, H. (1997). *Case studies in allied health ethics.* Upper Saddle River, NJ: Prentice Hall.

Veatch, R. M., & Haddad, A. M. (2008). *Case studies in pharmacy ethics* (2nd ed.). New York: Oxford University Press.

Welch, M. (1998). *Enhancing awareness and improving cultural competence in health care. A partnership guide for teaching diversity and cross-cultural concepts in heath professional training.* San Francisco: University of California.

Welsh, C. J. (2003). "Trapped": A mnemonic for taking a substance use history. *Academic Psychiatry, 27,* 289. http://dx.doi.org/10.1176/appi.ap.27.4.289

CHAPTER 15

Occupational Therapy Evaluation and Evidence-Based Practice

Jennifer S. Pitonyak, PhD, OTR/L, SCFES

Highlights

- What is evidence-based practice?
- How to engage in evidence-based practice
- A new evidence-based practice model for occupational therapy
- What are the data of occupational therapy practice?

Key Terms

Case studies
Correlation coeffecient
Correlation research
Descriptive or observational studies
Evidence-based practice
External validity
Impact factor
Internal validity
Meta-analysis

Nonexperimental studies
Qualitative research
Quantitative research
Quasi-experimental research
Randomized controlled trials
Respected opinion
Single-hierarchy models
Single-subject studies

This chapter discusses how evidence-based practice within occupational therapy influences the evaluation of clients. It begins with a history and description of traditional evidence-based practice and also presents current thinking in the profession on aligning evidence-based practice with theory-directed practice and the epistemology of the profession (Fleming-Castaldy & Gillen, 2013; Hinojosa, 2013; Tomlin & Borgetto, 2011).

From that base, the chapter presents ways to use data from evaluation and reevaluation to inform practice decisions and offers examples of evidence-based practice literature. Using evaluation data, an

occupational therapist can develop evidence needed to support his or her practice. The collection, organization, and examination of aggregate evaluation data build evidence for assessment methods and suggest specific interventions. The chapter concludes with a discussion on how to disseminate the evidence to promote evidence-based practice.

Occupational therapy students, therapists, assistants, educators, researchers, and policy makers must understand the importance of evidence-based practice for the profession. The objectives of this chapter are to describe the process of evidence-based practice and its relationship to occupational therapy evaluation; to examine traditional and emerging evidence-based practice models for usefulness in occupational therapy evaluation; and to apply evidence-based practice principles to occupational therapy evaluation through examples from the literature.

WHAT IS EVIDENCE-BASED PRACTICE?

Evidence-based practice in health care is a process that combines the current best-published evidence with practitioner expertise and client preferences when determining appropriate therapeutic interventions (Ilott, 2003; Law & Baum, 1998; Sackett, Rosenberg, Gray, Haynes, & Richardson, 1996; Straus, Richardson, Glasziou, & Haynes, 2010). There are various definitions of *evidence-based practice* in the literature, and most reflect this interaction among evidence; expertise; and client values, beliefs, and preferences. Sackett and his colleagues (1996) advised that the best evidence comes from combining clinical expertise and knowledge gained through practice with pertinent published clinical research.

The underlying concepts for evidence-based practice have evolved from the concept of *evidence-based medicine,* a phrase first coined during the 1980s at McMaster Medical School in Canada (Rosenberg & Donald, 1995). Supporters of evidence-based practice recognize that the ability to provide best care requires the integration of current best evidence, practitioner expertise, and client preferences (Law & MacDermid, 2008a; Lee & Miller, 2003; Sackett et al., 1996).

Evidence-based practice includes clinical reasoning and constant reflection, similar to the occupational therapy evaluation process. Before one can consider this relationship between evidence-based practice and evaluation, it is first necessary to understand what evidence-based practice is and how an occupational therapist can practice from an evidence-based perspective.

The occupational therapy process is a dynamic one that can vary, not only for each client–therapist partnership but also over the course of an individual intervention (Lee & Miller, 2003). Evidence-based practice requires therapists to be inquisitive; engage in self-directed, lifelong learning; be willing to consider evidence that conflicts with their current knowledge and beliefs; and be able to communicate research findings to clients and their families. Therapists need to select and examine the best available evidence in the form of published reviews or expert opinions. Further, as consumers of evidence, therapists need to be able to critically analyze existing research to determine whether findings translate to practice.

The occupational therapist begins engaging in evidence-based practice when he or she receives a referral to evaluate a client. The therapist uses procedural clinical reasoning to select assessment methods most commonly used for screening people with the referral problem. The screening further informs the therapist about which evidence-based and theory-directed assessments to use.

As the evaluation continues, the therapist develops a clear and searchable question related to client needs or the planned method of assessment. Once the therapist decides on the questions, he or she should search the literature for the most current and relevant evidence (Ilott, 2003; Rosenberg & Donald, 1995; Taylor, 1997). Evidence-based practice requires that a therapist be able to locate evidence quickly and easily (Dysart & Tomlin, 2002; Ilott, 2003; Lloyd-Smith, 1997). Searching databases for literature is a skill that improves with practice. A therapist is encouraged to use resources such as the reference librarians at public or university libraries and online tutorials.

After locating current and relevant literature, the therapist carefully reads it. While reading the published summaries, the therapist notes the information about the assessments and their use. The therapist combines the evidence reported and documented with his or her own clinical expertise.

While reading, the therapist examines each assessment and administration methods along with other information. One area to focus on is the information provided about the particular client issues and the client's (and family's) particular values, beliefs, and preferences (Ilott, 2003; Taylor, 1997). Evidence-based evaluation includes the use of assessment and administration methods that best match with the client's needs and therapist's identified theoretical perspective, rather than just the use of clinically available assessments.

Throughout the occupational therapy intervention process, the therapist continually evaluates the outcomes of intervention (Ilott, 2003). These occupational therapy intervention outcomes may be in such areas as client performance, quality of life, or intervention effectiveness. When assessing outcomes, the therapist must consider the accuracy of the assessments in measuring change.

Practicing from an evidence-based perspective has many advantages for occupational therapists. Perhaps the most important advantage is that evidence-based practice forces a therapist to upgrade his or her knowledge of current best practice (Taylor, 1997). Evidence-based practice helps therapists justify and demonstrate the effectiveness of their interventions to clients, families, and payers of health care services (Lloyd-Smith, 1997). Evidence-based practice allows for effective use of resources by enabling the occupational therapist and the client to focus efforts on interventions that have a greater likelihood of success (Taylor, 1997). The use of evidence-based practice helps an occupational therapist to identify assessments and interventions that have become standard practice but have not yet been recognized as best practice (Law & MacDermid, 2008b).

Tickle-Degnen (2002) identified several ways a therapist can use evidence-based practice during the early rapport-building stages of a therapist–client interaction, beginning with the initial evaluation of a client. As described earlier, it is important that a therapist explore the literature to identify the most appropriate, valid, and reliable assessments and administration methods to gather pertinent client information. During this exploration, the therapist focuses on the specific assessments used and how the therapist used them.

A therapist also might explore more descriptive or qualitative literature that provides information about the occupational desires, needs, and lifestyles of other people with similar diagnoses or characteristics as his or her clients. The therapist may find this information useful when using qualitative or nonstandardized methods of collecting data for the client's occupational profile.

Information obtained in the descriptive or qualitative literature may also be helpful as a point of discussion with the client to identify similarities and differences with the client's situation, while aiding rapport building by allowing the therapist an opportunity to show interest, knowledge, and awareness of others in similar situations. The therapist may also choose to share current understanding regarding the efficacy of therapeutic interventions as part of the client's education in the occupational therapy process.

> It is important for a therapist to explore the literature to identify the most appropriate, valid, and reliable assessments and administration methods to gather pertinent client information during an occupational therapy evaluation.

HOW TO ENGAGE IN EVIDENCE-BASED PRACTICE

In the traditional use of evidence-based practice, an occupational therapist bases decisions for evaluations, interventions, and outcomes on the best available published evidence, his or her clinical reasoning, and the client's response to the occupational therapy interventions. This section first presents traditional evidence-based practice models from medicine applied in occupational therapy and then examines a new evidence-based practice model that more closely aligns with the occupational therapy process.

The best evidence for practice is information obtained from peer-reviewed journals. Peer-reviewed publications provide expert evaluation of the material before dissemination; therefore, the reader knows that experts have evaluated the manuscript to determine that it has sufficient trustworthiness for publication. Within the realm of peer-reviewed publications, the best evidence for practice comes from journals with a high **impact factor** that establishes the journal's reputation. These research publications can use either quantitative or qualitative methods.

Therapists need evidence to support evaluation and treatment decisions. The relevance of research findings to practice depends on the direct applicability of the study, the design of the study, the method of intervention used within the study, and the number of persons studied. Common sense indicates that the closer a study is to the practice situation under question, the more applicable it will be. Studies that have the same population as the client or group in question will be more generalizable than those with populations with different conditions. Often the best available evidence may be in the literature of a related population or field, so a therapist needs to extrapolate the evidence from related studies that best fit the situation under consideration.

The more rigorous the design of the study, the more likely it is that a therapist can use the findings to support his or her practice decisions. Experimental studies with appropriate controls, interventions, and measures may provide a therapist with confidence in the study findings. A therapist, however, needs to consider the artificiality of controlled experiments against the reality of practice; therefore, he or she needs to understand the various research methods and the strengths and weaknesses of each.

A therapist can also obtain evidence-based support from empirical observations. They can range from clinical observations made in practice settings to tightly controlled observations in experimental research. Each type of observation has its own limitations. Generally, clinical observations are limited by small sample sizes and, more importantly, by the observer's biases. Similarly, there are limitations to observations in experimental research because of the strictly controlled environment of the study.

In the literature, experts have presented many hierarchies that rank the rigor of the various research methods and their applicability to practice (Helewa & Walker, 2000; Law & Philp, 2002; Lloyd-Smith, 1997; Sackett, 1989). The experts who have developed most of these hierarchies regard sophisticated quantitative research methods as providing more valid results. Figure 15.1 illustrates a commonly used hierarchy.

One characteristic that all hierarchies share is the basic structure of putting the expert deciding which research provides the most valid research evidence at the top and the less stringent or less applicable evidence below. Some experts in medicine base their hierarchies on scientists' studies in highly controlled laboratory settings. These studies take place in artificial environments and often use tissue samples or animals as subjects. Although these studies have the most rigor in terms of experimental validity, laboratory studies are rarely applicable to occupational therapy.

The hierarchy presented in Figure 15.1 was developed based on in vivo studies involving human beings. It was adapted from Lloyd-Smith (1997), who puts meta-analyses at the top and respected opinion at the base. The following sections describe in more detail the levels of evidence included in this hierarchy and strategies for evaluation of quantitative data.

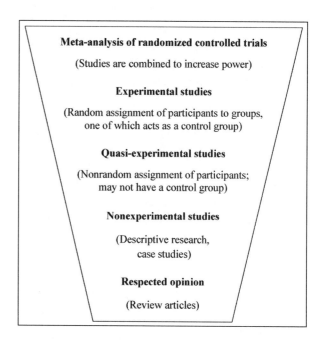

Figure 15.1. Hierarchy of support for evidence-based practice.

Note. From "Evidence-Based Practice and Occupational Therapy," by W. Lloyd-Smith, 1997, *British Journal of Occupational Therapy*, 60, 474–479. Adapted with permission.

How to Evaluate Quantitative Evidence

Respected opinion

The first level on the **quantitative research** hierarchy of evidence presented in Figure 15.1 is respected opinion. **Respected opinions** from knowledgeable people within a field can be a good start for clinical decision making when they are supported with appropriate scientific evidence to provide trustworthiness. In applied fields such as occupational therapy and psychology, research publication commonly lags behind the publication of theory and opinion. A therapist needs to be aware of the psychometrics published in assessment manuals. More importantly, a therapist needs to read reviews of assessments in journals and periodicals because the reviews may be more critical than the manuals.

When research studies about evaluation or assessments are not available, the best available evidence is that of published opinion, including published reviews. An example is a recent review article in the *American Journal of Occupational Therapy* that presented an in-depth analysis of driving assessments for use in evidence-based practice (Classen et al., 2009). Common places for finding reviews of assessments are the *Mental Measurement Yearbook* website (www.unl.edu/buros), the *Educational Testing Service* website (http://ets.org/tests/), and *StrokEngine Assess* website (http://strokengine.ca/assess/).

Nonexperimental studies

Moving up the hierarchy, the next level of evidence comprises studies characterized as **nonexperimental studies,** which are research studies that either have no manipulation or have an intervention that the researcher does not control. Such studies describe observation of an already occurring or ongoing event.

There are generally three types of studies classified as nonexperimental: (1) descriptive studies, (2) case studies, and (3) correlation research. **Descriptive or observational studies** describe an event or characteristic of a group. When examining these studies relative to evaluation, the therapist needs to consider the specific assessments used to determine outcomes. A recent example of descriptive evidence that informs assessment selection in occupational therapy is Kramer, Kielhofner, and Smith's (2010) study of the validity of the Child Occupational Self-Assessment (Keller, Kafkes, Basu, Federico, & Kielhofner, 2005).

Case studies, another type of nonexperimental research, are used to develop clinical knowledge. They are in-depth studies of one client and his or her disease course and response to treatment. Case studies are directly applicable to client care. However, because case studies use only one or a few participants, their generalizability to other clients or other environments is limited.

When reading a case study, the therapist needs to review the occupational therapy process, including the assessments used and how the treating therapist measured outcomes. Because of the nature of case studies, the therapist should be attentive to the methodology and interpretations of the author, and the reliability and validity of the assessments and process used. A good example of a case study is Kardos and White's (2006) case study demonstrating the use of assessments for the development of transition planning for a secondary school student with cognitive disabilities.

Correlation research examines relationships between variables, or in the situation of test development, correlation is used to establish interrater,

test–retest, or other types of reliability. The strength of the relationship between variables is measured by using a statistic called a **correlation coefficient.** A recent example of the use of correlation to establish test reliability in the *American Journal of Occupational Therapy* is the study of a new assessment for near-task home lighting for older adults with low vision (Perlmutter et al., 2013). It is important to understand that correlation research does not demonstrate that Variable A caused Variable B but that the variables are somehow linked, as is the case with test reliability.

Quasi-experimental research

The third level from the base of the hierarchy is **quasi-experimental research,** which involves manipulation of an independent variable and measurement of a dependent variable. Quasi-experimental studies do not randomly assign participants to groups; these studies may have only one group under study, or they may involve multiple groups. If more than one group is used, the groups are nonequivalent, because participants within the groups are not randomly assigned. With respect to evaluation, again, the therapist needs to attend to the specific assessments used and the measurement of the dependent variable.

The results of quasi-experimental studies generally have less internal validity than true experiments but, because they study preexisting groups, may have greater external validity or generalizability compared with true experiments (Portney & Watkins, 2009). These types of studies may have great applicability to practice. For example, Baum et al. (2008) studied the validity and reliability of the Executive Function Performance Test (Baum, Morrison, Hahn, & Edwards, 2003) in a matched-control study. In this quasi-experimental study, they demonstrated the use of an assessment for occupational therapy practice.

Experimental studies

The fourth level from the base of the hierarchy of evidence contains studies that use true experimental designs, commonly referred to as **randomized controlled trials (RCTs).** These studies are designed within experimental parameters, participants are randomly assigned to treatment or no-treatment groups, and independent and dependent variables are determined by the researcher.

Just as when reviewing quasi-experimental studies, the therapist needs to focus on the assessments used. Gutman, Kerner, Zombek, Dulek, and Ramsey (2009) presented an RCT demonstrating the effectiveness of an occupational therapy intervention for adults with psychiatric disabilities in which they use several assessments to evaluate participants before and after intervention. Similarly, Miller, Coll, and Schoen (2007) conducted a pilot RCT of the effectiveness of occupational therapy using a sensory integration approach, by using a diversity of pretest and posttest measures of behavior, sensory, and adaptive functioning.

Meta-analysis of randomized control trials

The top level in the quantitative research hierarchy consists of studies that use **meta-analysis,** a statistical procedure for combining data from multiple studies to determine the effect of the intervention. Unlike a review article, the meta-analysis does not merely summarize the results from individual studies. Combining individual RCTs increases the power of meta-analysis over that of a single study, improving the estimate of the effect size the intervention provides and the ability to generalize the results (Portney & Watkins, 2009).

Meta-analyses usually involve studies with the same target population and intervention, providing greater certainty of the effect of an intervention. Because meta-analyses pool data from many RCTs, they also increase the external validity of the results. The results are generalized more readily to multiple settings. Unfortunately, there are relatively few meta-analyses in the occupational therapy and health profession literature. In meta-analysis, because the concern lies with the variables of interest, the authors often do not identify or discuss assessments in great depth. Although meta-analytic studies are important pieces of evidence, they usually do not have much relevance to evidence-based practice in evaluation.

How to Evaluate Qualitative Evidence

Often, the therapist will not find published quantitative evidence to directly support his or her specific concerns. Another area in which to find evidence is the field of qualitative research. This section covers evaluation of qualitative studies for

evidence-based practice. Again, when reviewing qualitative literature, the therapist should review the assessments used to determine their appropriateness for the client's needs, reliability and validity of the data collected, and the manner in which the study authors used the assessments.

Qualitative research provides a therapist with evidence that helps him or her form relationships with clients and informs understanding of how clients live their lives and what they value. This understanding can guide the occupational therapist in how to evaluate a client to obtain the most pertinent information to guide client-centered practice (Hammell, 2004).

The occupational therapist needs to evaluate the various types of qualitative research, just like quantitative research, for trustworthiness and credibility. Unlike quantitative research, however, qualitative research does not have a hierarchy that ranks the rigor of the research. Nevertheless, many publications suggest how to evaluate qualitative research for evidence-based practice (Cohen & Crabtree, 2008; Devers, 1999; Dixon-Woods, Shaw, Agarwal, & Smith, 2004; Giacomini & Cook, 2000; Greenhalgh & Taylor, 1997; Henderson & Rheault, 2004; Popay & Williams, 1998).

> Qualitative research provides a therapist with evidence that helps him or her form relationships with clients and informs understanding of how clients live their lives and what they value.

The therapist needs to determine whether the research article addresses the therapist's clinical question about evaluation in some meaningful way. Often, qualitative research studies will address a broad query without extensive detail on evaluation. In the process of addressing the query, however, the authors may present ideas on how they gained access to the participants and built trust and rapport, which may be important when initiating or carrying out an evaluation. A therapist can use information from these examples to refine his or her methods of evaluating a client.

A major issue with qualitative research is the potential for bias. Qualitative researchers are the data-collection tool for their studies (Toma, 2006). When examining phenomena, the researcher decides which data are relevant and which to collect. Inductive reasoning drives data analysis. Qualitative researchers reflect upon their own personal perspectives, values, and interests and the way in which these factors influence the research process (Patton,

2002; Toma, 2006). The researcher addresses personal bias in the methods section with a discussion on reflexivity that demonstrates how researcher bias was handled in data collection and analyses.

In a qualitative study, Doig, Fleming, Cornwell, and Kuipers (2009) examined the use of a client-centered, goal-directed therapy from the perspective of adults with traumatic brain injury receiving care in a community-based setting. In their analysis, the researchers identified the importance of significant others and the treating occupational therapist. Further, Doig and colleagues described the use of the Canadian Occupational Performance Measure (COPM; Law et al., 2005) and goal attainment scaling in the evaluation and goal-setting process.

Doig and colleagues (2009) described several positive themes that emerged from semistructured interviews with the participant groups (i.e., clients, significant others, occupational therapists), including benefits resulting from the structure that was provided by goal-directed therapy, positive impact of clear goals on motivation, and a sense of goal ownership by clients. They outlined a process to ensure quality and rigor, with a specified number of interviews that the researcher and an assistant independently coded. In addition, the researchers had colleagues check to ensure that they had appropriately described and defined the new codes and categories.

Missing from Doig and colleagues' (2009) report, however, was a description of a reflective process wherein the researchers identified their perspectives and critically analyzed the influence these perspectives may have had on the data analysis process. An occupational therapist working with a similar population may choose to explore further the applicability of the COPM and goal attainment scaling in his or her practice but should seek out additional literature to learn a variety of perspectives on each assessment being considered.

A therapist should carefully read the qualitative research article conclusions. In this section, the qualitative researchers should present evidence from the outcomes and the literature to support their conclusions. Therefore, the presentation of the data should adequately describe each theme. The researchers also should describe how the theme was developed. Further, when reading such articles through the lens of an evaluator, the therapist should examine carefully the assessments used and their appropriateness given the study question.

Although qualitative studies may not use formal assessments, they provide rich data for the therapist to determine how to evaluate clients.

In general, an occupational therapist will find that qualitative research is more accessible and perhaps more directly related to practice. A therapist needs to remember, however, the individual nature of the reality addressed through qualitative research and carefully consider how the assessments were used within the studies.

A NEW EVIDENCE-BASED PRACTICE MODEL FOR OCCUPATIONAL THERAPY

The *Centennial Vision* of the American Occupational Therapy Association (2007) called for occupational therapy to be a science-driven and evidence-based profession, and scholars of the profession agree that translating evidence to practice is important for demonstrating the effectiveness of occupational therapy services (Fleming-Castaldy & Gillen, 2013; Hinojosa, 2013; Lin, Murphy, & Robinson, 2010; Thomas & Law, 2013). However, scholars have also voiced concern about definitive acceptance of research evidence in single-hierarchy evidence-based practice models (Hinojosa, 2013; Tomlin & Borgetto, 2011) over practitioner expertise and client response. For example, important qualitative constructs of our profession, such as client-centeredness, conflict with **single-hierarchy models** that rank true experimental designs over all other types of evidence.

Client-centered occupational therapy evaluation requires the therapist to select appropriate assessment methods supported not only by science but also by theory. Single-hierarchy evidence-based practice models are often inconsistent with the clinical reasoning of practitioners (Hinojosa, 2013; Tickle-Degnen & Bedell, 2003; Tomlin & Borgetto, 2011) and lack the ability to evaluate qualitative evidence. However, Hinojosa (2013) proposed several directions for action to bridge evidence-based and theory-directed practice, most

> Important qualitative constructs of our profession, such as client-centeredness, conflict with single-hierarchy models that rank true experimental designs over all other types of evidence. Client-centered occupational therapy evaluation requires the therapist to select appropriate assessment methods supported not only by science but also by theory.

importantly the need for an evidence-based model in occupational therapy that comprehensively evaluates evidence relevant to occupation.

Tomlin and Borgetto (2011) introduced a more comprehensive model of the research hierarchy to occupational therapy, the Research Pyramid, portrayed in Figure 15.2. The Research Pyramid more closely aligns with the philosophical underpinnings of the profession and addresses some of the limitations of single-hierarchy evidence-based practice models, one being the oversimplification and confounding of criteria of rigor (i.e., **internal validity**) and applicability (i.e., **external validity**). The ranking of evidence in single-hierarchy evidence-based practice models suggests that research designs with stronger internal validity also have stronger external validity.

Single-hierarchy models rank research designs, such as RCTs with high internal validity, as best evidence, yet statistically significant results in a controlled trial may not translate to meaningful or usable evidence in real-world situations. This assumption of single-hierarchy models fails to consider the limitations in generalizing findings of tightly controlled trials carried out with systematic procedures to diverse clinical and real-world situations.

Occupational therapy evaluation carried out in clinical and real-world settings requires both quantitative and qualitative evidence to fully inform occupational therapy decision making. As shown in Figure 15.2, the Research Pyramid addresses this concern with two orthogonal axes: (1) quantitative–qualitative and (2) internal–external validity. The Research Pyramid is constructed of three faces: (1) experimental research, (2) qualitative research, and (3) outcome research, providing a model that evaluates comprehensive forms of evidence and better aligns with clinical reasoning used during occupational therapy evaluation.

The Research Pyramid also addresses the limited consideration given to large-scale, population-based outcome studies in single-hierarchy models. Population-based outcome studies use observational methods and therefore lack the ability to randomly assign participants to various conditions. However, the inherently low internal validity of population-based outcome studies is tempered by the increased generalizability of this research design to real-life situations.

Ciro (2011) called for the profession to increase use of observational or epidemiological methods.

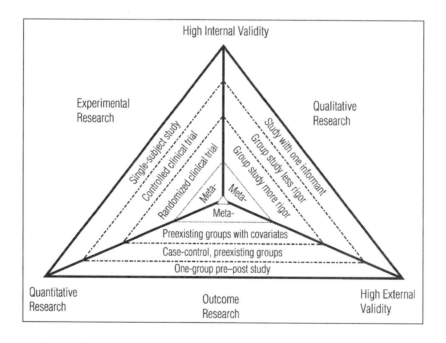

Figure 15.2. Research Pyramid.
Note. Meta = meta-analyses.
From "Research Pyramid: A New Evidence-Based Practice Model for Occupational Therapy," by G. Tomlin & B. Borgetto, 2011, *American Journal of Occupational Therapy, 65,* p. 191. Copyright © 2011 by the American Occupational Therapy Association. Used with permission.

Epidemiological research designs inform the understanding of various health conditions, which for occupational therapists means understanding occupational performance disabilities and related factors. Intervention effectiveness, the focus of single-hierarchy models that rank controlled trials as best evidence, is certainly important to occupational therapy; however, observational and qualitative research designs may offer better evidence for informing decision making in the overall occupational therapy process. Figure 15.2 illustrates the Research Pyramid's consideration of observational, or outcome, research.

WHAT ARE THE DATA OF OCCUPATIONAL THERAPY PRACTICE?

When neither quantitative nor qualitative evidence is available to support a therapist's practice, the best support for practice is practice itself. To use individual practice data as support for subsequent decisions, the therapist needs to know what data are available that support practice, how to evaluate the source of the data, how to compile the data, and how to disseminate his or her findings so others can benefit from them.

An evidence-based perspective on occupational therapy practice as it relates to evaluation can lead the occupational therapist to think about the data he or she generates through practice. The therapist must decide how to document outcomes and the efficacy of occupational therapy interventions. The therapist may begin to seek evidence that a particular intervention strategy, whether an old favorite or a new approach, is most effective in helping clients regain occupational performance.

When designing new programs, the therapist should conscientiously include evaluative outcome measures that will assist in the creation of clinical evidence to support practice. Administrators and third-party payers may have therapists justify the effectiveness of their interventions. Justifying the effectiveness of interventions and providing clinical evidence to support practice require the occupational therapist to identify the data that support practice and carefully consider what other data he or she should collect and analyze.

Occupational therapy practice is rich with potential areas of data collection to support

occupational therapy intervention, explore the therapeutic process, and understand better the lived experience of clients receiving occupational therapy services. This information can be relevant when analyzing the impact of occupational therapy intervention to help determine whether changes resulted specifically from occupational therapy intervention or from a combination of factors.

The sources of data are important in determining the impact of intervention and applicability of outcomes data. One example of a secondary analysis informing the lived experience of clients with multiple sclerosis is a recent study by Finlayson, Preissner, and Cho (2012) examining the degree to which age, gender, work status, or impairment moderated the outcomes of a fatigue management program. Thoughtful consideration of evaluation and reevaluation data can help the therapist produce outcomes data either in a prospective analysis of practice or in a retrospective chart review. Exhibit 15.1 includes questions a therapist can ask himself or herself when selecting an assessment and developing documentation strategies.

Determining the efficacy of intervention requires the therapist to look at the outcome measurement for intervention strategies. Depending on the goal of outcomes assessment, the occupational therapist may choose to collect data based on a specific guideline for intervention. For example, if the therapist uses the person–environment–occupation approach (Law et al., 1996), he or she may set out to collect specific data on the person's skills, abilities, experiences, or roles;

EXHIBIT 15.1. QUESTIONS TO ASK WHEN SELECTING ASSESSMENTS

Some evidence-based questions a therapist can use to guide selection of assessments and to develop strategies for documenting evaluation findings include
- What data are treatment decisions based on?
- Are the data from standardized assessments valid and reliable?
- Can the therapist generalize data collected from nonstandardized assessments to other clients whom the therapist sees or to other practice settings?
- Do evaluation and reevaluation results demonstrate that occupational therapy intervention was effective for a particular client or population?

environmental set-up, cues, barriers, or supports; the occupations the client engages in or wishes to engage in; and the relationship of all these components to occupational performance and occupational therapy intervention. The occupational therapist then can relate the results of his or her research back to the theoretical approach, further validating that approach as an appropriate guide to practice (Ottenbacher & Hinderer, 2001).

Using Data Generated From Practice

It is often difficult to apply the findings of studies to practice settings. It may be impossible to find any published literature that provides direct evidence for practice decisions. However, practice itself offers a rich opportunity to accumulate the data necessary to make informed decisions. Although it is difficult to conduct RCTs within the confines of clinical practice, two types of studies are feasible within the clinical setting and offer a therapist the ability to gather data through practice: (1) case studies and (2) single-subject designs. **Case studies** are a form of nonexperimental research, and **single-subject studies** qualify as quasi-experimental research.

Case studies often start with an interesting clinical problem. Unlike a single-subject study, case studies typically involve no systematic collection of baseline data before the implementation of intervention. Often a case study is retrospective; the therapist recognizes later that a case is interesting or unique or that a unique intervention produced optimal outcomes.

Case studies arise out of the general course of practice. Unlike research that the therapist undertakes for the sake of gaining new knowledge, case studies are the documentation of new knowledge that the therapist gained serendipitously through practice. For example, Carver (2009) presented a case study that describes the process of assisting a client with multiple brain injuries to learn to self-catheterize and the development of a custom piece of adaptive equipment for this task.

Case studies offer therapists a unique opportunity to provide evidence to the clinical community. A well-documented case study can provide evidence for practice and contribute to the generation of hypotheses for more formal research endeavors. By documenting cases in a systematic manner, a therapist can begin to amass the data necessary for larger, more experimentally valid research.

A typical single-subject study starts with the measurement of baseline data. Baseline data represent the state of the outcome variable, or target behavior, before any intervention. A therapist can obtain baseline data as part of the initial evaluation process. Then the therapist compares the baseline state of the target behavior to new data gathered after phases in the study during which the therapist applies or withdraws interventions. The therapist collects data over all phases of the study and can incorporate this data collection into reassessment practices. Data collection usually results from objective, quantitative evaluations. Data often address the frequency of occurrence of the target behavior in the presence or absence of the interventions.

> A well-documented case study can provide evidence for practice and contribute to the generation of hypotheses for more formal research endeavors. By documenting cases in a systematic manner, a therapist can begin to amass the data necessary for larger, more complex study.

Qualitative evidence from evaluation and reevaluation also can provide data for a single-subject study. These qualitative data can describe the roles a person has, how they are valued, and whether the roles or their value changes over the course of intervention. One strategy to collect this type of data may be through using the COPM during evaluation and reevaluation. Qualitative data can describe the process of an intervention and whether the client values it, thereby providing information on the likelihood of carryover of recommendations. Qualitative data also can provide important information about cultural values and beliefs that can affect occupational therapy outcomes, including those related to illness, disability, and role performance.

Gathering Data

An occupational therapist generates large volumes of data in day-to-day evaluation, treatment, reassessment, and reevaluation of clients, as well as through case studies and single-subject studies. To use these data to demonstrate outcomes and provide evidence for practice, a therapist needs to organize the data and ensure that the information obtained on individual clients is available for later use. The easiest and most efficient method of compiling data is to develop a database. With the use of readily available commercial software packages, setting up a database is relatively easy to do.

Determining important data

The first step in setting up a database is determining what data are important. In general, a database should start with the variables that describe the clients. The first descriptor should be a unique identification number for each person in the database. It is important to adhere to Health Insurance Portability and Accountability Act of 1996 regulations and protect the anonymity of clients when assigning identifiers. The use of patient numbers and Social Security numbers is inappropriate because these numbers can be connected easily to a client's private information. Therefore, the numbers used for a database should be unique and not connected to the client other than for the purpose of the database. A therapist must keep Social Security numbers, patient numbers, and other unique identifiers secure and separate from the overall database.

Once identifiers are determined, the next category of descriptive information is demographic data, such as age, race, gender, diagnosis, and medical history. The therapist needs to collect demographic data to describe the characteristics of the people in a given group. Demographic data are also important sources of potential confounding variables when attempting to determine the effectiveness of a treatment. Access to these data allows for analysis of the impact of demographic variables on the outcome of interest.

Collect information from assessments

The second step is to collect information generated from assessments used in the evaluation and reevaluation of individual clients. It is important that a therapist collect all the pertinent outcome information during evaluations and reevaluations. These data also need to be coded and recorded in the database. Use of standardized assessments ensures that the data collected are both valid and reliable, which strengthens the conclusions drawn from the data and aids in replication of the interventions.

When setting up a database, it is best to collect as much data as possible. It is better to have data available and not needed than to need the data and not have them. Therefore, a therapist should include all information possible pertaining to diagnosis and treatment—not just treatment provided by the occupational therapist, but concomitant treatments as well, including all medication. This information will be helpful in future analyses when explaining other possible causes for the outcomes. For example, Dunn, Carlson, Jackson, and Clark (2009) used personal information profiles from a previous qualitative research study to examine how clients with spinal cord injury responded after developing a low-grade pressure ulcer.

Databases provide valuable archival information. It is important to take sufficient time to set up a comprehensive and well-documented database; otherwise, the therapist will find himself or herself with data that are not clearly defined, not adequately documented, or too difficult to compile after the fact. Taking the time to plan and set up a well-thought-out database will ensure that, when it comes time to analyze and disseminate the data, the data will be in a useable form. Further, a clear record of exactly what information the therapist collected for each variable can be easily accessed without having to rely on human memory or information from other sources.

Disseminating Data

The knowledge base in any field is highly dependent on the dissemination of information in a public forum. In general, scientific knowledge progresses through the sharing of results, the critical evaluation of the results over time, and the replication of results in other settings. Without this cycle, therapists and researchers rely on outdated or erroneous information. Evidence-based practice is dependent on the public sharing of the newest and best available information for practice.

There are many levels in the dissemination of information. The first level consists of colleagues within the therapist's own institution or immediate community. This informal sharing of information can provide an initial level of feedback that helps a therapist refine ideas and processes. Journal clubs, brown bag lunches, and newsletters are ideal and low-pressure methods for initially bringing ideas into a public forum. However, the therapist should not stop at this level because peer reviews of articles focus on the content and not on analyzing the credibility of the study.

Once assured by colleagues that results are useful, the therapist has a professional and moral obligation to disseminate them to a wider forum. Publications and conference presentations are the two major avenues for disseminating new information. Publications provide the broadest dissemination and the greatest level of critical review. Conference presentations may be particularly effective if the proceedings of the conference are published. Although conference presentations move information to the public more quickly, they are not optimal because the level of critical review is not the same as a juried publication. Additionally, with a presentation, the audience is usually still limited and often biased toward a particular topic. However, conference presentations often provide interesting opportunities to discuss outcomes with colleagues, ways to potentially improve the study, and the experiences of other professionals with specific assessments.

Publication is the primary way of disseminating information to the public and ensuring that the information will be retrievable in the future. Publication can take the form of journal articles, books and book chapters, or magazines and newsletters. In general, journals serve the purpose of presenting new and interesting information, books and book chapters present reviews, and magazines and newsletters present new ideas.

Journals are of two types: peer-reviewed and non–peer-reviewed. Peer-reviewed journals require manuscripts undergo a process of evaluation by experts in the discipline who evaluate the manuscript based on the current level of knowledge in the field. Peer review ensures that the presented information has sufficient rigor, interest, and uniqueness to warrant dissemination. Non–peer-reviewed journals generally do not have the same rigor because manuscripts are reviewed only by an editor, who may not have expertise in the specific area.

SUMMARY

It is critical that occupational therapists engage in evidence-based practice that supports the philosophical underpinnings of the profession and informs decision making throughout the occupational therapy process. Comprehensive evidence-based practice models, such as the Research Pyramid,

evaluate and inform the quantitative and qualitative evidence necessary for occupational therapy evaluation. As the therapist gathers data on the client and chooses appropriate assessments, he or she can collect and provide information about the evidence of practice. The information gathered during effective practice can become the data for evidence-based practice. When the therapist uses the data from practice to provide evidence for practice, he or she not only aids practice but also, when disseminating findings, provides evidence to support the field of occupational therapy in general.

QUESTIONS

1. Describe the relationship between evidence-based practice and evaluation. How can a therapist use evaluation data to support evidence-based practice?
2. Choose 1 assessment, and use available evidence to support your decision to use this tool.
3. Choose 1 practice area, and identify the assessments commonly used in it. In your opinion, does evidence support the use of these assessments?
4. Think about a practice site where you have been. What data have you seen there that a therapist could collect to use for future evidence for practice?
5. Search an online database for evidence-based practice. Identify information in that database that might be useful to you in evaluation or assessment.

References

American Occupational Therapy Association. (2007). AOTA's *Centennial Vision* and executive summary. *American Journal of Occupational Therapy, 61,* 613–614. http://dx.doi.org/10.5014/ajot.61.6.613

Baum, C. M., Connor, L. T., Morrison, T., Hahn, M., Dromerick, A. W., & Edwards, D. F. (2008). Reliability, validity, and clinical utility of the Executive Function Performance Test: A measure of executive function in a sample of people with stroke. *American*

Journal of Occupational Therapy, 62, 446–455. http://dx.doi.org/10.5014/ajot.62.4.446

Baum, C. M., Morrison, T., Hahn, M., & Edwards, D. F. (2003). *Test manual: Executive Function Performance Test.* St. Louis: Washington University.

Carver, M. D. (2009). Adaptive equipment to assist with one-handed intermittent self-catheterization: A case study of a patient with multiple brain injuries. *American Journal of Occupational Therapy, 63*, 333–336. http://dx.doi.org/10.5014/ajot.63.3.333

Ciro, C. (2011). Enhancing our collective research acumen by using an epidemiological perspective. *American Journal of Occupational Therapy, 65*, 594–598. http://dx.doi.org/10.5014/ajot.2001.000703

Classen, S., Levy, C., McCarthy, D., Mann, W. C., Lanford, D., & Waid-Ebbs, J. K. (2009). Traumatic brain injury and driving assessment: An evidence-based literature review. *American Journal of Occupational Therapy, 63*, 580–591. http://dx.doi.org/10.5014/ajot.63.5.580

Cohen, D. J., & Crabtree, B. F. (2008). Evaluative criteria for qualitative research in health care: Controversies and recommendations. *Annals of Family Medicine, 6*, 331–339. http://dx.doi.org/10.1370/afm.818

Devers, K. J. (1999). How will we know "good" qualitative research when we see it? Beginning the dialogue in health services research. *Health Services Research, 34*, 1153–1188.

Dixon-Woods, M., Shaw, R. L., Agarwal, S., & Smith, J. A. (2004). The problem of appraising qualitative research. *Quality and Safety in Health Care, 13*, 223–225. http://dx.doi.org/10.1136/qshc.2003.008714

Doig, E., Fleming, J., Cornwell, P. L., & Kuipers, P. (2009). Qualitative exploration of a client-centered, goal-directed approach to community-based occupational therapy for adults with traumatic brain injury. *American Journal of Occupational Therapy, 63*, 559–568. http://dx.doi.org/10.5014/ajot.63.5.559

Dunn, C. A., Carlson, M., Jackson, J. M., & Clark, F. A. (2009). Response factors surrounding progression of pressure ulcers in community-residing adults with spinal cord injury. *American Journal of Occupational Therapy, 63*, 301–309. http://dx.doi.org/10.5014/ajot.63.3.301

Dysart, A. M., & Tomlin, G. S. (2002). Factors related to evidence-based practice among U.S. occupational therapy clinicians. *American Journal of Occupational Therapy, 56*, 275–284. http://dx.doi.org/10.5014/ajot.56.3.275

Finlayson, M., Preissner, K., & Cho, C. (2012). Outcome moderators of a fatigue management program for people with multiple sclerosis. *American Journal of Occupational Therapy, 66*, 187–197. http://dx.doi.org/10.5014/ajot.2012.003160

Fleming-Castaldy, R. P., & Gillen, G. (2013). Ensuring that education, certification, and practice are evidence based. *American Journal of Occupational Therapy, 67*, 364–369. http://dx.doi.prg/10.5014/ajot.2013.006973

Giacomini, M. K., & Cook, D. J., for the Evidence-Based Medicine Working Group. (2000). Users' guides to the medical literature: XXIII. Qualitative research in health care B. What are the results and how do they help me care for my patients? Evidence-Based Medicine Working Group. *JAMA, 284*, 478–482. http://dx.doi.org/10.1001/jama.284.3.357

Greenhalgh, T., & Taylor, R. (1997). Papers that go beyond numbers (qualitative research). *British Medical Journal, 315*, 740–743. http://dx.doi.org/10.1136/bmj.315.7110.740

Gutman, S. A., Kerner, R., Zombek, I., Dulek, J., & Ramsey, C. A. (2009). Supported education for adults with psychiatric disabilities: Effectiveness of an occupational therapy program. *American Journal of Occupational Therapy, 63*, 245–254. http://dx.doi.org/10.5014/ajot.63.3.245

Hammell, K. W. (2004). Dimensions of meaning in the occupations of daily life. *Canadian Journal of Occupational Therapy, 71*, 296–305. http://dx.doi.org/10.1177/000841740407100509

Health Insurance Portability and Accountability Act of 1996. Pub. L. 104–191, 45 C.F.R. § 160, 164. Retrieved from http://www.hhs.gov/ocr/hipaa

Helewa, A., & Walker, J. M. (2000). *Critical evaluation of research in physical rehabilitation: Towards evidence-based practice.* Philadelphia: W. B. Saunders.

Henderson, R., & Rheault, W. (2004). Appraising and incorporating qualitative research in evidence-based practice. *Journal of Physical Therapy Education, 18*, 35–40.

Hinojosa, J. (2013). The evidence-based paradox. *American Journal of Occupational Therapy, 67*, e18–e23. http://dx.doi.org/10.5014/ajot.2013.005587

Ilott, I. (2003). Challenging the rhetoric and reality: Only an individual and systemic approach will work for evidence-based occupational therapy. *American Journal of Occupational Therapy, 57*, 351–354. http://dx.doi.org/10.5014/ajot.57.3.351

Kardos, M. R., & White, B. P. (2006). Evaluation options for secondary transition planning. *American Journal of Occupational Therapy, 60*, 333–339. http://dx.doi.org/10.5014/ajot.60.3.333

Keller, J., Kafkes, A., Basu, S., Federico, J., & Kielhofner, G. (2005). *Child Occupational Self-Assessment.* Chicago: MOHO Clearinghouse.

Kramer, J. M., Kielhofner, G., & Smith, E. V., Jr. (2010). Validity evidence for the Child Occupational Self Assessment. *American Journal of Occupational Therapy, 64*, 621–632. http://dx.doi.org/10.5014/ajot.2010.08142

Law, M., Baptiste, S., Carswell, A., McColl, M. A., Polatajko, H., & Pollock, N. (2005). *Canadian Occupational Performance Measure* (4th ed.). Ottawa: CAOT Publications.

Law, M., & Baum, C. (1998). Evidence-based occupational therapy. *Canadian Journal of Occupational Therapy, 65,* 131–135. http://dx.doi.org/10.1177/000841749806500301

Law, M., Cooper, B., Strong, S., Stewart, D., Rigby, P., & Letts, L. (1996). The Person–Environment–Occupation model: A transactive approach to Occupational performance. *Canadian Journal of Occupational Therapy, 63,* 9–23. http://dx.doi.org/10.1177/000841749606300103

Law, M., & MacDermid, J. (Eds.). (2008a). *Evidence-based rehabilitation: A guide to practice* (2nd ed.). Thorofare, NJ: Slack.

Law, M., & MacDermid, J. (2008b). Introduction to evidence-based practice. In M. Law & J. MacDermid (Eds.), *Evidence-based rehabilitation: A guide to practice* (pp. 3–14). Thorofare, NJ: Slack.

Law, M., & Philp, I. (2002). Evaluating the evidence. In M. Law (Ed.), *Evidence-based rehabilitation* (pp. 97–107). Thorofare, NJ: Slack.

Lee, C. J., & Miller, L. T. (2003). The process of evidence-based clinical decision making in occupational therapy. *American Journal of Occupational Therapy, 57,* 473–477. http://dx.doi.org/10.5014/ajot.57.4.473

Lin, S. H., Murphy, S. L., & Robinson, J. C. (2010). Facilitating evidence-based practice: Process, strategies, and resources. *American Journal of Occupational Therapy, 64,* 164–171. http://dx.doi.org/10.5014/ajot.64.1.164

Lloyd-Smith, W. (1997). Evidence-based practice and occupational therapy. *British Journal of Occupational Therapy, 60,* 474–479.

Miller, L. J., Coll, J. R., & Schoen, S. A. (2007). A randomized controlled pilot study of the effectiveness of occupational therapy for children with sensory modulation disorder. *American Journal of Occupational Therapy, 61,* 228–238. http://dx.doi.org/10.5014/ajot.61.2.228

Ottenbacher, K. J., & Hinderer, S. R. (2001). Evidence-based practice: Methods to evaluate individual patient improvement. *American Journal of Physical Medicine and Rehabilitation, 80,* 786–796. http://dx.doi.org/10.1097/00002060-200110000-00014

Patton, M. Q. (2002). *Qualitative Research and Evaluation Methods* (3rd ed.). Thousand Oaks, CA: Sage.

Perlmutter, M. S., Bhorade, A., Gordon, M., Hollingsworth, H., Engsberg, J. E., & Baum, M. C. (2013). Home lighting assessment for clients with low vision. *American Journal of Occupational Therapy, 67,* 674–682. http://dx.doi.org/10.5014/ajot.2013.006692

Popay, J., & Williams, G. (1998). Qualitative research and evidence-based healthcare. *Journal of the Royal Society of Medicine, 91*(Suppl. 35), 32–37. http://dx.doi.org/10.1177/0141076898091S3508

Portney, L. G., & Watkins, M. P. (2009). *Foundations of Clinical Research: Applications to Practice* (3rd ed.). Upper Saddle River, NJ: Prentice Hall Health.

Rosenberg, W., & Donald, A. (1995). Evidence based medicine: An approach to clinical problem-solving. *British Medical Journal, 310,* 1122–1126. http://dx.doi.org/10.1136/bmj.310.6987.1122

Sackett, D. L. (1989). Rules of evidence and clinical recommendations on the use of antithrombotic agents. *Chest, 95*(Suppl.), 2S–4S. http://dx.doi.org/10.1378/chest.95.2.2S

Sackett, D. L., Rosenberg, W. M. C., Gray, J. A. M., Haynes, R. B., & Richardson, W. S. (1996). Evidence based medicine: What it is and what it isn't. *British Journal of Medicine, 312,* 71–72. http://dx.doi.org/10.1136/bmj.312.7023.71

Straus, S. E., Richardson, W. S., Glasziou, P., & Haynes, R. B. (2010). *Evidence-based medicine: How to practice and teach EBM* (4th ed.). Edinburgh, Scotland: Churchill Livingstone.

Taylor, M. C. (1997). What is evidence-based practice. *British Journal of Occupational Therapy, 60,* 470–474.

Thomas, A., & Law, M. (2013). Research utilization and evidence-based practice in occupational therapy: A scoping study. *American Journal of Occupational Therapy, 67,* e55–e65. http://dx.doi.org/10.5014/ajot.2013.006395

Tickle-Degnen, L. (2002). Client-centered practice, therapeutic relationship, and the use of research evidence. *American Journal of Occupational Therapy, 56,* 470–474. http://dx.doi.org/10.5014/ajot.56.4.470

Tickle-Degnen, L., & Bedell, G. (2003). Heterarchy and hierarchy: A critical appraisal of the "levels of evidence" as a tool for clinical decision making. *American Journal of Occupational Therapy, 57,* 234–237. http://dx.doi.org/10.5014/ajot.57.2.234

Toma, J. D. (2006). Approaching rigor in applied qualitative research. In C. F. Conrad & R. C. Serlin (Eds.), *The SAGE handbook for research in education* (pp. 405–423). Thousand Oaks, CA: SAGE.

Tomlin, G., & Borgetto, B. (2011). Research Pyramid: A new evidence-based practice model for occupational therapy. *American Journal of Occupational Therapy, 65,* 189–196. http://dx.doi.org/10.5014/ajot.2011.000828

CHAPTER 16

Additional Uses of Evaluation Data

Virginia Stoffel, PhD, OT, BCMH, FAOTA
Nikhil Tomar, MS

Highlights

- Promoting the profession
- Outcomes measurement for occupational therapy
- Retrospective chart reviews, systematic reviews, and scoping reviews of the literature
- Clinical research methods using small numbers of participants
- Fieldwork evaluation: preparing evidence-informed practitioners
- Program development and evaluation.

Key Terms

Clinical trials
Comparative Effectiveness Research approach
Effectiveness
Efficacy
Meta-analysis
Outcomes-oriented approach

Outcomes research
Participation
Progress
Scoping reviews
Single-subject research methods
Systematic review

This chapter considers uses of evaluation data beyond those specific to clinical practice. In day-to-day clinical practice, the focus is on individual client needs and the processes used, including screening, determination of level of functional performance on the basis of the results of specific assessments, intervention planning, and so forth. Beyond meeting clinical practice needs, evaluation data provide critical information for the occupational therapist in the roles of program manager, outcomes evaluator, and researcher. These applications of data then relate directly back to clinical practice as therapists use the data to develop, improve, or even discontinue specific intervention programs and provide the evidence that guides clinical decision making. In addition, therapists can use program outcomes data to highlight reports to external groups, such as grant funders or policy leaders from community agencies.

This chapter provides an overview of the use of evaluation data for three purposes. First, it discusses using evaluation data for outcomes measurement, including evidence that supports standardized and systematic assessments in clinical use. In this section, the use of data shows how they can guide practice, including data-based retrospective chart reviews and systematic and scoping reviews of the literature. Second, the chapter summarizes the use of small clinical research studies that support evaluation processes, specifically single-subject designs. Third, the chapter presents how therapists can use data in program development and evaluation.

PROMOTING THE PROFESSION

Earlier chapters in this text include substantial information to guide new therapists or update seasoned therapists with the skills needed to conduct evaluations using a variety of assessments in a variety of situations. These assessments should reflect theoretical premises and should be psychometrically sound, administered in uniform or standardized formats, and interpreted accurately. Knowledge obtained using these assessments is key to the profession's continued efforts to improve evaluation procedures to provide the best information to clients and their families, colleagues, and health care payers and regulators.

Occupational therapists' efforts to be conscientious and competent help develop and promote the profession when evaluation data are recorded in a way that not only benefits the individual recipients of services but also clearly and succinctly communicates the outcomes of interventions. Further, the therapist advances the profession when he or she evaluates the effectiveness of intervention programs for those outside of the profession. Given the demands of accountability in the health care environment of the 21st century, occupational therapists must embrace the systematic use of sound evaluation data to report outcomes and evaluate programs.

OUTCOMES MEASUREMENT FOR OCCUPATIONAL THERAPY

The goals of health care are to extend life and "ensure optimal quality of life" (Oldridge, 1996, p. 95). *Outcomes measurement* is "a comprehensive and integrated system of assessments to measure the efficiency and effectiveness of health care services and interventions" (Barr, Schumacher, & Ohman,

2003, p. 1) to reach those goals. Barr and colleagues pose four questions in outcomes assessment:

1. Are the services and therapies provided improving the client's status, at least preventing or slowing further deterioration of the client's conditions?
2. Are our treatments effective (do they work), and are they efficient (do they use only the necessary resources)?
3. Are clients better because they receive these services?
4. Have we made a difference in clients' end results or "outcomes"? (p. 1)

Occupational therapists should ask themselves these questions when providing services to clients. In outcomes measurement, the therapist's interest extends to groups of clients or populations. Because health care outcomes are increasingly defined by functional indicators (Clifton, 2005b), that is, what the person being served defines as better, the contributions from the occupational therapist can be substantial because occupational therapy addresses the aspects of living that improve quality of life, participation, and well-being.

Predictably determining the outcomes of occupational therapy services, often to maintain credibility in the competitive health care market-

> The focus on functional indicators as health care outcomes underscores the substantial contributions of the occupational therapist, who addresses a client's ability to participate in and to live an improved quality of life.

place, has been discussed in the literature since the 1980s. The American Occupational Therapy Association (AOTA), in partnership with the American Occupational Therapy Foundation, embraced this goal as a mandate when it provided funds to create the Center for Outcomes Research and Education at the University of Illinois at Chicago (Kielhofner, Hammel, Finlayson, Helfrich, & Taylor, 2004). The development of an entity devoted to outcomes research and education was an important step toward establishing a tradition of outcomes research in the profession.

More recently, the AOTA *Centennial Vision* (AOTA, 2007; Stoffel, 2011) adopted an outcomes-driven professional "road map" for the future that includes the development of a national database for occupational therapy clinical outcomes. The first step toward achieving this goal was the adoption of the Boston University Activity Measure for Post-Acute Care (AM–PAC) as a primary tool to gather functional improvement data for the measurement of occupational therapy outcomes (AOTA, 2009). Another clinical outcomes–related goal from the AOTA *Centennial Vision* is the preparation of all future occupational therapists to have competencies in using outcome measures and interpreting outcomes data (AOTA, 2007). It is clear that occupational therapy shares the goal of sound outcomes measurement with colleagues across the spectrum of health professions, including medicine, dentistry, nursing, physical therapy, and psychology.

Outcomes-Oriented Approach

Occupational therapists agree that clinical outcomes research is important for present and future practice, but they seldom engage in such efforts, primarily because of insufficient knowledge of research methods and institutional barriers to conducting outcomes research (Bowman, 2006; Bowman & Llewellyn, 2002). It is important to clarify the nature of outcomes research as compared with clinical trials research. Ellek (1996) described **outcomes research** as examining "the effectiveness of treatment as it is administered under real-life circumstances, where patients as well as the treatment itself are likely to have some variances" (p. 886), vs. **clinical trials,** which are conducted under strict protocols and ideal conditions with little variation.

A thorough discussion of the structure and processes of outcomes research is beyond the scope of this chapter, but an overview will be provided. Therapists are encouraged to gain additional graduate, postprofessional education to develop research skills. However, each therapist can adopt an outcomes-oriented approach to clinical practice by drawing on the best available practice evidence, including standardized assessments in evaluation, and using consistent methods for reporting data.

The increased emphasis on intervention outcomes in the profession in the past decade reflects issues and trends in all of health care for the past 20 years (Baum, 2011; Coster, 2008; Law, Baum, & Dunn, 2005). The involvement of each therapist in acquiring the information necessary to determine the outcomes of occupational therapy interventions is key to building the body of evidence to support practice.

What are occupational therapy outcomes?

It is worth considering at this point what might be measured as occupational therapy outcomes. The *Occupational Therapy Practice Framework: Domain and Process* (3rd ed.; *Framework;* AOTA, 2014) defines *outcomes* as vital to health. In addition, outcomes must address the characteristics of intervention and must result in client satisfaction and improved ability to function. As described in the introduction of the *Framework,* the primary outcome of the profession is that practitioners support the health of a person so that he or she can engage in occupation (AOTA, 2014). This idea includes two outcomes that are common across the provision of health care—health and participation (World Health Organization [WHO], 2001)—and one that is unique to occupational therapy—engagement in occupation. The *Framework* lists seven categories of outcomes:

1. Occupational performance in areas of occupation (activities of daily living [ADLs], instrumental activities of daily living [IADLs], rest and sleep, education, work, play, leisure, and social participation that are measured as improved or enhanced)
2. Occupational performance
3. Health and wellness
4. Quality of life
5. Prevention
6. Participation
7. Role competence.

Other aspects of the domain of occupational therapy as described in the *Framework* (AOTA, 2014), particularly performance skills and client factors, suggest more outcomes to be measured. Examples of performance skills include motor skills such as posture, coordination, and bending; sensory–perceptual skills specific to tasks, such as locating, visualizing, and discerning sensory input; and communication and social skills such as gesturing, maintaining physical space with others, and taking turns. Examples of client factors that might be measured as outcomes include values such as honesty and fairness; the mental functions of orientation, memory, motivation, and attention; sensory functions and pain; and neuromusculoskeletal and movement-related functions. The *Framework* provides specific definitions to operationalize the outcomes of most occupational therapy interventions.

The emphasis on function and participation implicit in occupational therapy outcomes within the areas of occupation is consistent with models of outcome measurement found in the rehabilitation literature. The focus in rehabilitation has moved away from pathology and impairment models toward those that emphasize function and well-being (Clifton, 2005a). Barr and colleagues (2003) provided an overview of the history of outcomes measurement, including the Nagi disability model (Nagi, 1964), the *International Classification of Functioning, Disability and Health* (ICF; WHO, 2001), and the Wilson–Cleary outcomes model (Wilson & Cleary, 1995). All models move from the measurement of outcomes at the level of pathology to measurement of function and performance in society. The concepts addressed by these models, broadly used in medical rehabilitation, are consistent with desired outcomes in the domain of occupational therapy service.

Implementing an outcomes-oriented approach

An **outcomes-oriented approach** begins with the belief that data are important to guiding clinical practice and that a therapist is well-suited to gather, record, and report data. An outcomes-oriented approach is a dynamic system in which data provide feedback about the impact (outcome) of an individual intervention as well as information about the process and effect of the intervention (program evaluation).

A therapist can model an outcomes-oriented approach after the process of outcomes research. Kielhofner, Hammel, and colleagues (2004) suggested that the first step in outcomes research is identifying client needs. Baum (2011) suggested that in addition to identifying needs and level of care, outcome data can also inform the kinds of services that

> An outcomes-oriented approach is a dynamic system in which data provide feedback about the impact (outcome) of an individual intervention as well as information about the process and effect of the intervention (program evaluation).

will meet the person's need for movement, communication, and performance essential to quality of life.

Identifying Needs of Client Populations

Assessing an individual client's needs is the primary focus of this text; in an outcomes-oriented approach to client needs, the evaluation process is both population focused and individual focused. Evaluation data are not only gathered and maintained for an individual client, they are also stored in a database (commercial or facility specific) for the purpose of determining and documenting the needs of the population to which the individual client belongs (e.g., older adults with hip fractures with impairment in dressing, fourth graders with handwriting deficits, adults with mental illness with employment needs).

The identification of outcome measures can be daunting; a PubMed search of "outcomes assessment in occupational therapy" yielded almost 3,250 refereed publications that used standardized outcome assessments. Use of the www.rehabmeasures.org website is one way to find appropriate tools as well as to access excellent educational materials that help the learner to better understand an evidence-based approach to selecting appropriate standardized measures for a given person or population. The National Institutes of Health (NIH) website offers the NIH Toolbox for Neurological and Behavioral Function (with potential items in the domains of cognition, emotion, motor, and sensation) at http://www.nihtoolbox.org/Pages/default.aspx. Item access at the NIH website and assessment access through the rehabmeasures website have made the search process related to health and well-being outcomes efficient for all health professionals.

Allen Heinemann (Rehabilitation Institute of Chicago, 2010) developed the contents of the Rehabilitation Measures Database (www.rehabmeasures.org) under a grant from the U.S. Department of Education and Rehabilitation Institute of Chicago, Center for Rehabilitation Outcomes Research. The Northwestern University, Feinberg School of Medicine, Department of Medical Social Sciences Informatics group developed the website. The database is dynamic and, when accessed in November 2013, had 200 outcome measures in the database, offering links to the source of each assessment, in-depth reviews of each assessment, and easily searched properties.

The full reviews first covered assessments for stroke and spinal cord injury, then expanded to acquired brain injury, arthritis, cardiac conditions, cerebral palsy, multiple sclerosis, pain, traumatic brain injury, and vestibular disorders. Areas of assessment include ADLs, IADLs, attention, depression and mental health, life participation, social relationships, vision, and perception. This dynamic database continues to grow and expand to include more conditions as well as areas of occupational function and participation.

Earlier, Law and colleagues (2005) organized more than 100 outcome measures according to the categories of the current *ICF* (WHO, 2001), including measurement of participation; play, work, ADLs, IADLs, and leisure performance; occupational roles and balance; community integration and social support; and environmental factors.

Following are some familiar standardized measures for reporting individual and population evaluation data in occupation-based outcomes:

- The FIM™ (Uniform Data System for Medical Rehabilitation [UDSMR], 1997) has been used in dozens of studies to report the status of daily living activities for people with disabilities in rehabilitation programs.
- The Functional Independence Measure for Children (WeeFIM; UDSMR, 1993) was used to describe outcomes of 814 pediatric patients in inpatient rehabilitation (Chen, Heinemann, Bode, Granger, & Mallinson, 2004). The FIM and WeeFIM measures maintain databases through the UDSMR, located at the Center for Functional Assessment Research at the State University of New York–Buffalo, to which subscribers submit information and have access to large pools of data for outcomes prediction, communication, information, and management.
- The Canadian Occupational Performance Measure (COPM; Law et al., 1998) has been reviewed for its contribution to outcomes research in 33 different studies (Carswell et al., 2004).

Several assessments that have been used to measure outcomes in pediatrics and school-based practice include

- Pediatric Evaluation of Disability Index (PEDI; Haley, Coster, Ludlow, Haltiwanger, & Andrellos, 1992),
- Beery–Buktenica Developmental Test of Visual–Motor Integration (VMI; Beery, Buktenica, & Beery, 2004),
- Peabody Developmental Motor Scales–2 (PDMS–2; Folio & Fewell, 2000), and
- School Function Assessment (Coster, Deeney, Haley, & Haltiwinger, 1998).

A growing area of assessments measuring community participation includes

- Community Participation Indicators (CPI; Heinemann et al., 2011),
- Participation Measure for Post Acute Care (PM–PAC; Gandek, Sinclair, Jette, & Ware, 2007), and
- Craig Handicap Assessment Reporting Technique (CHART; Whiteneck, Charlifue, Gerhart, Overholser, & Richardson, 1992).

Participation, defined as "involvement in a life situation" (WHO, 2002), is an important concept in understanding disability; inclusion of participation within intervention strategies is warranted to create effective outcome measures that can assist occupational therapists to evaluate the effect of disability on the client's participation in personal and social contexts at a population level. Such measurement provides knowledge of the effect of a particular intervention on clients' participation, which affects program development and program evaluation. Salter, Foley, Jutai, and Teasell (2007) reported that only 6% of the assessments used in 491 stroke intervention clinical trials included measures of participation.

Only in the recent past have outcome measures such as the CPI, CHART, and PM–PAC been developed solely to measure participation. Development and use of effective participation measures should be advocated in both research and practice to reflect core values of occupational therapy in client evaluation, intervention planning, and outcome reporting (Dunford, Bannigan, & Wales, 2013; Whiteneck, 2010; Wolf, 2011). See Chapter 7, "Contextual Evaluation to Support Participation," for additional information on measures of participation.

Using Standardized Measures of Outcomes

In an outcomes-oriented approach, the use of standardized measures of outcomes is critical both to the process of individual evaluation (i.e., identifying the client's needs) and to the systematic accumulation of evaluation data for information about client populations. The following are examples of studies that used standardized measures to record occupation-based outcomes for individual participants; the data can be applied to similar client groups and the instruments can be considered for clinical applications:

- The impact of occupational therapy services on 37 kindergarteners' fine motor and emergent literacy outcomes (Bazyk et al., 2009) was measured using the VMI, PDMS–2, and three subtests of the Observation Survey of Early Literacy Achievement (Clay, 1993) and Approximations to Text (Pappas, 1993).
- The outcome of individualized occupational therapy intervention for people with psychotic conditions was compared with usual care for 44 adults in a United Kingdom city (Cook, Chambers, & Coleman, 2009). Outcomes measures included the Social Functioning Scale (Birchwood, Smith, Cochrane, Wetton, & Copestake, 1990) and the Scale for the Assessment of Negative Symptoms (Andreasen, 1983).
- The relationships among sensory processing, classroom behavior, and educational outcomes were examined for 28 children with autism spectrum disorders using the Short Sensory Profile (Ashburner, Ziviani, & Rodger, 2008; McIntosh, Miller, Shyu, & Dunn, 1999).
- The outcomes of augmenting a traditional occupational therapy and physical therapy treatment program in occupational health service clinics in Vermont using the Worker-Based Outcomes Assessment System tool were reported for 136 participants with work-related musculoskeletal disorders (Ross, Callas, Sargent, Amick, & Rooney, 2006).
- The outcomes of rehabilitation were identified for 125 inner-city older women (Lysack, Neufeld, Mast, MacNeill, & Lichtenberg, 2003) using the FIM (UDSMR, 1997), the Geriatric Depression Scale (Sheikh & Yesavage, 1986), the Mattis Dementia Rating (Mattis, 1988), and the Charlson Index of Co-Morbidity (Charlson, Pompei, Ales, & MacKenzie, 1987).
- The progress made by 44 preschool children in fine motor skills and related functional outcomes was assessed in a multisite study (Case-Smith, 1998) using standardized instruments, including subtests from the Sensory Integration and Praxis Test (Ayres, 1989) and Southern California Sensory Integration Tests (Ayres, 1972), the Developmental Test of Visual Perception (DTVP; Hammill, Pearson, & Voress, 1993), the Sensory Profile (Dunn & Westman, 1997), the PDMS–2, and the PEDI.
- The effectiveness of a rehabilitation program on quality of life and symptom severity for 47 participants with chronic fatigue syndrome (Taylor, 2004) was examined using the Chronic Fatigue Syndrome Symptom Rating Form (Jason et al., 1997) and the Quality of Life Index (Ferrans & Powers, 1985).

These studies are examples of studies that used standardized outcomes measures so results can be interpreted and generalized to the same clinical populations. The assessments used can provide the evaluation data necessary to plan interventions unique to an individual client and to contribute to a body of evidence that guides practice with an identified clinical population.

This process—the generating of evidence about the impact of services in a particular area of practice—is the third step in outcomes research (Kielhofner, Hammel, et al., 2004). Readers can consult the articles describing these studies for more information about how they can use these standardized assessments in their own practice with the same clinical populations.

Using standardized measurement assessments to gather evaluation data is critical to following an outcomes-oriented approach. The characteristics of the assessments and methods used, both qualitative and quantitative, determine the success of a program in making a difference in client outcomes. Qualities of standardized assessments are reviewed in several chapters earlier in this text.

The occupational therapy and rehabilitation literature report ongoing development of instruments and measurement techniques (Baker, Jacobs, & Tickle-Degnen, 2003; Baum & Edwards, 2008; Baum et al., 2008; Cup, Scholte op Reimer, Thijssen, & van Kuyk-Minis, 2003; Darzins, Imms, & Di Stefano, 2013; Fang, Hsiung, Yu, Chen, & Wang, 2002; Goverover & Hinojosa, 2004; Hartman-Maeir, Harel, & Katz, 2009; Hotchkiss et al., 2004; Huebner, Custer, Freudenberger, & Nichols, 2006; Jang, Chern, & Lin, 2009; Jong, van Nes, & Lindeboom, 2012; Katz, Golstand, Traub Bar-Ilan, & Parush, 2007; Lindstrom-Hazel, Kratt, & Bix, 2009; Passmore, 2004; Reker et al., 2005; Stagnitti & Unsworth, 2004). Authors have discussed the development of functional assessments and the outcomes of occupational therapy interventions since the 1980s. Gutman (2008), editor-in-chief of the *American Journal of Occupational Therapy*, recently wrote that the development of assessments is a research priority of the profession, noting that it is consistent with the AOTA (2007) *Centennial Vision*.

With the explosion of new standardized assessments in the past decade, the selection of appropriate measures for one's clinical situation can be daunting. Criteria for the selection of outcome measures have been suggested (Barr et al., 2003; Clifton, 2005a; Coster, 2013; MacDermid & Michlovitz, 2008). These sources recommend against using assessments that are locally developed (i.e., institution based) because they do not meet standards for validity, reliability, and consistent administration. Criteria for selection of outcome measures include

- The therapist must define the scope of the clinical population receiving services. The clinical population must match the population for whom an assessment was developed.
- The scores of the population are distributed across the full range of the assessment so that the therapist can differentiate among them and detect improvement or deterioration.
- The scoring system must be sensitive enough to detect changes.
- The domains or concepts that the therapist wants to measure should be included in the

assessment, whether they are reported as separate domains or a summary score.
- The assessment must report appropriate indicators of intrarater, interrater, and internal reliability.
- The assessment must report appropriate indicators of content, convergent, discriminate, and construct validity.
- The assessment must be feasible to administer (in terms of time and cost), with clear directions for administration.
- The assessment must be acceptable to the client population, with minimal discomfort.
- The assessment must help guide clinical practice for the client and aid in goal setting (MacDermid & Michlovitz, 2008).
- The assessment must measure the outcomes of interest to the groups or stakeholders interested in the outcomes data, including measuring program effectiveness.

Law and colleagues (2005) offered a selection process for the identification of suitable outcome measures. Their "decision-making process that occupational therapists can use to guide the measurement of occupational performance" (p. 33) is

1. Identification of occupational performance issues by the client, often gained through interview or other self-report method;
2. Identification of occupational performance issues for this client by another individual or group who may be involved in caregiving or other critical support roles;
3. Further assessment of specific occupational performance areas (e.g., IADLs, work) using appropriate measures;
4. Assessment of environmental conditions and occupational performance attributes such as client factors, performance skills, and performance patterns;
5. Selection of specific outcome measures that meet the criteria listed above, with an emphasis on clinical utility and compilation of other useful data (i.e., will contribute to evaluation of the program or services); and
6. Implementation of the assessment process and interpretation of the results (Law et al., 2005).

Identifying Who Is Interested in Outcomes Data

The data that result from outcomes measurement are of interest to at least three constituent groups or stakeholders: (1) clients, (2) providers, and (3) payers or regulators. Clients include people who receive occupational therapy services and their families and caregivers, facilities and agencies that offer occupational therapy services, and other communities who receive or may benefit from occupational therapy services. Providers are therapists, therapy students doing fieldwork, and other health professionals. Payers or regulators include public and private insurance programs and state and federal regulatory groups that set standards and policies for practice and reimbursement. Table 16.1 identifies these constituents and provides examples of the uses of outcome measurement by each.

Role of Qualitative Data in Outcomes

Many of the standardized assessment instruments noted earlier provide quantitative information necessary for uses identified by providers, payers, and regulators. Qualitative evaluation data also provide important information that initially can identify client needs and expectations. After intervention services, qualitative measures can provide the evaluation data for subjective outcomes such as satisfaction and quality of life from the client's perspective. Clients value the interpersonal and communication skills of providers, and the effect of these skills on a client's compliance and motivation in therapy cannot be overestimated (Clifton, 2005a). For providers, the subjective outcomes of satisfaction with intervention services and quality of life after services can be important predictors of the success of an intervention.

Table 16.1. Constituents of Outcomes Measurement

Constituent Group	Description	Uses of Evaluation Data
Clients	Individual persons (e.g., patients, clients, residents, students, consumers) Families and caregivers Groups (e.g., agencies, facilities, communities, neighborhoods) who are affected by occupational therapy services	Monitoring success of interventions Making predictions for status at discharge, return home, or location to another facility or program Illustrating need for continuation of services Providing program development and evaluation (i.e., groups)
Providers	Occupational therapists and occupational therapy assistants Other health care professionals (e.g., physical therapists, psychologists, nurses, physicians, speech–language therapists) Facilities and agencies (e.g., hospitals, skilled nursing facilities, outpatient rehabilitation programs, schools)	Monitoring success of interventions Making qualitative and quantitative comparison of clinical performance by individual providers, programs, departments, facilities (i.e., quality assurance) Providing risk management assessment Monitoring cost-effectiveness and cost-containment measures Providing program development and evaluation
Payers and regulators	Public health programs (e.g., Medicare, Medicaid) Private insurance companies Federal, state, and local regulatory boards (e.g., Agency for Healthcare Quality and Research, state licensing boards)	Developing policies and professional standards by regulatory boards Establishing reimbursement guidelines and policies Determining reimbursable services

Examples of studies that used qualitative approaches to gather information about client needs include an ethnography of the occupational needs of patients in a hospice program (Jacques & Hasselkus, 2004); narrative interviews about the influence of chronic lower back pain on the motives for occupational performance (Satink, Winding, & Jonsson, 2004); phenomenological interviews and observation to uncover how people with dementia respond to the problems and changes they experience in everyday occupations (Nygard & Ohman, 2002); phenomenological interviews with older adults with multiple sclerosis (Finlayson, 2004); phenomenological analysis of how people with multiple sclerosis and their significant others cope (Boland, 2011); and an interview study of people with chronic pain and their performance of occupations (Aegler & Satink, 2009).

The study by Finlayson (2004) illustrates application of a theoretical framework—the determinants of health framework—to explore and understand factors that may influence a client's health-related concerns. By applying a theoretical framework in the evaluation process, a therapist can collect data on important outcomes of services from the client's perspective. The therapist can use qualitative techniques alongside standardized quantitative measures to get more comprehensive and accurate information from a client group. In the Finlayson study, each participant was interviewed twice, first from a phenomenological perspective and second to clarify information from the first interview and administer standardized quantitative assessments. The qualitative results identified areas of health concern—outcomes important to the client group (e.g., staying mobile and independent)—that may not have emerged from quantitative instruments.

Other qualitative studies provide outcome expectations from the perspective of clients and family members that typically include participation in meaningful occupations and participation in society (well-being and quality of life). A study by Cohn, Miller, and Tickle-Degnen (2000) identified parents' priorities for therapy for children with sensory modulation disorders. Interviews revealed child-focused and parent-focused "hopes for therapy outcomes" (p. 36) that resulted in proposed interventions to meet those outcome expectations.

Another study used a longitudinal qualitative design to describe the outcomes of an individualized adaptation-based intervention for low-income older adults with multiple chronic illnesses returning to the community (Spencer, Hersch, Eschenfelder, Fournet, & Murray-Gerzik, 1999). Outcome expectations were obtained from the older adult participants, family members, and occupational therapists providing services. The authors noted the importance of recognizing multiple outcome expectations in planning interventions.

Erdner, Magnusson, and Lützén (2012) interviewed persons with long-term mental illness living in the community, exploring their relationships at work and at home. Findings indicated that the interviewees were cognizant of social norms but could not integrate them into their daily lives. Thus, they had difficulty maintaining satisfying relationships with others. Qualitative data-collection techniques have much to offer in terms of identifying client needs and outcomes related to well-being and quality of life.

Qualitative data have also been useful in predicting intervention outcomes. Simmons, Crepeau, and White (2000) found that narrative information from the COPM used in combination with the FIM "enhances accuracy in prediction of outcomes for rehabilitative services for persons in adult physical disabilities settings" (p. 471). Kielhofner, Braveman, et al. (2004) reported the outcomes of a vocational program for people with AIDS. They found that evaluative data from an occupation-based narrative interview, the Occupational Performance History Interview II (Kielhofner, Mallinson, Forsyth, & Lai, 2001), were closely associated with outcomes and helped predict future behaviors related to successful and unsuccessful outcomes in the areas of employment, return to school, and volunteerism.

Databases as Resources of Outcome-Related Data

In addition to the evaluation data that occupational therapists can acquire in clinical settings, there is information beyond the immediate clinical environment that is crucial to the success of our clients, programs, and agencies and facilities: nonclinical knowledge (Clifton, 2005b). Government agencies, nonprofit agencies, educational institutions, and professional associations are excellent resources for health care goals, standards of practice, outcomes expectations, and other information that is useful in outcomes measurement and management. Some government agencies and other resources are listed here:

- The U.S. Department of Health and Human Services (www.hhs.gov) has established strategic objectives for the health of the country for the past 30 years with initiatives focused on "healthy people." Healthy People 2020 (http://www.healthypeople.gov/2020/default. aspx) has extensive databases and statistics.
- The Centers for Disease Control and Prevention (ww.cdc.gov) houses the National Center for Health Statistics, which promotes the development of prevention and intervention programs for a wide range of health conditions and provides extensive educational resources.
- NIH (www.nih.gov) establishes funding priorities for health-related research and administers federal funds. The many agencies under the NIH umbrella maintain extensive databases of health information resources.
- The National Institute on Disability and Rehabilitation Research (www.ed.gov/about/offices/ list/osers/nidrr/index.html), under the umbrella of the U.S. Department of Education, Office of Special Education and Rehabilitation Services, funds rehabilitation research, advocates for people with disabilities, and houses disability databases through the National Rehabilitation Information Clearinghouse.
- The Agency for Healthcare Research and Quality (www.ahrq.gov) oversees quality-of-care research, provides clinical practice guidelines, and has extensive policy statements and databases related to outcomes.
- The Substance Abuse and Mental Health Services Administration (www.samhsa.gov) focuses on programs and services for people of all ages who are at risk for mental illness or substance use disorders. Its Office of Applied Studies houses an extensive database of results from the National Survey on Drug Use and Health, which is conducted annually to determine national behavioral health practices and issues.

- The Institute of Medicine (www.iom.edu) develops information, policy statements, and recommendations on various health issues.
- The American Heart Association (www.heart. org) provides public education and research funding and promotes hospital-based quality improvement guidelines for cardiovascular care.
- The State University of New York–Buffalo Center for Functional Assessment Research houses the UDSMR (www.udsmr.org/Web-Modules/UDSMR/Com_CFAR.aspx), which maintains the FIM and WeeFIM databases.
- The Virginia Commonwealth University Traumatic Brain Injury Model System (http:// www.tbi.pmr.vcu.edu) supports education, reports research on traumatic brain injury, and provides links to databases.
- AOTA (www.aota.org) establishes standards of practice, hosts an evidence-based resource directory that includes databases, and provides links to related Internet sites.
- The American Physical Therapy Association (www.apta.org) establishes standards of practice and productivity standards and provides links to research-related sites.
- The NIH Patient Reported Outcomes Measurement Information System (www.assess mentcenter.net) provides several valid and reliable measures of patient-reported outcomes such as satisfaction with participation in social roles, physical functions, ability to participate in social roles and activities, and well-being.

Electronic Health Record and the Affordable Care Act

In 2009, the Institute of Medicine emphasized an analysis of treatment effectiveness between interventions, known as a *Comparative Effectiveness Research (CER) approach,* an aim that is not always addressed through randomized controlled trials (RCTs; Hoffman & Podgurski, 2011). CER was also adopted by the Patient Protection and Affordable Care Act of 2010 (Hoffman & Podgurski, 2011). The use of electronic health records (EHRs) has been recommended to enable physicians and other health care providers to make better decisions by implementing CER on large EHR databases.

Using EHRs to make personalized comparisons of treatment effectiveness to develop individualized interventions based on a pool of individuals sharing similar characteristics (such as clinical and demographic; Hoffman & Podgurski, 2011) is an idea that can be replicated by occupational therapy practitioners developing a database using standardized measures of outcomes.

Occupational therapy practitioners have long advocated for client-centered intervention strategies (Law, 1998; Sumsion, 2006). Using standardized outcome assessments to compare treatment effectiveness between two intervention strategies can help identify those best suited for a particular client.

AOTA is developing a national database for occupational therapy outcomes using evaluation data from AM–PAC through CREcare (Stoffel, 2011) and an electronic patient record and documentation system (AOTA, 2007). Using information from the database and electronic records can enable occupational therapy practitioners to evaluate treatment effectiveness and therefore use effective intervention strategies. Electronic documentation, once secured appropriately, allows easy access and sharing of information with other practitioners and researchers, forming a nexus of information that can be used nationwide to effectively implement individualized or client-centered interventions.

Mental Health Outcomes

Measurement of mental and behavioral health services outcomes deserves its own discussion. Occupational therapists who work in mental health programs will work toward the same desired occupational therapy services outcomes as their colleagues in rehabilitation and other practice areas as noted throughout this chapter—occupational performance, satisfaction, role competence, and so forth, as articulated in the *Framework* (AOTA, 2014). The mental health professionals with whom an occupational therapist works—psychologists, social workers, counselors, psychiatrists—use primarily verbal methods of intervention (in addition to psychotropic medications) and have identified changes in everyday life or function as an important outcome of counseling, psychotherapy, and

related verbal therapies in the past decade (Kazdin, 1999; Lyons, Howard, Mahoney, & Lish, 1997).

The psychology and counseling literature has discussed the efficacy and effectiveness of medications and psychotherapy (Howard, Moras, Brill, Martinovich, & Lutz, 1996). *Efficacy* is whether an intervention works under experimental conditions; *effectiveness* is whether the intervention works in practice. A third concept, *progress,* asks whether an intervention works for a particular patient. Howard and colleagues suggested that researchers and payers or regulators are concerned with efficacy and effectiveness, clinical providers with effectiveness, and clients with progress.

The measurement of therapeutic outcomes in psychology and treatment has historically emphasized the statistical significance of outcomes (i.e., whether a client's postintervention score on an outcome measure was statistically different from a preintervention as established by a normative group; Howard et al., 1996; Kazdin, 1999; Thompson, 2002). In the 1980s, Jacobson and colleagues developed an approach, a metric called the Reliable Change Index (RCI), deemed to have both clinical relevance and sound psychometrics for determining whether the magnitude of change from treatment effects was statistically reliable (Jacobson, Roberts, Berns, & McGlinchey, 1999).

The RCI has received considerable attention and modification since its original inception (Ogles, Lunnen, & Bonesteel, 2001), including the development and comparison of different RCI indices (Maassen, Bossema, & Brand, 2009; Waldorf, Wjedl, & Schottke, 2009). Although the RCI is described as measuring "clinical significance," the significance refers to a cutoff score that "can be used to categorize clients as recovered or not recovered" (Jacobson et al., 1999, p. 301) and that "does not include information regarding the clinical importance of the change" (Ottenbacher, Hsu, Granger, & Fiedler, 1996, p. 1231). The concept of "practical significance" refers to the statistical magnitude of the effect of an intervention outcome on a population; this concept should not be confused with the effect of therapy on outcomes related to daily life skills that have practical value.

The concept of clinical significance in psychotherapy and counseling, as elucidated by Kazdin (2001), seems most closely related to the outcomes that one might expect from occupational therapy intervention: "differences in the everyday lives of the clients" (p. 456). Kazdin suggested that the current outcome measures used in psychotherapy and counseling measure symptoms rather than impairment, do not include the client's perspectives on what is important to be successful in therapy, and do not address the relationship between "clinical significance" as defined by a metric such as the RCI and client functioning in everyday life. Kazdin proposed that psychology and the other counseling professions identify the constructs that "capture the impact of treatment" (p. 458) and how that impact might be "evident in everyday life" (p. 458). He also suggested a need for a measure or measures that assess these constructs.

An occupational therapist who practices in a mental health setting might offer the paradigm of the domain of occupational therapy to counseling and psychology colleagues as an excellent starting point for defining the constructs of everyday life. Outcome measures identified in this chapter—for example, the COPM, which has a large body of literature supporting its application across clinical populations—could be used to launch a discussion about occupational therapy professionals as functional specialists. An occupational therapist has much to teach his or her mental health colleagues about the conceptualization of daily functioning and measuring the outcomes of mental health intervention.

RETROSPECTIVE CHART REVIEWS, SYSTEMATIC REVIEWS, AND SCOPING REVIEWS OF THE LITERATURE

The amount of evaluation data stored in medical and educational records potentially can yield millions of pieces of information about occupational therapy services. Step 4 in the outcomes research process proposed by Kielhofner, Hammel, and colleagues (2004)—accumulating and evaluating evidence about specific occupational therapy services for the purposes of understanding clinical practice and outcomes measurement—can be accomplished with retrospective chart reviews.

Retrospective cohort studies occasionally appear in the occupational therapy literature, with more seen in recent years. The advantage of retrospective reviews is the availability of large sample sizes for data analysis—sample sizes that would be unfeasible to secure in prospective studies. Fulks and Harris (1995) analyzed the scores on the Miller Assessment for Preschoolers (Miller, 1993) of 54 children who were prenatally exposed to drugs, to determine whether a distinct clinical profile existed. The authors noted that prospective studies of this population of children, although more desirable if multiple outcome measures could be used, are difficult, given the drug addiction and unreliability of the mothers. Gathering the information retrospectively provides at least a glimpse into the needs and potential interventions for this clinical population.

Ivarsson, Söderback, and Stein (2000) reported a retrospective content analysis of 64 occupational therapy records documenting services for people with psychoses in Sweden. This analysis provided insights into treatment goals, the content of occupational therapy interventions, and the client-centered approach of the therapists. The findings demonstrated a need for a standardized measure of therapy outcomes; fewer than 5% of the items analyzed addressed the outcomes of occupational therapy. Chua, McCluskey, and Smead's (2012) retrospective analysis of 441 cases of the factors that affect driving assessments poststroke found that strongest predictors of initial driving assessment outcome were off-road assessment scores, age, gender, and time poststroke. Retrospective chart reviews thus not only provide a better understanding of a practice area, but also identify gaps in documentation of services and the need for standardized measures in a practice area.

Researchers evaluated Cognitive Orientation to Daily Occupational Performance, an intervention for children, during the final phase of its development (Polatajko, Mandich, Miller, & Macnab, 2001). Data from the outcomes of earlier studies of the intervention were compiled in a retrospective chart audit to see whether the intervention did, in fact, have "clinical replicability" (i.e., consistency) in terms of treatment effects. This compilation of data provided valuable information about the replicability of the intervention without the complexities associated with multiple-site research.

The large number of cases that researchers can analyze in retrospective chart reviews is illustrated in two studies (Chen et al., 2004; Ottenbacher et al., 2004). Chen and colleagues analyzed the records of therapy services and functional assessments of 814 pediatric patients who received inpatient rehabilitation over 3 years at 12 facilities using the admission and discharge ratings of the WeeFIM. This study had the advantages of a large sample size and a standardized assessment that yields consistent data.

Large retrospective studies are feasible only if data have been reported in this manner, as illustrated by the report by Ottenbacher and colleagues (2004) in which data were analyzed from 744 inpatient medical rehabilitation hospitals and centers on 148,807 patient records across 5 impairment groups over 7 years in a retrospective cohort study. This volume of data is only available for review when consistent data reporting measures are used; in this case, the FIM was the primary functional outcome measure, along with length of stay, living setting after discharge, and mortality. The most remarkable result from this study—an increase in mortality rates over 7 years from 1% to 4.7%—has considerable credibility because of the volume of cases analyzed, a criterion that could be met only with retrospective review.

More recent studies using retrospective data analysis include identification of the sensory processing and behavioral problems of young children with fetal alcohol spectrum disorders (Franklin, Deitz, Jirikowic, & Astley, 2008) and, by occupational therapists, the identification of the primary use of "prefunctional" activities (65.77%) compared with functional activities during inpatient stroke rehabilitation (Smallfield & Karges, 2009). Retrospective data can provide insights into client characteristics and assessment and intervention protocols, provided that data are collected in a systematic manner that lends itself to further analysis.

Qualitative data also can be analyzed retrospectively, as illustrated by the following studies. Retrospective analysis of data from the COPM on 38 mothers of children with disabilities found that the children's occupational performance was challenging emotionally and they lacked sufficient social contact (Donovan, VanLeit, Crowe, & Keefe, 2005). A retrospective analysis of naturalistic home video of infants with disabilities demonstrated the first categorization of levels of object play in the home environment (Baranek et al., 2005).

Another retrospective analysis of home videos (Freuler, Baranek, Watson, Boyd, & Bulluck, 2012)

revealed that in children with autism spectrum disorder, precursors of extreme sensory features emerge early, with hyporesponsiveness remaining stable. On the other hand, hyperresponsiveness and sensory seeking were less stable. Support for the theory underlying a sensory integrative approach was determined after a retrospective analysis of parent interview data and assessment data for a single child with sensory processing problems (Schaaf & Nightlinger, 2007). In 2011, Brauer, Hay, and Francisco's study revealed that occupational therapy services are an important part of the rehabilitation of people with traumatic brain injury. Finally, Pearce, Smead, and Cameron's (2012) retrospective cohort study supported the idea that a multidisciplinary driver assessment would be appropriate to assess driver safety for people poststroke.

Other types of reviews that use evaluation data and contribute to our understanding of occupational therapy practice include meta-analysis and systematic reviews of the literature. Researchers have used both of these strategies in the last decade to provide more resources for evidence-based practice in many clinical arenas.

Meta-analysis is a systematic review of research evidence that uses statistical procedures for combining data from several studies to analyze the effectiveness of specific treatment interventions (Clifton, 2005a). Operational definitions and procedures for inclusion of studies are explicit to ensure that the same interventions are being reviewed, and analysis is typically done on comparison studies (experimental designs). Meta-analyses are important procedures in step 4 of the outcomes research process (Kielhofner, Hammel, et al., 2004), analyzing evidence for a specific occupational therapy practice area. They are important because they provide the evidence needed for practice and fulfill the expectations of an outcomes-oriented approach in handling data. They also are restricted to areas of practice that have generated enough research studies of sufficient quality to be analyzed.

Examples of meta-analysis studies reported in the occupational therapy literature include a review of the effect of alternative keyboard designs on the acquisition of upper-extremity musculoskeletal disorders (Baker & Cidboy, 2006); analysis of the co-occurrence of communication disorders with motor impairments in children with language disorders (Rechetnikov & Maitra,

2009); the effectiveness of physical, psychological, and functional interventions in treatment of multiple sclerosis (Baker & Tickle-Degnen, 2001); the effectiveness of occupational therapy–related treatments for persons with Parkinson's disease (Murphy & Tickle-Degnen, 2001); the effectiveness of occupational therapy for persons with dementia (Kim, Yoo, Jung, Park, & Park, 2012); a comparison of constraint-induced movement therapy and traditional rehabilitation for patients with upper-extremity dysfunction (Shi, Tian, Yang, & Zhao, 2011); and a review of research on sensory integration treatment (Vargas & Camilli, 1999).

When insufficient numbers of research studies exist to apply the statistical procedures of a meta-analysis, a **systematic review** that completes a comprehensive literature search for relevant studies on a specific topic can be done (Brown & Burns, 2001; Murphy, Robinson, & Lin, 2009). A systematic literature review has a clear clinical topic of interest and selection standards for the relevant literature, evaluates the quality of the studies using predetermined criteria, and yields conclusions to guide clinical practice decisions. It is another helpful approach in evaluating intervention outcomes and providing evidence for practice.

The Systematic Process for Investigating and Describing Evidence-Based Research, or SPIDER (Classen et al., 2008), is a tool that helps researchers assess the value of primary studies for potential use in systematic literature reviews. The tool was determined to have strong content and criterion validity and significant correlations between quality indicators and the overall quality score. The SPIDER can be found as an appendix in the above reference.

Some systematic literature reviews of interest to an occupational therapist are a review of assessments that predict driving performance of people with traumatic brain injury (Classen et al., 2009), an analysis of the research to support the use of splinting for people with carpometacarpal osteoarthritis (Egan & Brousseau, 2007), a review of the impact of high- and low-technology modifications to automobiles on the driving performance of older adults (Arbesman & Pellerito, 2008), a review of outcomes of interventions for people with substance-use disorders (Stoffel & Moyers, 2004), a review of occupational therapy interventions that improve leisure and social participation for older adults with low vision (Berger, McAteer, Schreier,

& Kaldenberg, 2013), a review of occupational therapy that promotes motor performance for children from birth to age 5 years (Case-Smith, Frolek Clark, & Schlabach, 2013), and a review of the use of yoga to reduce anxiety (Chugh-Gupta, Baldassarre, & Vrkljan, 2013).

AOTA has developed resources to address the profession's need to have access to research to support clinical decision making. The steps of identifying evidence to support practice have been articulated in journal articles, and AOTA has developed a section on the AOTA website for evidence-based practice and research that includes articles, an evidence-based practice resource directory, evidence bytes, critically appraised topics and papers, "Evidence Perks" (a quarterly column), and an evidence brief series on a wide range of topics.

Another resource to identify evidence for occupational therapy practice comes from Australia, where a team of occupational therapists has developed a web-based evidence resource called OTseeker (Bennett et al., 2003). OTseeker (www.otseeker.com), available at no cost to users, is a database that contains abstracts of systematic reviews and RCTs relevant to occupational therapy. In the database, trials are critically appraised and rated to assist the occupational therapist in evaluating validity and interpretability. These ratings will help the therapist judge the quality and usefulness of trials for informing clinical interventions. In one database, OTseeker provides occupational therapists with fast and easy access to trials from a wide range of sources (Bennett et al., 2003).

Some other evidence-focused resources with helpful information for occupational therapists include the five databases of the Cochrane Library, which are available through institutional subscription: (1) OTDBASE (www.otdbase.org), available with individual and institution subscriptions; (2) PEDro (www.pedro.org.au) and (3) RehabDATA (www.naric.com/research), which are both available for free on the web; and (4) OT CATS (www.otcats.com) and (5) Critically Appraised Topics in Rehabilitation Therapy (https://qspace.library.queensu.ca/handle/1974/213), which also are both available for free on the Web.

These evidence-focused resources, among many others, make the information needed to understand and support best practice increasingly accessible and understandable. Opportunities are limited for the typical occupational therapist to participate in the efforts needed to conduct retrospective reviews of charts and evaluation data, systematic reviews of the literature, meta-analyses, outcomes research, and so forth. However, occupational therapists need to recognize the value of the evaluation data that are acquired every day and the methods necessary to make that data available to advance the profession's knowledge base, so that each occupational therapist can be part of the ongoing efforts of the profession to provide the highest quality services with the most desired outcomes to our clients.

Scoping reviews have been advocated by the National Institute for Health Research and involve "synthesis and analysis of a wide range of research and non-research material to provide greater conceptual clarity about a specific topic or field of evidence" (Davis, Drey, & Gould, 2009, p. 1386). Scoping reviews or studies may share some conceptual foundation but are different from systematic reviews. Systematic reviews have focused research questions and include predetermined study designs with quality assessment. Scoping reviews can be conducted to

- Examine the extent, range, and nature of research activity;
- Determine the value of undertaking a systematic review;
- Identify research gaps in the existing literature; and
- Summarize and disseminate research findings (Arksey & O'Malley, 2005; Davis et al., 2009).

Although scoping reviews address broader topics and can include in the analysis a range of study designs with no quality assessment (Boyd & Bastian, 2011), the basic framework guiding a scoping review involves

- "Identifying the research question,
- Identifying relevant studies,
- Selecting studies,
- Charting the data, and
- Summarizing and reporting the results" (Arksey & O'Malley, 2005, p. 21).

A rise in scoping reviews has been seen in occupational therapy literature in the recent past.

Thomas and Law (2013) performed a scoping review addressing research use and evidence-based practice in occupational therapy. They suggested that client-centered practice, case application, and peer consultations facilitate evaluation and integration of research evidence in clinical practice. Another scoping study reviewed use of home health services in occupational therapy (Craig, 2012). A scoping review addressing occupational therapy interventions for chronic diseases was also undertaken (Hand, Law, & McColl, 2011). Scoping reviews can assist occupational therapy practitioners in collecting evidence regarding clinical implications of various occupation-based interventions along with recent advancements that are documented in the literature but widely dispersed.

CLINICAL RESEARCH METHODS USING SMALL NUMBERS OF PARTICIPANTS

The strategies described in this chapter for using evaluation data to build evidence and knowledge about occupational therapy services—retrospective chart reviews, meta-analysis, and systematic reviews of the literature—depend upon the availability of large bodies of data and literature to be successful. However, some research methodologies can be applied in the clinical setting and are within the range of accomplishment for most occupational therapists and, if used, could make important contributions to the profession's knowledge base. **Single-subject research methods,** in particular, provide the "opportunity for the therapist to evaluate treatment procedures within the context of clinical care, and to share insights about patient behavior and response that are typically ignored or indiscernible using traditional group research approaches" (Portney & Watkins, 2009, p. 271).

Single-subject research studies have appeared in the occupational therapy literature on a regular basis, with some examples from recent years including a study of the effects of an occupational therapy intervention emphasizing sensory integration with 5 preschool children with autism (Case-Smith & Bryan, 1999), an examination of the effectiveness of using a weighted vest for increasing attention to a fine motor task and decreasing self-stimulatory behaviors in preschool children with pervasive developmental disorders (Fertel-Daly, Bedell, & Hinojosa, 2001), and a study on the effects of traditional and computer-aided instruction on promoting independent skin care in adults with paraplegia (Pellerito, 2003).

Patrick, Mozzoni, and Patrick (2000) suggested that single-subject designs are the best approach to use when "confronted with questions of effectiveness and clinical decision making in the absence of sufficient development of standards of care" (p. 60) that are based on research and empirical findings. This view concurs with the position of Portney and Watkins (2009), who suggested that "the clinician, working in the practice setting, is uniquely qualified to perform these [single-subject] studies. This is especially true in terms of the importance of clinical replication" (p. 271). This observation reinforces the important role of the typical occupational therapist in contributing to the knowledge base of the profession through systematic and careful documentation of occupational therapy services. Both of the references presented in this paragraph are good resources for more information about single-subject research methods and determining their suitability for implementation in one's practice setting.

FIELDWORK EVALUATION: PREPARING EVIDENCE-INFORMED PRACTITIONERS

Occupational therapy students participate in fieldwork opportunities, as directed by their respective sites, to gain clinical experience while reflecting on their academic learning. During the process, many graduate students are guided by their fieldwork supervisors to develop interventions while keeping outcome measures in mind. Gathering data through fieldwork experiences can be used in a variety of ways to benefit both student learning and the clinical setting, such as carrying out small research projects (de Jongh, 2012; Shordike & Howell, 2002) and preparing students for future professional employment (Aiken, Menaker, & Barsky, 2001; Beltran, Scanlan, Hancock, & Luckett, 2007; Crowe & Mackenzie, 2002; Rodger et al., 2007.).

Training students to use standardized outcomes measurement can assist in producing professionals who seek and use evidence-based practices.

In addition to advancing student education, fieldwork experience can also benefit fieldwork supervisors. Fieldwork supervisors have noted that supervising students enables them to develop clinical reasoning skills, keep their skills current, and improve team development (Thomas et al., 2007). Client and self-evaluation during fieldwork experience can thus benefit both students and clinicians in developing clinical expertise and gathering data for program development while ensuring a science-driven and evidence-based approach for clinical practice. In 2013, the AOTA Board of Directors approved priorities for 2014 that included emphasis on science-driven and evidence-based practice (AOTA, 2013).

PROGRAM DEVELOPMENT AND EVALUATION

Another important use of evaluation data is the development and evaluation of occupational therapy service programs. In the competitive health care marketplace of the 21st century, all occupational therapists and occupational therapy assistants need to consider potential new service areas of practice. New practice areas emerge in occupational therapy because a therapist sees the need for occupation-based prevention and intervention services across wide spectrums of the population.

Examples of new service areas that have emerged in the past decade are backpack awareness education programs, older adult driver awareness campaigns and driver rehabilitation programs, low-vision services, and technology and assistive device development and consulting. Efforts have been directed toward the development of service programs in the community, including hospice care, horticultural programs for people with psychiatric disabilities, and violence prevention in schools.

Ideas for new programs can be operationalized only with data to support the need for a new initiative. Two texts on occupational therapy services in community settings (Fazio, 2007; Scaffa & Reitz, 2013) provide detailed outlines for planning, implementation, and evaluation of new programs. They are invaluable resources for expanding occupational therapy services in familiar practice arenas as well as in new areas of practice that previously had not been considered.

In addition to these texts, articles about innovative programs with new and familiar clinical populations can serve as models for program development and evaluation. Some examples are the implementation and evaluation of an online program to manage fatigue, which was developed from a standard face-to-face format (Ghahari, Packer, & Passmore, 2009), development of a program to manage stress for people living in impoverished conditions in South Africa (Crouch, 2008), the conversion of a face-to-face group energy conservation program to a group teleconference format for people with multiple sclerosis (Finlayson, 2005), a social participation program for children with Asperger syndrome (Carter et al., 2004), the development of programs for underserved clinical populations using participatory action research (Taylor, Braveman, & Hammel, 2004), programs for persons with chronic rheumatic disease (Bailey, Starr, Alderson, & Moreland, 1999; Samuelson & Ahlmén, 2000), a program for refugee high school students (Copley, Turpin, Gordon, & McLaren, 2011), a program of telerehabilitation for children with autism (Gibbs & Toth-Cohen, 2011), and training for adults with severe intellectual disabilities to engage in the virtual environment (Lotan, Yalon-Chamovitz, & Weiss, 2010).

The application of systematic screening and evaluation procedures for a risk appraisal for older adults (identified through the research literature on evidence for practice) allowed one therapist to educate older adults about fitness and promote a community wellness program (Toto, 2001). This occupational therapist adopted an outcomes-oriented approach, used resources for evidence to support practice, implemented use of a standardized assessment protocol in her program, met the needs of older adults in her community, and promoted the value of occupations and the profession of occupational therapy. In this example, the evaluation data helped to provide the best possible occupational therapy services to the clients.

SUMMARY

Can evaluation data change practice? The use of evaluation data in a systematic manner can be used to shape and change not just practice but also the profession. Evaluation data can be used for outcomes measurement to support the use of standardized assessments in clinical use. Data-based retrospective chart reviews and systematic reviews of the literature can be used to guide practice. Small clinical research studies, such as single-subject designs, can support evaluation processes. Finally, the collection of evaluation data can be effectively used in program development and evaluation and to improve practice.

QUESTIONS

1. How does the use of standardized assessments relate to determining outcomes measures?
2. Choose an occupational therapy topic, and research it using 3 of the databases discussed in this chapter. What did you find? Did it change your understanding of your chosen topic?
3. How do quantitative outcomes data differ from qualitative outcomes data? Give an example of a topic that would be appropriate for each type of data.
4. Think about areas of practice that you have been exposed to or in which you have worked. Identify a topic that would be appropriate for a single case study.
5. Explain how program development and evaluation relate to outcomes data.
6. Explain how the development of new arenas of practice relates to outcomes data.
7. Overall, how do you think the proliferation of increased outcomes data will affect the profession of occupational therapy?

References

Aegler, B., & Satink, T. (2009). Performing occupations under pain: The experience of persons with chronic pain. *Scandinavian Journal of Occupational Therapy, 16,* 49–56. http://dx.doi.org/10.1080/11038120802512425

Aiken, F., Menaker, L., & Barsky, L. (2001). Fieldwork education: The future of occupational therapy depends on it. *Occupational Therapy International, 8,* 86–95. http://dx.doi.org/10.1002/oti.135

American Occupational Therapy Association. (2007). AOTA's *Centennial Vision* and executive summary.

American Journal of Occupational Therapy, 61, 613–614. http://dx.doi.org/10.5014/ajot.61.6.613

American Occupational Therapy Association. (2009). *Q&A: AOTA's endorsement of outcomes measurement tool. AOTA Partners with Cedaron Medical Inc., to develop electronic patient record and documentation system* [Press release]. Retrieved on from http://www.aota.org/News/Media/PR/2009-Press-Releases/ElectronicRecords.aspx

American Occupational Therapy Association. (2013). *AOTA FY2014* Centennial Vision *priorities: Boldly navigating a changing world.* Retrieved from http://www.aota.org/en/aboutaota/get-involved/bod/news/2013/2014-priorities.aspx

American Occupational Therapy Association. (2014). Occupational therapy practice framework: Domain and process (3rd ed.). *American Journal of Occupational Therapy, 68*(Suppl. 1), S1–S48. http://dx.doi.org/10.5014/ajot.2014.682006

Andreasen, N. C. (1983). *The Scale for the Assessment of Negative Symptoms (SANS): Conceptual and theoretical foundations.* Iowa City: University of Iowa.

Arbesman, M., & Pellerito, J. M., Jr. (2008). Evidence-based perspective on the effect of automobile-related modifications on the driving ability, performance, and safety of older adults. *American Journal of Occupational Therapy, 62,* 173–186. http://dx.doi.org/10.5014/ajot.62.2.173

Arksey, H., & O'Malley, L. (2005). Scoping studies: Towards a methodological framework. *International Journal of Social Research Methodology, 8,* 19–32. http://dx.doi.org/10.1080/1364557032000119616

Ashburner, J., Ziviani, J., & Rodger, S. (2008). Sensory processing and classroom emotional, behavioral, and educational outcomes in children with autism spectrum disorder. *American Journal of Occupational Therapy, 62,* 564–573. http://dx.doi.org/10.5014/ajot.62.5.564

Ayres, J. (1972). *Southern California sensory integration tests manual.* Los Angeles: Western Psychological Services.

Ayres, J. (1989). *Sensory integration and praxis tests.* Los Angeles: Western Psychological Services.

Bailey, A., Starr, L., Alderson, M., & Moreland, J. (1999). A comparative evaluation of a fibromyalgia rehabilitation program. *Arthritis Care and Research, 12,* 336–340. http://dx.doi.org/10.1002/1529-0131(199910)12:5<336::AID-ART5>3.0.CO;2-E

Baker, N. A., & Cidboy, E. L. (2006). The effect of three alternative keyboard designs on forearm pronation, wrist extension, and ulnar deviation: A meta-analysis. *American Journal of Occupational Therapy, 60,* 40–49. http://dx.doi.org/10.5014/ajot.60.1.40

Baker, N. A., Jacobs, K., & Tickle-Degnen, L. (2003). A methodology for developing evidence about meaning in occupation: Exploring the meaning of working. *OTJR: Occupation, Participation and Health, 23,* 5–66.

Baker, N. A., & Tickle-Degnen, L. (2001). The effectiveness of physical, psychological, and functional interventions in treating clients with multiple sclerosis: A meta-analysis. *American Journal of Occupational Therapy, 55,* 324–331. http://dx.doi.org/10.5014/ajot.55.3.324

Baranek, G. T., Barnett, C. R., Adams, E. M., Wolcott, N. A., Watson, L. R., & Crais, E. R. (2005). Object play in infants with autism: Methodological issues in retrospective video analysis. *American Journal of Occupational Therapy, 59,* 20–30. http://dx.doi.org/10.5014/ajot.59.1.20

Barr, J., Schumacher, G., & Ohman, S. (2003). *Outcomes assessment and health-related quality of life measurement.* Boston: National Education and Research Center for Outcomes Assessment in Healthcare (NERCOA), Northeastern University.

Baum, C. M. (2011). Fulfilling the promise: Supporting participation in daily life. *Archives of Physical Medicine and Rehabilitation, 92,* 169–175. http://dx.doi.org/10.1016/j.apmr.2010.12.010

Baum, C. M., Connor, L. T., Morrison, T., Hahn, M., Dromerick, A. W., & Edwards, D. F. (2008). Reliability, validity, and clinical utility of the Executive Function Performance Test: A measure of executive function in a sample of people with stroke. *American Journal of Occupational Therapy, 62,* 446–455. http://dx.doi.org/10.5014/ajot.62.4.446

Baum, C. M., & Edwards, D. (2008). *Activity card sort* (2nd ed.). Bethesda, MD: AOTA Press.

Bazyk, S., Michaud, P., Goodman, G., Papp, P., Hawkins, E., & Welch, M. A. (2009). Integrating occupational therapy services in a kindergarten curriculum: A look at the outcomes. *American Journal of Occupational Therapy, 63,* 160–171. http://dx.doi.org/10.5014/ajot.63.2.160

Beery, K. E., Buktenica, N. A., & Beery, N. A. (2004). *Developmental test of visual–motor integration* (5th ed.). Minneapolis: Pearson Assessments.

Beltran, R. O., Scanlan, J. N., Hancock, N., & Luckett, T. (2007). The effect of first year mental health fieldwork on attitudes of occupational therapy students towards people with mental illness. *Australian Occupational Therapy Journal, 54,* 42–48. http://dx.doi.org/10.1111/j.1440-1630.2006.00619.x

Bennett, S., Hoffmann, T., McCluskey, A., McKenna, K., Strong, J., & Tooth, L. (2003). Introducing OT-seeker (Occupational Therapy Systematic Evaluation of Evidence): A new evidence database for occupational therapists. *American Journal of Occupational Therapy, 57,* 635–638. http://dx.doi.org/10.5014/ajot.57.6.635

Berger, S., McAteer, J., Schreier, K., & Kaldenberg, J. (2013). Occupational therapy interventions to improve leisure and social participation for older adults with low vision: A systematic review. *American Journal of Occupational Therapy, 67,* 303–311. http://dx.doi.org/10.5014/ajot.2013.005447

Birchwood, M., Smith, J., Cochrane, R., Wetton, S., & Copestake, S. (1990). The Social Functioning Scale. The development and validation of a new scale of social adjustment for use in family intervention programmes with schizophrenic patients. *British Journal of Psychiatry, 157,* 853–859. http://dx.doi.org/10.1192/bjp.157.6.853

Boland, P. (2011). *Coping and multiple sclerosis: Individuals with multiple sclerosis and their significant others* (Unpublished master's thesis), University of Otago, Dunedin, New Zealand.

Bowman, J. (2006). Challenges to measuring outcomes in occupational therapy: A qualitative focus group study. *British Journal of Occupational Therapy, 69,* 464–472.

Bowman, J., & Llewellyn, G. (2002). Clinical outcomes research from the occupational therapist's perspective. *Occupational Therapy International, 9,* 145–166. http://dx.doi.org/10.1002/oti.162

Boyd, A., & Bastian, M. (2011). *What is a scoping study?* Retrieved from http://www.methods.manchester.ac.uk/events/whatis/scopingstudy.pdf

Brauer, J., Hay, C. C., & Francisco, G. (2011). A retrospective investigation of occupational therapy services received following a traumatic brain injury. *Occupational Therapy in Health Care, 25,* 119–130. http://dx.doi.org10.3109/07380577.2011.570420

Brown, G. T., & Burns, S. A. (2001). The efficacy of neurodevelopmental treatment in paediatrics: A systematic review. *British Journal of Occupational Therapy, 64*(5), 235–244.

Carswell, A., McColl, M. A., Baptiste, S., Law, M., Polatajko, H., & Pollock, N. (2004). The Canadian Occupational Performance Measure: A research and clinical literature review. *Canadian Journal of Occupational Therapy, 71,* 210–222. http://dx.doi.org/10.1177/000841740407100406

Carter, C., Meckes, L., Pritchard, L., Swensen, S., Wittman, P. P., & Velde, B. (2004). The Friendship Club: An after-school program for children with Asperger syndrome. *Family and Community Health, 27,* 143–150. http://dx.doi.org/10.1097/00003727-200404000-00007

Case-Smith, J. (1998). Outcomes research using a collaborative multi-site model. *Journal of Rehabilitation Outcomes Measurement, 2*(6), 9–17.

Case-Smith, J., & Bryan, T. (1999). The effects of occupational therapy with sensory integration emphasis on preschool-age children with autism. *American Journal of Occupational Therapy, 53,* 489–497. http://dx.doi.org/10.5014/ajot.53.5.489

Case-Smith, J., Frolek Clark, G. J., & Schlabach, T. L. (2013). Systematic review of interventions used in occupational therapy to promote motor performance for children ages birth–5 years. *American Journal of Occupational Therapy, 67,* 413–424. http://dx.doi.org/10.5014/ajot.2013.005959

Charlson, M. E., Pompei, P., Ales, K. L., & MacKenzie, C. R. (1987). A new method of classifying prognostic comorbidity in longitudinal studies: Development and validation. *Journal of Chronic Diseases, 40,* 373–383. http://dx.doi.org/10.1016/0021-9681(87)90171-8

Chen, C. C., Heinemann, A. W., Bode, R. K., Granger, C. V., & Mallinson, T. (2004). Impact of pediatric rehabilitation services on children's functional outcomes. *American Journal of Occupational Therapy, 58,* 44–53. http://dx.doi.org/10.5014/ajot.58.1.44

Chua, M., McCluskey, A., & Smead, J. M. (2012). Retrospective analysis of factors that affect driving assessment outcomes after stroke. *Australian Occupational Therapy Journal, 59,* 121–130. http://dx.doi.org/10.1111/j.1440-1630.2012.01005.x

Chugh-Gupta, N., Baldassarre, F. G., & Vrkljan, B. H. (2013). A systematic review of yoga for state anxiety: Considerations for occupational therapy. *Canadian Journal of Occupational Therapy—Revue Canadienne d'Ergothérapie, 80*(3), 150–170. Retrieved from http://ovidsp.ovid.com/ovidweb.cgi?T=JS&PAGE=reference&D=prem&NEWS=N&AN=24224228

Classen, S., Levy, C., McCarthy, D., Mann, W. C., Lanford, D., & Waid-Ebbs, J. K. (2009). Traumatic brain injury and driving assessment: An evidence-based literature review. *American Journal of Occupational Therapy, 63,* 580–591. http://dx.doi.org/10.5014/ajot.63.5.580

Classen, S., Winter, S., Awadzi, K. D., Garvan, C. W., Lopez, E. D., & Sundaram, S. (2008). Psychometric testing of SPIDER: Data capture tool for systematic literature reviews. *American Journal of Occupational Therapy, 62,* 335–348. http://dx.doi.org/10.5014/ajot.62.3.335

Clay, M. M. (1993). *Observation survey of early literacy achievement.* Portsmouth, NH: Heinemann Educational.

Clifton, D. W., Jr. (2005a). How to locate sources of disability-related data. In D. W. Clifton, Jr. (Ed.), *Physical rehabilitation's role in disability management: Unique perspectives for success* (pp. 229–238). St. Louis: Elsevier/Saunders.

Clifton, D. W., Jr. (2005b). Outcomes management. In D. W. Clifton, Jr. (Ed.), *Physical rehabilitation's role in disability management: Unique perspectives for success* (pp. 207–228). St. Louis: Elsevier/Saunders.

Cohn, E., Miller, L. J., & Tickle-Degnen, L. (2000). Parental hopes for therapy outcomes: Children with sensory modulation disorders. *American Journal of Occupational Therapy, 54,* 36–43. http://dx.doi.org/10.5014/ajot.54.1.36

Cook, S., Chambers, E., & Coleman, J. H. (2009). Occupational therapy for people with psychotic conditions in community settings: A pilot randomized controlled trial. *Clinical Rehabilitation, 23,* 40–52. http://dx.doi.org/10.1177/0269215508098898

Copley, J., Turpin, M., Gordon, S., & McLaren, C. (2011). Development and evaluation of an occupational therapy program for refugee high school students. *Australian Occupational Therapy Journal, 58,* 310–316. http://dx.doi.org/10.1111/j.1440-1630.2011.00933.x

Coster, W. J. (2008). Embracing ambiguity: Facing the challenge of measurement (Eleanor Clarke Slagle Lecture). *American Journal of Occupational Therapy, 62,* 743–752. http://dx.doi.org/10.5014/ajot.62.6.743

Coster, W. J. (2013). Making the best match: Selecting outcome measures for clinical trials and outcome studies. *American Journal of Occupational Therapy, 67,* 162–170. http://dx.doi.org/10.5014/ajot.2013.006015

Coster, W. J., Deeney, T., Haley, S. M., & Haltiwanger, J. (1998). *School Function Assessment.* San Antonio, TX: Psychological Corporation.

Craig, D. G. (2012). Current occupational therapy publications in home health: A scoping review. *American Journal of Occupational Therapy, 66,* 338–347. http://dx.doi.org/10.5014/ajot.2012.003566

Crouch, R. B. (2008). A community-based stress management programme for an impoverished population in South Africa. *Occupational Therapy International, 15,* 71–86. http://dx.doi.org/10.1002/oti.246

Crowe, M. J., & Mackenzie, L. (2002). The influence of fieldwork on the preferred future practice areas of final year occupational therapy students. *Australian Occupational Therapy Journal, 49,* 25–36. http://dx.doi.org/10.1046/j.0045-0766.2001.00276.x

Cup, E. H., Scholte op Reimer, W. J., Thijssen, M. C., & van Kuyk-Minis, M. A. (2003). Reliability and validity of the Canadian Occupational Performance Measure in stroke patients. *Clinical Rehabilitation, 17,* 402–409. http://dx.doi.org/10.1191/0269215503cr635oa

Darzins, S., Imms, C., & Di Stefano, M. (2013). Measurement properties of the Personal Care Participation Assessment and Resource Tool: A systematic review. *Disability and Rehabilitation, 35,* 265–281. http://dx.doi.org/10.3109/09638288.2012.690819

Davis, K., Drey, N., & Gould, D. (2009). What are scoping studies? A review of the nursing literature. *International Journal of Nursing Studies, 46,* 1386–1400. http://dx.org/doi:10.1016/j.ijnurstu.2009.02.010

de Jongh, J. C. (2012). Undergraduate occupational therapy students' engagement in qualitative research: Identifying research problems and questions through reflection while in a community fieldwork setting. *South African Journal of Occupational Therapy, 42,* 35–39.

Donovan, J. M., VanLeit, B. J., Crowe, T. K., & Keefe, E. B. (2005). Occupational goals of mothers of children with disabilities: Influence of temporal, social, and emotional contexts. *American Journal of Occupational Therapy, 59,* 249–261. http://dx.doi.org/10.5014/ajot.59.3.249

Dunford, C., Bannigan, K., & Wales, L. (2013). Measuring activity and participation outcomes for children and youth with acquired brain injury: An occupational therapy perspective. *British Journal of Occupational Therapy, 76,* 67–76. http://dx.doi.org/10.4276/030802213X13603244419158

Dunn, W., & Westman, K. (1997). The Sensory Profile: The performance of a national sample of children without disabilities. *American Journal of Occupational Therapy, 51,* 25–34. http://dx.doi.org/10.5014/ajot.51.1.25

Egan, M. Y., & Brousseau, L. (2007). Splinting for osteoarthritis of the carpometacarpal joint: A review of the evidence. *American Journal of Occupational Therapy, 61,* 70–78. http://dx.doi.org/10.5014/ajot.61.1.70

Ellek, D. (1996). Policy implications of outcomes research. *American Journal of Occupational Therapy, 50,* 886–889. http://dx.doi.org/10.5014/ajot.50.10.886

Erdner, A., Magnusson, A., & Lützén, K. (2012). Basic attitudes toward life expressed by persons with long-term mental illness living in a Swedish community. *Issues in Mental Health Nursing, 33,* 387–393. http://dx.doi.org/10.3109/01612840.2012.661520

Fang, C. T., Hsiung, P. C., Yu, C. F., Chen, M. Y., & Wang, J. D. (2002). Validation of the World Health Organization quality of life instrument in patients with HIV infection. *Quality of Life Research, 11,* 753–762. http://dx.doi.org/10.1023/A:1020870402019

Fazio, L. S. (2007). *Developing occupation-centered programs for the community: A workbook for students and professionals* (2nd ed.). Upper Saddle River, NJ: Prentice Hall.

Ferrans, C. E., & Powers, M. J. (1985). Quality of life index: Development and psychometric properties. *ANS. Advances in Nursing Science, 8,* 15–24. http://dx.doi.org/10.1097/00012272-198510000-00005

Fertel-Daly, D., Bedell, G., & Hinojosa, J. (2001). Effects of a weighted vest on attention to task and self-stimulatory behaviors in preschoolers with pervasive developmental disorders. *American Journal of Occupational Therapy, 55,* 629–640. http://dx.doi.org/10.5014/ajot.55.6.629

Finlayson, M. (2004). Concerns about the future among older adults with multiple sclerosis. *American Journal of Occupational Therapy, 58*, 54–63. http://dx.doi.org/10.5014/ajot.58.1.54

Finlayson, M. (2005). Pilot study of an energy conservation education program delivered by telephone conference call to people with multiple sclerosis. *NeuroRehabilitation, 20*, 267–277.

Folio, M., & Fewell, R. R. (2000). *Peabody Developmental Motor Scales* (2nd ed.). Austin, TX: Pro-Ed.

Franklin, L., Deitz, J., Jirikowic, T., & Astley, S. (2008). Children with fetal alcohol spectrum disorders: Problem behaviors and sensory processing. *American Journal of Occupational Therapy, 62*, 265–273. http://dx.doi.org/10.5014/ajot.62.3.265

Freuler, A., Baranek, G. T., Watson, L. R., Boyd, B. A., & Bulluck, J. C. (2012). Precursors and trajectories of sensory features: Qualitative analysis of infant home videos. *American Journal of Occupational Therapy, 66*, e81–e84. http://dx.doi.org/10.5014/ajot.2012.004465

Fulks, M. L., & Harris, S. R. (1995). Children exposed to drugs in utero: Their scores on the Miller Assessment for Preschoolers. *Canadian Journal of Occupational Therapy, 62*, 7–15. http://dx.doi.org/10.1177/000841749506200103

Gandek, B., Sinclair, S. J., Jette, A. M., & Ware, J. E., Jr. (2007). Development and initial psychometric evaluation of the Participation Measure for Post-Acute Care (PM–PAC). *American Journal of Physical Medicine and Rehabilitation, 86*, 57–71. http://dx.doi.org/10.1097/01.phm.0000233200.43822.21

Ghahari, S., Packer, T. L., & Passmore, A. E. (2009). Development, standardisation and pilot testing of an online fatigue self-management program. *Disability and Rehabilitation, 31*, 1762–1772. http://dx.doi.org/10.1080/09638280902751956

Gibbs, V., & Toth-Cohen, S. (2011). Family-centered occupational therapy and telerehabilitation for children with autism spectrum disorders. *Occupational Therapy in Health Care, 25*, 298–314. http://dx.doi.org/10.3109/07380577.2011.606460

Goverover, Y., & Hinojosa, J. (2004). Interrater reliability and discriminant validity of the deductive reasoning test. *American Journal of Occupational Therapy, 58*, 104–108. http://dx.doi.org/10.5014/ajot.58.1.104

Gutman, S. (2008). From the Desk of the Editor—Research priorities of the profession. *American Journal of Occupational Therapy, 62*, 499–501. http://dx.doi.org/10.5014/ajot.62.5.499

Haley, S. M., Coster, W. J., Ludlow, L., Haltiwanger, J., & Andrellos, P. (1992). *Pediatric Evaluation of Disability Inventory (PEDI)*. Boston: Trustees of Boston University.

Hammill, D. D., Pearson, N. A., & Voress, J. K. (1993). *Developmental Test of Visual Perception* (2nd ed.). Austin, TX: Pro-Ed.

Hand, C., Law, M., & McColl, M. A. (2011). Occupational therapy interventions for chronic diseases: A scoping review. *American Journal of Occupational Therapy, 65*, 428–436. http://dx.doi.org/10.5014/ajot.2011.002071

Hartman-Maeir, A., Harel, H., & Katz, N. (2009). Kettle Test—A brief measure of cognitive functional performance. Reliability and validity in stroke rehabilitation. *American Journal of Occupational Therapy, 63*, 592–599. http://dx.doi.org/10.5014/ajot.63.5.592

Heinemann, A. W., Lai, J. S., Magasi, S., Hammel, J., Corrigan, J. D., Bogner, J. A., & Whiteneck, G. G. (2011). Measuring participation enfranchisement. *Archives of Physical Medicine and Rehabilitation, 92*, 564–571. http://dx.doi.org/10.1016/j.apmr.2010.07.220

Hoffman, S., & Podgurski, A. (2011). Improving health care outcomes through personalized comparisons of treatment effectiveness based on electronic health records. *Journal of Law, Medicine and Ethics, 39*, 425–436.

Hotchkiss, A., Fisher, A., Robertson, R., Ruttencutter, A., Schuffert, J., & Barker, D. B. (2004). Convergent and predictive validity of three scales related to falls in the elderly. *American Journal of Occupational Therapy, 58*, 100–103. http://dx.doi.org/10.5014/ajot.58.1.100

Howard, K. I., Moras, K., Brill, P. L., Martinovich, Z., & Lutz, W. (1996). Evaluation of psychotherapy. Efficacy, effectiveness, and patient progress. *American Psychologist, 51*, 1059–1064. http://dx.doi.org/10.1037/0003-066X.51.10.1059

Huebner, R. A., Custer, M. G., Freudenberger, L., & Nichols, L. (2006). The Occupational Therapy Practice Checklist for adult physical rehabilitation. *American Journal of Occupational Therapy, 60*, 388–396. http://dx.doi.org/10.5014/ajot.60.4.388

Ivarsson, A., Söderback, I., & Stein, F. (2000). Goal, intervention and outcome of occupational therapy in individuals with psychoses. Content analysis through chart review. *Occupational Therapy International, 7*, 21–41. http://dx.doi.org/10.1002/oti.105

Jacobson, N. S., Roberts, L. J., Berns, S. B., & McGlinchey, J. B. (1999). Methods for defining and determining the clinical significance of treatment effects: Description, application, and alternatives. *Journal of Consulting and Clinical Psychology, 67*, 300–307. http://dx.doi.org/10.1037/0022-006X.67.3.300

Jacques, N. D., & Hasselkus, B. R. (2004). The nature of occupation surrounding dying and death. *OTJR: Occupation, Participation and Health, 24*, 44–53.

Jang, Y., Chern, J.-S., & Lin, K.-C. (2009). Validity of the Loewenstein occupational therapy cognitive assessment in people with intellectual disabilities. *American Journal of Occupational Therapy, 63*, 414–422. http://dx.doi.org/10.5014/ajot.63.4.414

Jason, L. A., Ropacki, M. T., Santoro, N. B., Richman, J. A., Heatherly, W., . . . Plioplys, S. (1997). A screening instrument for chronic fatigue syndrome: Reliability and validity. *Journal of Chronic Fatigue Syndrome, 3*, 39–59.

Jong, A. M., van Nes, F. A., & Lindeboom, R. (2012). The Dutch Activity Card Sort institutional version was reproducible, but biased against women. *Disability and Rehabilitation, 34*, 1550–1555. http://dx.doi.org/10.3109/09638288.2011.647232

Katz, N., Golstand, S., Traub Bar-Ilan, R. T., & Parush, S. (2007). The Dynamic Occupational Therapy Cognitive Assessment for Children (DOTCA-Ch): A new instrument for assessing learning potential. *American Journal of Occupational Therapy, 61*, 41–52. http://dx.doi:10.5014/ajot.61.1.41

Kazdin, A. E. (1999). The meanings and measurement of clinical significance. *Journal of Consulting and Clinical Psychology, 67*, 332–339. http://dx.doi.org/10.1037/0022-006X.67.3.332

Kazdin, A. E. (2001). Almost clinically significant ($p < .10$): Current measures may only approach clinical significance. *Clinical Psychology: Science and Practice, 8*, 455–462. http://onlinelibrary.wiley.com/doi/10.1093/clipsy.8.4.455/abstract

Kielhofner, G., Braveman, B., Finlayson, M., Paul-Ward, A., Goldbaum, L., & Goldstein, K. (2004). Outcomes of a vocational program for persons with AIDS. *American Journal of Occupational Therapy, 58*, 64–72. http://dx.doi.org/10.5014/ajot.58.1.64

Kielhofner, G., Hammel, J., Finlayson, M., Helfrich, C., & Taylor, R. R. (2004). Documenting outcomes of occupational therapy: The center for outcomes research and education. *American Journal of Occupational Therapy, 58*, 15–23. http://dx.doi.org/10.5014/ajot.58.1.15

Kielhofner, G., Mallinson, T., Forsyth, K., & Lai, J. S. (2001). Psychometric properties of the second version of the Occupational Performance History Interview (OPHI–II). *American Journal of Occupational Therapy, 55*, 260–267. http://dx.doi.org/10.5014/ajot.55.3.260

Kim, S. Y., Yoo, E. Y., Jung, M. Y., Park, S. H., & Park, J. H. (2012). A systematic review of the effects of occupational therapy for persons with dementia: A meta-analysis of randomized controlled trials. *NeuroRehabilitation, 31*, 107–115. http://dx.doi.org/10.3233/NRE-2012-0779

Law, M. C. (Ed.). (1998). *Client-centered practice in occupational therapy.* Thorofare, NJ: Slack.

Law, M., Baptiste, S., Carswell, A., McColl, M. A., Polatajko, H., & Pollock, N. (1998). *Canadian Occupational Performance Measure* (3rd ed.). Ottawa: Canadian Association of Occupational Therapists Publications.

Law, M., Baum, C., & Dunn, W. (2005). *Measuring occupational performance: Supporting best practice in occupational therapy* (2nd ed.). Thorofare, NJ: Slack.

Lindstrom-Hazel, D., Kratt, A., & Bix, L. (2009). Interrater reliability of students using hand and pinch dynamometers. *American Journal of Occupational Therapy, 63*, 193–197. http://dx.doi.org/10.5014/ajot.63.2.193

Lotan, M., Yalon-Chamovitz, S., & Weiss, P. L. T. (2010). Virtual reality as means to improve physical fitness of individuals at a severe level of intellectual and developmental disability. *Research in Developmental Disabilities, 31*, 869–874. http://dx.doi.org/10.1016/j.ridd.2010.01.010

Lyons, J. S., Howard, K. I., Mahoney, M. T., & Lish, J. D. (1997). *The measurement and management of clinical outcomes in mental health.* New York: John Wiley & Sons.

Lysack, C. L., Neufeld, S., Mast, B. T., MacNeill, S. E., & Lichtenberg, P. A. (2003). After rehabilitation: An 18-month follow-up of elderly inner-city women. *American Journal of Occupational Therapy, 57*, 298–306. http://dx.doi.org/10.5014/ajot.57.3.298

Maassen, G. H., Bossema, E., & Brand, N. (2009). Reliable change and practice effects: Outcomes of various indices compared. *Journal of Clinical and Experimental Neuropsychology, 31*, 339–352. http://dx.doi.org/10.1080/13803390802169059

MacDermid, J., & Michlovitz, S. (2008). Incorporating outcomes measures in evidence-based practice. In M. Law & J. MacDermid (Eds.), *Evidence-based rehabilitation: A guide to practice* (2nd ed., pp. 63–94). Thorofare, NJ: Slack.

Mattis, S. (1988). *Dementia Rating Scale: Professional manual.* Odessa, FL: Psychological Assessment Resources.

McIntosh, D., Miller, L., Shyu, V., & Dunn, W. (1999). Development and validation of the Short Sensory Profile. In W. Dunn (Ed.), *The Sensory Profile examiner's manual* (pp. 59–73). San Antonio, TX: Psychological Corporation.

Miller, L. J. (1993). *Miller Assessment for Preschoolers.* San Antonio, TX: Psychological Corporation.

Murphy, S. L., Robinson, J. C., & Lin, S. H. (2009). Conducting systematic reviews to inform occupational therapy practice. *American Journal of Occupational Therapy, 63*, 363–368. http://dx.doi.org/10.5014/ajot.63.3.363

Murphy, S., & Tickle-Degnen, L. (2001). The effectiveness of occupational therapy-related treatments for persons with Parkinson's disease: A meta-analytic review. *American Journal of Occupational Therapy, 55*, 385–392. http://dx.doi.org/10.5014/ajot.55.4.385

Nagi, S. Z. (1964). A study in the evaluation of disability and rehabilitation potential: Concepts, methods, and procedures. *American Journal of Public Health and the Nation; Health, 54,* 1568–1579.

Nygard, L., & Ohman, A. (2002). Managing changes in everyday occupations: The experience of persons with Alzheimer's disease. *OTJR: Occupation, Participation and Health, 22,* 70–81.

Ogles, B. M., Lunnen, K. M., & Bonesteel, K. (2001). Clinical significance: History, application, and current practice. *Clinical Psychology Review, 21,* 421–446. http://dx.doi.org/10.1016/S0272-7358(99)00058-6

Oldridge, N. B. (1996). Outcomes measurement: Health state preferences and economic evaluation. *Assistive Technology, 8,* 94–102. http://dx.doi.org/10.1080/10400435.1996.10132279

Ottenbacher, K. J., Hsu, Y., Granger, C. V., & Fiedler, R. C. (1996). The reliability of the functional independence measure: A quantitative review. *Archives of Physical Medicine and Rehabilitation, 77,* 1226–1232. http://dx.doi.org/10.1016/S0003-9993(96)90184-7

Ottenbacher, K. J., Smith, P. M., Illig, S. B., Linn, R. T., Ostir, G. V., & Granger, C. V. (2004). Trends in length of stay, living setting, functional outcome, and mortality following medical rehabilitation. *JAMA, 292,* 1687–1695. http://dx.doi.org/10.1001/jama.292.14.1687

Pappas, C. (1993). Is narrative "primary"? Some insights from kindergarteners' pretend readings of stories and information books. *Journal of Reading Behavior, 25,* 97–129. http://dx.doi.org/10.1080/10862969309547803

Passmore, A. (2004). A measure of perceptions of generalized self-efficacy adapted for adolescents. *OTJR: Occupation, Participation and Health, 24,* 64–71.

Patrick, P. D., Mozzoni, M., & Patrick, S. T. (2000). Evidence-based care and the single-subject design. *Infants and Young Children, 13,* 60–73. http://dx.doi.org/10.1097/00001163-200013010-00009

Pearce, A. M., Smead, J. M., & Cameron, I. D. (2012). Retrospective cohort study of accident outcomes for individuals who have successfully undergone driver assessment following stroke. *Australian Occupational Therapy Journal, 59,* 56–62. http://dx.doi.org/10.1111/j.1440-1630.2011.00981.x

Pellerito, J. M., Jr. (2003). The effects of traditional and computer-aided instruction on promoting independent skin care in adults with paraplegia. *Occupational Therapy International, 10,* 1–19. http://dx.doi.org/10.1002/oti.174

Polatajko, H. J., Mandich, A. D., Miller, L. T., & Macnab, J. J. (2001). Cognitive Orientation to Daily Occupational Performance (CO–OP): Part II—The evidence. *Physical and Occupational Therapy in Pediatrics, 20,* 83–106. http://dx.doi.org/10.1080/J006v20n02_06.

Portney, L. G., & Watkins, M. P. (2009). *Foundations of clinical research: Applications to practice* (3rd ed.). Upper Saddle River, NJ: Prentice-Hall.

Rechetnikov, R. P., & Maitra, K. (2009). Motor impairments in children associated with impairments of speech or language: A meta-analytic review of research literature. *American Journal of Occupational Therapy, 63,* 255–263. http://dx.doi.org/10.5014/ajot.63.3.255

Rehabilitation Institute of Chicago. (2010). *Rehabilitation Measures Database.* Retrieved from www.rehabmeasures.org

Reker, D. M., Reid, K., Duncan, P. W., Marshall, C., Cowper, D., Stansbury, J., & Warr-Wing, K. L. (2005). Development of an integrated stroke outcomes database within Veterans Health Administration. *Journal of Rehabilitation Research and Development, 42,* 77–91. http://dx.doi.org/10.1682/JRRD.2003.11.0164

Rodger, S., Thomas, Y., Dickson, D., McBryde, C., Broadbridge, J., Hawkins, R., & Edwards, A. (2007). Putting students to work: Valuing fieldwork placements as a mechanism for recruitment and shaping the future occupational therapy workforce. *Australian Occupational Therapy Journal, 54,* S94–S97. http://dx.doi.org/10.1111/j.1440-1630.2007.00691.x

Ross, R. H., Callas, P. W., Sargent, J. Q., Amick, B. C., & Rooney, T. (2006). Incorporating injured employee outcomes into physical and occupational therapists' practice: A controlled trial of the Worker-Based Outcomes Assessment System. *Journal of Occupational Rehabilitation, 16,* 607–629. http://dx.doi.org/10.1007/s10926-006-9060-1

Salter, K. L., Foley, N. C., Jutai, J. W., & Teasell, R. W. (2007). Assessment of participation outcomes in randomized controlled trials of stroke rehabilitation interventions. *International Journal of Rehabilitation Research. Internationale Zeitschrift fur Rehabilitationsforschung. Revue Internationale de Recherches de Readaptation, 30,* 339–342. http://dx.doi.org/10.1097/MRR.0b013e3282f144b7

Samuelson, U. K., & Ahlmén, E. M. (2000). Development and evaluation of a patient education program education program for persons with systemic sclerosis (scleroderma). *Arthritis Care and Research, 13,* 141–148. http://dx.doi.org/10.1002/1529-0131(200006)13:3<141::AID-ANR3>3.0.CO;2-M

Satink, T., Winding, K., & Jonsson, H. (2004). Daily occupations with or without pain: Dilemmas in occupational performance. *OTJR: Occupation, Participation and Health, 24,* 144–150.

Scaffa, M., & Reitz, S. M. (Eds.). (2013). *Occupational therapy in community-based practice settings* (2nd ed.). Philadelphia: F. A. Davis.

Schaaf, R. C., & Nightlinger, K. M. (2007). Occupational therapy using a sensory integrative approach: A case study of effectiveness. *American Journal of Occupational Therapy, 61,* 239–246. http://dx.doi:10.5014/ajot.61.2.239

Sheikh, J. I., & Yesavage, J. A. (1986). Geriatric Depression Scale (GDS): Recent evidence and development of a shorter version. *Clinical Gerontologist, 5,* 165–173. http://dx.doi.org/10.1300/J018v05n01_09

Shi, Y. X., Tian, J. H., Yang, K. H., & Zhao, Y. (2011). Modified constraint-induced movement therapy versus traditional rehabilitation in patients with upper-extremity dysfunction after stroke: A systematic review and meta-analysis. *Archives of Physical Medicine and Rehabilitation, 92,* 972–982. http://dx.doi.org/10.1016/j.apmr.2010.12.036

Shordike, A., & Howell, D. (2002). The reindeer of hope: An occupational therapy program in a homeless shelter. *Education for Occupational Therapy in Health Care, 15,* 57–68. http://dx.doi.org/10.1080/J003v15n01_07

Simmons, D. C., Crepeau, E. B., & White, B. P. (2000). The predictive power of narrative data in occupational therapy evaluation. *American Journal of Occupational Therapy, 54,* 471–476. http://dx.doi.org/10.5014/ajot.54.5.471

Smallfield, S., & Karges, J. (2009). Classification of occupational therapy intervention for inpatient stroke rehabilitation. *American Journal of Occupational Therapy, 63,* 408–413. http://dx.doi.org/10.5014/ajot.63.4.408

Spencer, J., Hersch, G., Eschenfelder, V., Fournet, J., & Murray-Gerzik, M. (1999). Outcomes of protocol-based and adaptation-based occupational therapy interventions for low-income elderly persons on a transitional unit. *American Journal of Occupational Therapy, 53,* 159–170. http://dx.doi.org/10.5014/ajot.53.2.159

Stagnitti, K., & Unsworth, C. (2004). The test–retest reliability of the child-initiated pretend play assessment. *American Journal of Occupational Therapy, 58,* 93–99. http://dx.doi.org/10.5014/ajot.58.1.93

Stoffel, V. (2011). *Report of the vice president* (AOTA Vice President's Reports on the *Centennial Vision*). Retrieved from https://www.aota.org/-/media/Corporate/Files/AboutAOTA/Centennial/Commission/VP%20report%20ABM%202-15-11April.pdf

Stoffel, V. C., & Moyers, P. A. (2004). An evidence-based and occupational perspective of interventions for persons with substance-use disorders. *American Journal of Occupational Therapy, 58,* 570–586. http://dx.doi.org/10.5014/ajot.58.5.570

Sumsion, T. (Ed.). (2006). *Client-centred practice in occupational therapy: A guide to implementation* (2nd ed.). New York: Churchill Livingstone/Elsevier.

Taylor, R. R. (2004). Quality of life and symptom severity for individuals with chronic fatigue syndrome: Findings from a randomized clinical trial. *American Journal of Occupational Therapy, 58,* 35–43. http://dx.doi.org/10.5014/ajot.58.1.35

Taylor, R. R., Braveman, B., & Hammel, J. (2004). Developing and evaluating community-based services through participatory action research: Two case examples. *American Journal of Occupational Therapy, 58,* 73–82. http://dx.doi.org/10.5014/ajot.58.1.73

Thomas, A., & Law, M. (2013). Research utilization and evidence-based practice in occupational therapy: A scoping study. *American Journal of Occupational Therapy, 67,* e55–e65. http://dx.doi.org/10.5014/ajot.2013.006395

Thomas, Y., Dickson, D., Broadbridge, J., Hopper, L., Hawkins, R., Edwards, A., & McBryde, C. (2007). Benefits and challenges of supervising occupational therapy fieldwork students: Supervisors' perspectives. *Australian Occupational Therapy Journal, 54,* S2–S12. http://dx.doi.org/10.1111/j.1440-1630.2007.00694.x

Thompson, B. (2002). "Statistical," "practical," and "clinical": How many kinds of significance do counselors need to consider? *Journal of Counseling and Development, 80,* 64–71. http://dx.doi.org/10.1002/j.1556-6678.2002.tb00167.x

Toto, P. E. (2001). Moving toward evidence-based practice. *Gerontology Special Interest Section Quarterly, 24,* 4.

Uniform Data System for Medical Rehabilitation. (1993). *Guide for the Uniform Data Set for Medical Rehabilitation for Children (WeeFIM) (Version 4.0).* Buffalo: State University of New York.

Uniform Data System for Medical Rehabilitation. (1997). *Guide for the Uniform Data Set for Medical Rehabilitation (including the FIM™ instrument) (Version 5.1).* Buffalo: State University of New York.

Vargas, S., & Camilli, G. (1999). A meta-analysis of research on sensory integration treatment. *American Journal of Occupational Therapy, 53,* 189–198. http://dx.doi.org10.5014/ajot.53.2.189

Waldorf, M., Wjedl, K. H., & Schottke, H. (2009). In the concordance of three reliable change indexes: An analysis applying the dynamic Wisconsin Card Sorting Test. *Journal of Cognitive Education and Psychology, 8,* 63–80. http://dx.doi.org/10.1891/1945-8959.8.1.63

Whiteneck, G. G. (2010). Issues affecting the selection of participation measurement in outcomes research and clinical trials. *Archives of Physical Medicine and Rehabilitation, 91*(Suppl.), S54–S59. http://dx.doi.org/10.1016/j.apmr.2009.08.154

Whiteneck, G. G., Charlifue, S. W., Gerhart, K. A., Overholser, J. D., & Richardson, G. N. (1992). Quantifying handicap: A new measure of long-term rehabilitation outcomes. *Archives of Physical Medicine and Rehabilitation, 73,* 519–526.

Wilson, I. B., & Cleary, P. D. (1995). Linking clinical variables with health-related quality of life. *JAMA, 273, 59–65.*

Wolf, T. J. (2011). Rehabilitation, disability, and participation research: Are occupational therapy researchers addressing cognitive rehabilitation after stroke? *American Journal of Occupational Therapy, 65,* e46–e59. http://dx.doi:10.5014/ajot.2011.002089

World Health Organization. (2001). *International classification of functioning, disability and health.* Geneva: Author.

World Health Organization. (2002). Towards a common language for functioning, disability and health. In *International classification of functioning, disability, and health (ICF)* (pp. 1–22). Geneva: Author.

Subject Index

Citation Index